# Magnesium Alloys for Biomedical Applications

Magnesium alloys have enormous potential for use in biomedical implants. *Magnesium Alloys for Biomedical Applications* delves into recent advances and prospects for implementation and provides scientific insights into current issues posed by Mg alloy materials. It provides an overview of research on their mechanical and tribological characteristics, corrosion tendencies, and biological characteristics, with a particular emphasis on biomedical implants.

- Details the fundamentals of Mg alloys as well as necessary surface modifications of Mg alloys for biomedical use.
- Discusses emerging Mg alloys and their composites.
- Covers mechanical, tribological, and chemical properties, as well as fatigue and corrosion.
- Highlights emerging manufacturing methods and advancements in new alloy design, composite manufacturing, unique structure design, surface modification, and recyclability.
- Helps readers identify appropriate Mg-based materials for their applications and select optimal improvement methods.
- Summarizes current challenges and suggests a roadmap for future research.

Aimed at researchers in materials and biomedical engineering, this book explores the many breakthroughs achieved with these materials and where the field should concentrate to ensure the development of safe and reliable Mg alloy-based implants.

# Magnesium Alloys for Biomedical Applications

## Advances and Challenges

Edited by
Deepak Kumar and Nooruddin Ansari

**CRC Press**
Taylor & Francis Group
Boca Raton London New York

CRC Press is an imprint of the
Taylor & Francis Group, an **informa** business

Cover image: © Shutterstock

First edition published 2024
by CRC Press
2385 NW Executive Center Drive, Suite 320, Boca Raton FL 33431

and by CRC Press
4 Park Square, Milton Park, Abingdon, Oxon, OX14 4RN

CRC Press is an imprint of Taylor & Francis Group, LLC

---

**Library of Congress Cataloging-in-Publication Data**

---

Names: Kumar, Deepak, PhD, editor. | Ansari, Nooruddin, editor.
Title: Magnesium alloys for biomedical applications : advances and challenges /
edited by Deepak Kumar and Nooruddin Ansari.
Description: First edition. | Boca Raton, FL : CRC Press, 2024. | Includes
bibliographical references and index.
Identifiers: LCCN 2023050327 | ISBN 9781032508818 (hardback) |
ISBN 9781032509587 (paperback) | ISBN 9781003400462 (ebook)
Subjects: MESH: Magnesium--chemistry | Alloys--chemistry | Biocompatible
Materials--chemistry | Materials Testing--methods
Classification: LCC R857.M3 | NLM QT 37.5.M4 | DDC
610.28--dc23/eng/20240126
LC record available at https://lccn.loc.gov/2023050327

---

ISBN: 978-1-032-50881-8 (hbk)
ISBN: 978-1-032-50958-7 (pbk)
ISBN: 978-1-003-40046-2 (ebk)

DOI: 10.1201/9781003400462

Typeset in Times
by KnowledgeWorks Global Ltd.

# Contents

**Chapter 3**   Role of Alloying Elements on Biomedical Performance
            of Mg Alloys ............................................................................. 62

*Qazi Junaid Ashraf and G.A. Harmain*

**Chapter 6**    Surface Modification of Mg Alloys: An Insight into Friction

*Sufian Raja, Farazila Yusof, Ridha bin Muhamad, Mohd Fadzil
Jamaludin, MD.F. Khan, Mohd Bilal Naim Shaikh, Sajjad Arif
and Mohammad Azad Alam*

**Chapter 7**

*Fatima Jalid and Aravi Muzaffar*

# List of Figures and Tables

# About the Editors

**Dr. Deepak Kumar** boasts an impressive academic journey. He obtained his B.Tech. in Mechanical Engineering from Uttar Pradesh Technical University, India, in 2013 and went on to earn his M.Tech. in Mechanical System Design from the National Institute of Technology, Srinagar, India, in 2016. During his Master's program, he had the privilege of being a visiting student at the esteemed Indian Institute of Technology, Delhi, and his dedication was rewarded with a Gold Medal for his Master of Technology achievement. In 2021, Dr. Kumar achieved a significant milestone by completing his doctorate from the Materials Science and Engineering Department at the Indian Institute of Technology, Delhi, India. His academic excellence was further showcased when he participated in a summer camp organized by the University of Tokyo, Japan, in 2019, where he received recognition for his innovative ideas. Moreover, he secured best presentation and paper awards in India for IEEE and AIP conferences. Driven by his passion for research and learning, he traveled to Germany after being awarded a travel scholarship by the Government of India, enabling him to attend an international conference. Dr. Kumar's contributions to the field are notable, as evidenced by his publication record. He has authored 36 papers in prestigious SCI journals and presented 6 conference proceedings. Notably, several articles are currently under review in renowned SCI journals. His doctoral dissertation delved into the nanoscale mechanical and tribological behavior of magnesium alloys. He conducted comprehensive investigations into the fundamental mechanisms of friction, wear, and deformation under both dry and lubricated conditions. Using a unique AFM setup, he probed the in situ tribofilm development mechanisms, particularly in localized regions/phases of magnesium alloy under distinct lubricative conditions. Additionally, Dr. Kumar has explored the mechanical and tribological properties of titanium alloys and high-entropy alloys (HEAs). His expertise extends to the field of corrosion, where he has conducted research on Ni-Ti shape memory alloys. Following the completion of his Ph.D. in the Department of Materials Science and Engineering at IIT Delhi, Dr. Kumar continued to expand his research horizons. He has investigated nanomechanical and tribological characteristics of 3D printed medium entropy alloys. Currently, Dr. Kumar serves as a postdoctoral research associate in the Department of Mechanical Engineering at Carnegie Mellon University, USA, a position he has held since September 2021. His work involves the development of thin conductive film, integration of these methods with devices using clean room technology, characterizing device behavior through a novel, in-house-built controlled characterization platform, and analyzing the results to unravel the mechanisms governing performance limits and failure modes.

**Dr. Nooruddin Ansari** earned his B. Tech. in Mechanical Engineering from Jamia Millia Islamia, India, in 2014, followed by an M. Tech. in Industrial and Production Engineering from Aligarh Muslim University, India, in 2017, where he was awarded the Silver Medal for his Master of Technology. In 2021, he successfully completed his doctorate from the Materials Science and Engineering Department at the Indian

Institute of Technology, Delhi, India. In 2018, he represented India as an Indian Youth Delegate in China, fostering collaborations in education. Dr. Ansari has an impressive publication record, with 12 papers in renowned SCI journals and 2 conference proceedings. His doctoral research focused on the thermomechanical processing and deformation behavior of Mg-Y alloys with varying Y concentrations. This involved the development of lightweight Mg-Y alloys through casting and hot rolling, as well as an exploration of recrystallization and deformation behavior at both room and high temperatures. Additionally, he has devoted attention to the mechanical behavior of steel, Al, and Ti alloys.

Presently, Dr. Ansari serves as Postdoctoral Research Associate in the Department of Mechanical Engineering at Texas A & M University, Qatar. His current work focuses on the development of steels, Ti, Al, and Mg alloys through additive manufacturing, with a focus on investigating their mechanical and corrosion behavior across different environments.

# Contributors

**Akbar Ahmad**
School of Mechatronics Engineering
Symbiosis Skills and Professional
    University
Pune, India

**Mohammad Azad Alam**
Department of Mechanical Engineering
Universiti Teknologi PETRONAS
Seri Iskandar, Malaysia

**Sajjad Arif**
Department of Mechanical Engineering
ZHCET
Aligarh Muslim University
Aligarh, India

**Qazi Junaid Ashraf**
Department of Mechanical Engineering
University of Kashmir, Zakura Campus
Srinagar, India
and
National Institute of Technology
Srinagar, India

**Shivprakash Barve**
School of Mechanical Engineering
Dr. Vishwanath Karad MIT World
    Peace University
Pune, India

**Shubrajit Bhaumik**
Department of Mechanical Engineering
Amrita School of Engineering
Amrita Vishwa Vidyapeetham
Chennai, India

**Umer Masood Chaudry**
Department of Mechanical Engineering
Incheon National University
Incheon, Republic of Korea
and
Research Institute for Engineering and
    Technology
Incheon, Republic of Korea

**Vivudh Gupta**
Department of Mechanical Engineering
Government College of Engineering &
    Technology
Jammu, India

**G.A. Harmain**
Department of Mechanical Engineering
National Institute of Technology
    Srinagar
Srinagar, India

**Dineshkumar Harursampath**
Department of Aerospace Engineering
NMCAD Lab.
Indian Institute of Science
Bengaluru, India

**Fatima Jalid**
Department of Chemical Engineering
National Institute of Technology
Srinagar, India

**Mohd Fadzil Jamaludin**
Centre of Advanced Manufacturing and
    Material Processing (AMMP Centre)
University of Malaya
Kuala Lumpur, Malaysia

**Tea-Sung Jun**
Department of Mechanical Engineering
Incheon National University
Incheon, Republic of Korea
and
Research Institute of Engineering &
    Technology
Incheon, Republic of Korea

**Gourav Khajuria**
Department of Mechanical Engineering
Government College of Engineering &
    Technology
Jammu, India

**Md. F. Khan**
Department of Mechanical Engineering
College of Engineering
King Faisal University
Al-Ahsa, Saudi Arabia

**Vinyas Mahesh**
Department of Mechanical Engineering
National Institute of Technology
Silchar, India

**Badar Zaman Minhas**
Department of Materials Science &
    Engineering
Institute of Space Technology
Islamabad, Pakistan

**Manoj Mugale**
Cleveland State University
Cleveland, USA

**Ridha bin Muhamad**
Department of Mechanical Engineering,
    Faculty of Engineering
Centre of Advanced Manufacturing
    and Material Processing
    (AMMP Centre)
University of Malaya
Kuala Lumpur, Malaysia

**Aravi Muzaffar**
Department of Metallurgical and
    Materials Engineering
National Institute of Technology
Srinagar, India

**Viorel Paleu**
Mechanical Engineering Faculty
Gheorghe Asachi Technical University
    of Iaşi
Iaşi, Romania

**Pralhad Pesode**
School of Mechanical Engineering
Dr. Vishwanath Karad MIT World
    Peace University
Pune, India

**Sumit Pramanik**
Department of Mechanical Engineering
College of Engineering & Technology
SRM Institute of Science & Technology
Chennai, India

**Sufian Raja**
Department of Mechanical Engineering,
    Faculty of Engineering
University of Malaya
Kuala Lumpur, Malaysia

**Muhammad Atiq Ur Rehman**
Department of Materials Science &
    Engineering
Institute of Space Technology
Islamabad, Pakistan

**Mohd Bilal Naim Shaikh**
Department of Mechanical Engineering
ZHCET
Aligarh Muslim University
Aligarh, India

**Virendra Pratap Singh**
Department of Mechanical Engineering
National Institute of Technology Mizoram
Aizawl, India
and
Department of Mechanical Engineering
IES College of Technology
Bhopal, India

**Hafiz Muhammad Rehan Tariq**
Department of Mechanical Engineering
Incheon National University
Incheon, Republic of Korea

**Kamlendra Vikram**
Department of Mechanical Engineering
College of Engineering & Technology
SRM Institute of Science & Technology
Chennai, India

**Sagar V. Wankhede**
School of Mechatronics Engineering
Symbiosis Skills and Professional
 University
Pune, India

**Farazila Yusof**
Department of Mechanical Engineering,
 Faculty of Engineering
and
Centre of Advanced Manufacturing
 and Material Processing (AMMP
 Centre)
and
Centre for Foundation Studies in
 Science
University of Malaya
Kuala Lumpur, Malaysia

# 1 Magnesium Alloys for Biomedical Applications

## Scope and Opportunities

*Gourav Khajuria and Vivudh Gupta*
Department of Mechanical Engineering, Government
College of Engineering & Technology, Jammu, India

## 1.1 INTRODUCTION

Tissue engineering is a multidisciplinary area dedicated to the regeneration of vital human tissues. Although living organs have inherent self-healing abilities, the extent of healing differs between tissues and can be compromised by the extent of injury [1–5]. Tissue engineering is the formation of bioengineered tissues in vitro and the modification of cell growth and function in vivo by the implantation of appropriate cells extracted from donor tissue and biocompatible scaffolds [2, 6–9]. Tissue engineering combines material and cell transplantation principles to create tissues and promote regeneration. The strategy was devised to bridge the gap between the enhancing number of patients due to end-stage failures and the limited number of donated organs [3, 10–13]. Tissue engineering is a branch of biomedical engineering discipline that integrates biology and ecological system with engineering to create tissues or cellular products outside the living body or to make use of gained knowledge to better manage the repair/reconstruction of tissues within the living body [12–15].

Biomaterials are an integral part of tissue engineering. The biodegradability, chemistry, and porosity of biomaterials used in tissue engineering must be controlled to promote optimum properties like cell adhesion and deposition of extracellular matrix materials by cells [10, 16]. The utilization of biocompatible materials for the development of implants has increased manifolds with the purpose to improve patients' health. Usage of such implants is commonly observed in the field of orthopedics (spinal fixation, bone fixation, tendon/ligament/cartilage replacement, etc.). Various biomaterials' properties that make them useful for medical applications include their ductility, high strength, fracture toughness, wear resistance, and corrosion resistance. Commonly used examples of implant materials include Co-Cr alloys, stainless steel, titanium alloys, magnesium alloys, etc. [17].

Biomaterials are used in a wide variety of industries for a variety of applications. There are many materials that can be used to create biomaterials, including metals, ceramics, polymers, glass, and living cells/tissues [18–20]. The basic function of a biomaterial implant is to replace the damaged biological part in the body so that it

DOI: 10.1201/9781003400462-1

can perform its basic function well in coordination with other biological tissues and organs. Biomaterials should have biocompatible composition so that adverse chemical reactions can be avoided. Moreover, such materials should also offer excellent degradation resistance in terms of corrosion, biological, and wear resistance. Also, these biomaterials should have sufficient strength to withstand fluctuations arisen due to cyclic loads. Furthermore, in order to minimize resorption in bones, low modulus is required. Minimum wear in these implant materials result in minimum generation of debris as well [21]. Less wear debris accounts for presence of less foreign particles in the physiological system that hamper the working of various tissues. Present-day research studies show that there has been a substantial increase in the manufacturing methods of implants. Fabrication techniques like fused deposition modelling, investment casting, and vapor smoothing have also been in practice for the development of implant materials [22]. Moreover, it is evident from Figure 1.1 that research articles published in the field of biomaterials and biomedical magnesium alloys are continuously enhancing year-wise.

3D printing techniques have been extensively used for the development of the same. The life of the implant materials is generally hampered by corrosion. For prolonging the life of biomaterials, various coatings and surface modification techniques have been employed. For instance, ZrN/Cu coating has been successfully employed by the researchers on stainless steel and titanium materials for biomedical

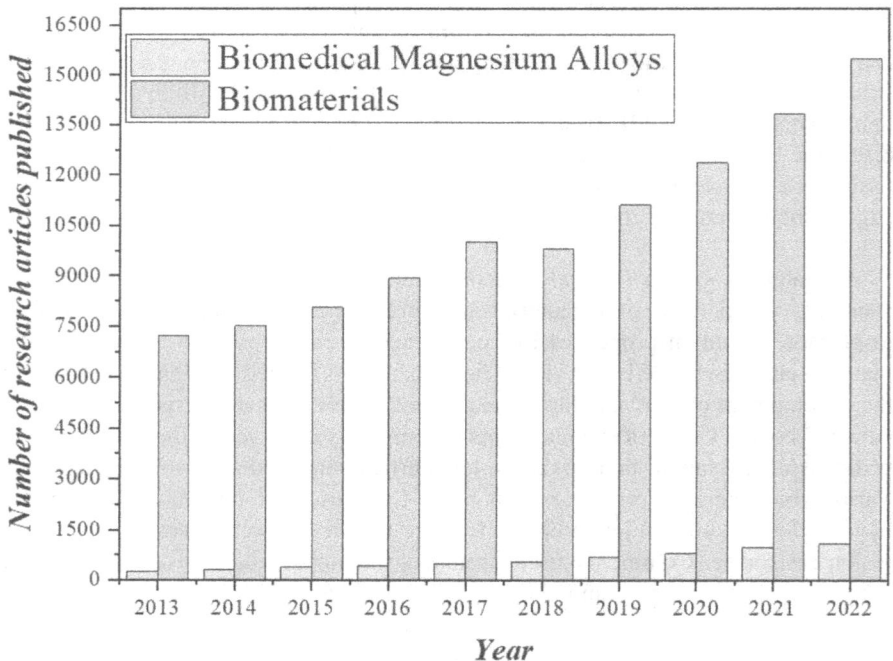

**FIGURE 1.1** Yearwise distribution of research articles in biomaterials and biomedical magnesium alloys. (From ScienceDirect.)

purposes [23]. Coating techniques include thermal spraying, sputter coating, dip coating, sol–gel technique, electrophoretic deposition, pulsed layer deposition, biomimetic coating, etc. [24].

Different types of corrosion that affect conventional materials utilized for biomaterials development include pitting, crevice, stress corrosion cracking, corrosion fatigue, fretting, galvanic, and selective leaching. By-products arising out of corrosion of implant materials can cause dermatitis, anemia, ulcers, disturbance in central nervous system, Alzheimer's disease, etc.

The surface modification technique is one of the prominent solutions to reducing corrosion, thereby enhancing the life span of biomaterials [25]. Electrical discharge machining (EDM) process is also one of the potential choices for the surface modification of titanium alloys utilized for different orthopedic applications. In EDM process variants, powder-mixed EDM process is significantly used for modifying the surface of any material [26]. The complete structure of this chapter is shown in Figure 1.2.

## 1.1.1 Metal-based Biomaterials

Due to the increasing number of cardiovascular, orthopedic, dental, and neurological diseases that require implants and surgeries, metals are utilized at every stage, and there is a growing demand for biocompatible and biodegradable metals such as stainless steel, gold, chromium, titanium, cobalt, nitinol, and silver [27].

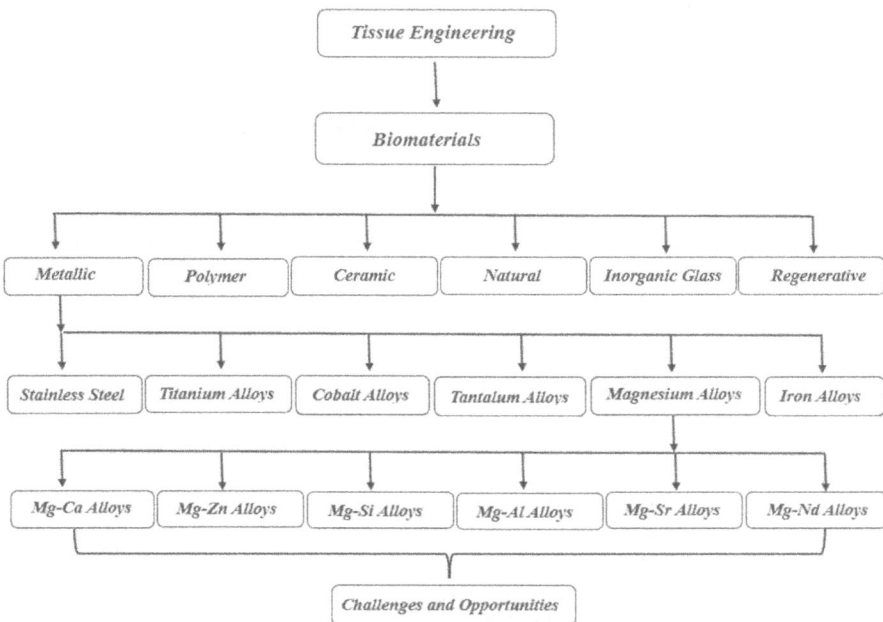

**FIGURE 1.2** The schematic diagram depicting the complete structure of this chapter.

### 1.1.2 POLYMER-BASED BIOMATERIALS

Polymeric biomaterials are used in a variety of medical applications, including vascular grafts, implants applications, dressings, catheters, sutures, ligament repair, meshes, stents, tendon repair, and cardiac surgery valves. Polymeric (plastic) materials used in these areas can be synthetic or natural. For example, proteins, cellulose, deoxyribonucleic acid (DNA), ribonucleic acid (RNA), silk, wool, etc. are common among natural polymers derived from both plant and animal resources [27].

### 1.1.3 CERAMIC-BASED BIOMATERIALS

Bioceramics have specific properties such as chemical stability, stiffness, wear resistance, and hardness, and are biocompatible. The biocompatibility of bioceramics varies depending on the composition of the ceramic oxides (alumina, hydroxyapatite, zirconia, etc.), which are chemically inactive in the human body, and on the biodissolvable materials, which are to be finally replaced by the human tissues after carrying out repair work. These biomaterials are widely used in implants for teeth and bones, surgical crowns, and arthroplasty surgery (Table 1.1) [28].

### 1.1.4 NATURAL BIOMATERIALS

Natural biomaterials can be classified into chitin, hyaluronic acid, cellulose, silk, gelatin, chitosan, and fibrin. They are commonly used to replace and restore the function and structure of injured organs, as drug delivery systems, and as medical biases similar to surgical sutures [18, 20, 27].

### TABLE 1.1
### List of Biomaterials and Its Characteristics and Applications

| S. No. | Biomaterials | Characteristics | Applications | References |
|---|---|---|---|---|
| 1. | Metal | Ductile, high wear resistance, impact resistance, low biocompatibility and corrosion resistance in physiological environment, mechanical properties different from biological tissues | Plates and wires, joint prostheses, dental implants, cranial plaques, artificial hip joints, knee joints, screw, plates | Kumar [29] dos Santos [30] Niinomi [31] Minnath [32] |
| 2. | Polymer | Low density, easy to produce, easily degradable | Sutures, arteries, tendons, veins, artificial, implants | Love [33] Dutta [34] Chen [35] |
| 3. | Ceramic | High biocompatibility, corrosion resistance, low thermal and electrical conductivity, low impact strength, difficult in manufacturing implants | Medical equipment and tools, coatings, bone filling | Punj et al. [36] Moshiri et al. [37] Migonney [38] |

### 1.1.5 Inorganic Glass-based Biomaterials

Certain glasses are used in medical devices such as biotechnology, IR detection, and high-power mid-infrared laser delivery. Inorganic bioactive biomaterials are used to replace bone hard tissue, bone tissue engineering, and dental restorations [27].

### 1.1.6 Regenerative Biomaterials

The significant applications of regenerated biomaterials in tissue engineering are what propel the market for these materials. Tissue engineering uses cells and biomaterials with some engineering to create products. Until recently, prosthetics were the only application for regenerative biomaterials. However, they are also used for the development of biomaterial scaffolds, wound healing, and tissue engineering for the heart, liver, cornea, bone, and blood vessels. Regenerative biomaterials are primarily used in tissue engineering to build bones and joints. This market niche is growing as a result of technological developments (nanotechnology-based tissue engineering) [18, 37].

Metallic biomaterials are natural or artificial and have potentially been used as implants to replace or repair lost/damaged hard tissues or diseased biological structures of living bodies to reinstate the structure–function. Metallic biomaterials play a vital role in the replacement of failed hard tissues and other damaged/lost tissues, i.e., surgical applications, artificial hip joints, dental applications, artificial knee joints, etc. Metallic biomaterials have excellent biocompatibility, good mechanical properties, corrosion resistance, thermal conductivity, and sufficient fatigue strength to rigorous conditions, lightweight, and wear resistance properties which seek attention and are used in various biomedical applications. The current (metallic) materials used in biomedical implants behave almost neutrally inside the body. Such non-biodegradable bio-passive implants either remain in place (where there is a risk of loosening, fracturing, and tissue inflammation) or are removed after healing (where there is an increased risk of surgery, discomfort for the patient, and cost). These biomaterials aid to enhance the quality of life. These biomaterials are used as implant applications due to their properties, i.e., nontoxic, nonmagnetic, and inflammatory or nonallergic reactions in the living bodies [38–41]. Various characteristics of biomaterials have been summed up in Figure 1.3. The most commonly used examples of implant materials include Co-Cr alloys, stainless steel, titanium alloys, magnesium alloys, etc. (Table 1.2) [17].

Stainless steel-316L alloy has good mechanical strength and corrosion resistance and has various biomedical applications, i.e., femoral heads and stems. Titanium alloys have majority of biomedical applications due to their outstanding characteristics such as good biocompatibility, high immunity to corrosion low density, low Young's modulus, better corrosion resistance, etc., Titanium alloys are widely used in the replacement of damaged hard tissues, i.e., dental implants, artificial bones and joints, hip joints, knee joints, etc. Cobalt-based alloys have good mechanical properties and corrosion resistance in chloride environment [39–43].

Magnesium-, iron-, and zinc-based alloys are biodegradable and biocompatible, and they also have excellent mechanical properties. These alloys are mainly used

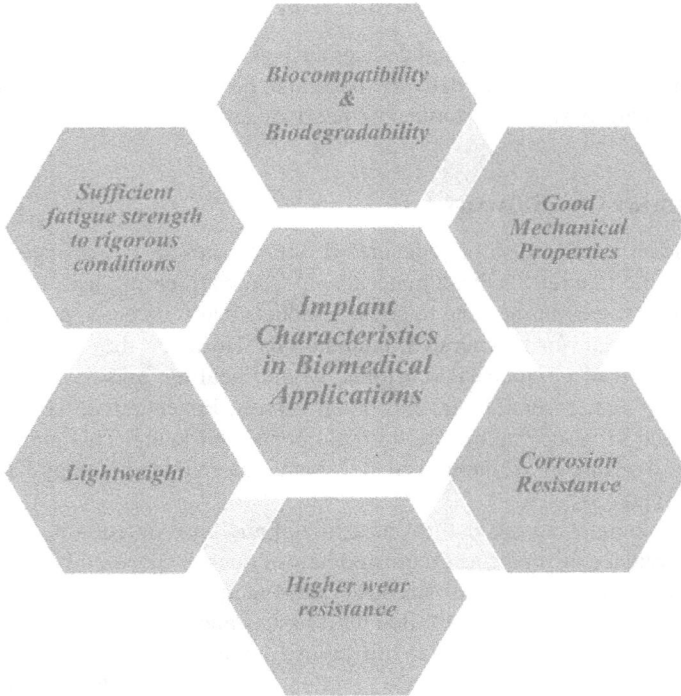

**FIGURE 1.3**   Diagram depicting the implant characteristics in biomedical applications.

in cardiovascular and orthopedic implants applications. Mg-based alloys have very limited applications due to their rapid corrosion rates in physiological environments. There are many techniques to reduce the effect of corrosion in implant applications, i.e., improve mechanical properties, surface modifications, heat treatments, coatings, etc. [42, 43].

This chapter primarily focuses on the recent advancements in major areas of magnesium-based alloy biomaterials such as orthopedics, ophthalmology, cardiovascular, neuronal, etc.

Additionally, this chapter particularly emphasizes on the tissue engineering aspect of biomaterials for the replacement/restoration of tissues.

Magnesium has become a popular substitute for materials used in permanent implants because of its improved biodegradability, greater mechanical strength than polymeric biodegradable materials, and biocompatibility [51–54]. It is evident that Mg-based alloys are an implant material for both orthopedic and cardiovascular applications. Mg-based alloys as an implant material reduce the risk of long-term noncompatible interaction with tissues and eliminate the need for a second procedure to remove/repair the implant, thereby minimizing complications.

The difficulty with using magnesium implants extensively is their rapid rate of degradation, which consequently lowers their mechanical strength to support the surgical site. The methods that can result in the improved corrosion resistance of

## TABLE 1.2
## Different Examples of Implant Materials

| S. No. | Material | Examples | Implant Applications of Biomaterials | References |
|---|---|---|---|---|
| 1. | Stainless steel | 316L SS | Surgical implants, stent, artificial valve, bone fixation, artificial joints, orthodontic wire, filling, plates screw in craniofacial, artificial ear drum | Prasad et al. [44] dos Santos [30] Hermawan et al. [45] |
| 2. | Titanium and its alloys | Ti, Ti$_6$Al$_4$V Ti- Ni Ti-6Al-7Nb Ti-20 Cr-0.2 Si Ti-20Pd-5Cr Ti-5Al-2.5Fe Ti-Al-Nb etc. | Dental applications, surgical applications, femoral stems, femoral components, tibial bones, femoral head and cup, artificial hip joints, artificial bones, orthodontic wire, filling, knee implants, bones screw and plates, stent, artificial valve, bone fixation, artificial joints, plates screw in craniofacial | Niinomi [29] dos Santos [30] Gupta et al. [46] Stadlinger et al. [47] Subramani et al. [48] Dvorský et al. [49] |
| 3. | Cobalt-based alloys | Co-Cr-Mo Co-Ni-Cr-Mo-W-Fe Co-20Cr- 15W-10Ni Co- 28Cr-6Mo alloys | Artificial hip joints, repairing soft tissues, i.e., stents, femoral stems and femoral components, artificial valve, plates screw in craniofacial, bone fixation, orthodontic wire, filling, artificial joints | dos Santos [30] Hermawan et al. [45] Aherwar et al. [50] |
| 4. | Tantalum-based biomaterials | Tantalum and titanium-tantalum alloys | Osteoporosis (bone implants), surgical implants, heart pacemakers, implanted automated defibrillators and hearing aids, hip arthroplasty components | Dos Santos [30] Niinomi [31] Hermawan et al. [45] |
| 5. | Magnesium alloys | Mg-Ca alloy Mg- Zn-Mn-Ca alloy WE43 | Stent (cardiovascular), bone implants, orthopedic | Kamrani et al. [51] Yang et al. [52] Kumar et al. [53] Amukarimi and Mozafari [54] |
| 6. | Iron-based alloys | Fe-Mn-Ca alloy Fe-Mn alloy | Orthopedic and cardiovascular implants | Prasad et al. [44] |

Mg implants are alloy development, surface treatment, and design modification of implants.

Magnesium alloys have properties somewhat similar to bone tissues. Such properties are capable of suppressing stress-shielding effect which is commonly observed in implant materials having a high modulus of elasticity. High corrosion rate is the major drawback associated with the usage of magnesium alloys occurring due to the release of hydrogen, which in turn complicates the healing process [52–54].

Nowadays, magnesium alloys have also been in practice for the development of biodegradable Mg-based composites meant for biomedical applications [53]. Over a period of time, with a view to improving the mechanical properties of magnesium for biomedical purposes, it has been alloyed with certain elements to form Mg-based alloys such as Mg-Sr alloys, Mg-Ca alloys, Mg-Zn alloys, etc. [20]. Biodegradability, biocompatibility, and improved mechanical properties of magnesium over biodegradable polymer materials have made it a potential alternative material for implants [54].

Magnesium-based implants are absorbed by the body tissues after carrying out their basic function [55]. Magnesium is basically less toxic in nature, aids in enhanced bone formation, provides shelter against oxidative stresses, etc. [56]. The properties of magnesium alloys are greatly affected by grain size, morphologies, and constituent phase distribution. Microstructural modification can be done through processing routes, heat treatment, alloying different elements and, in turn, improving the physical, mechanical, tribological, and corrosion properties of Mg-based alloys. Use of coatings and the inclusion of reinforcements as filler materials are also known to improve the properties of such alloys [57, 58].

Various factors which are taken into consideration while evaluating the performance of magnesium alloys include alloying design, modification of the surface, and in vivo and in vitro performance of magnesium while repairing hard tissues [59]. Some major issues associated with magnesium alloys include their enhanced corrosion rates owing to hydrogen generation, maintenance of mechanical properties including rigidity, and roughness value of magnesium implant resulting in higher initial degradation and thus affecting cell adherence along with cell viability [60, 61]. Magnesium as an implant material can reduce the long-term problem of noncompatible interaction with human tissues and eradicates the need for a new procedure to remove the implant, thereby minimizing drawbacks [52–54].

## 1.2 MAGNESIUM ALLOYS: ADVANCEMENTS AND APPLICATIONS

In order to attain biocompatibility and biodegradability of the Mg alloys, some nutritional elements have been viewed as primary alternatives for alloying purposes (Table 1.3). These also improve strength, which differs from already existing designed Mg alloys. It is suitable for use in hard-tissue engineering because of its mechanical qualities, particularly its strength and elasticity modulus, which are quite similar to those of natural bone. Furthermore, proper processing procedure has a significant effect on the mechanical properties of Mg-based alloys, including heat treatment, surface deformation, and plastic deformation. The worn-out products affect tissue and human metabolism. Magnesium element has been alloyed with different elements such as calcium, zinc, silicon, aluminum, strontium, neodymium, etc. [20, 52–54] and hence are classified as follows.

**TABLE 1.3**

**Biocompatibility and Mechanical Properties of Magnesium Alloy Elements**

| S. No. | Magnesium Alloys | Features | References |
|---|---|---|---|
| 1. | Mg-Ca-based alloys | • Noncytotoxic<br>• Reduces metabolic disorder<br>• Enhances the Ca content to increase corrosion resistance and grain refinement<br>• Strength increases and plasticity reduces,<br>• Promotes the bone healing process | Zheng et al. [65]<br>Jähn et. al. [66]<br>Mohamed et al. [67] |
| 2. | Mg-Al-based alloys | • Neurotoxic<br>• Damages muscle fibers<br>• Increases corrosion resistance<br>• Increases strength and plasticity | Agarwal et al. [68]<br>Maier et al. [55]<br>Mirza et al. [69] |
| 3. | Mg-Sr-based alloys | • Noncytotoxic<br>• Promotes bone formation<br>• The strength increases with increasing Sr content<br>• Promotes osteoblast maturations | Dong et al. [70]<br>Yang et al. [71] |
| 4. | Mg-Zn-based alloys | • Good biocompatibility<br>• Noncytotoxic<br>• Solid solution strengthening<br>• Strength increases<br>• Important trace element in human body | Philip et al. [72]<br>Becerra et al. [73]<br>Duley [74] |
| 5. | Mg-Mn-based alloys | • Cytotoxic and neurotoxic<br>• Decreases tensile strength and elongation<br>• Increases yield strength and corrosion resistance | Cho et al. [75]<br>Liu et al. [76] |

## 1.2.1 Mg-Ca Alloys

Calcium is an important bone element and essential for human health. Because Mg-Ca alloy has a density that is similar to that of human bone, it has greater advantages as a material for bone implants. When Ca is added in the right amount, it has the ability to refine grains, inhibits inter-grain boundary compounds, improves the density of the oxide film, and increases the corrosion resistance of Mg alloys. Mg alloys with a Ca content of 1–10 wt% were created, and their corrosion resistance was examined. Electrochemical tests revealed that Mg-based Ca alloys with 5–10 wt% Ca content had notably lower corrosion resistance than those with 1 wt% Ca content. It was also discovered that the addition of Ca (0.2 wt%) reduced the potential difference between the phases, which in turn reduced the degradation rates of the as-cast Mg-4Zn-based alloy (30%). According to studies, adding more Ca to Mg-Ca alloys improves the $Mg_2Ca$ phase, compression strength, and the hardness elastic modulus, but detracts from plasticity, corrosion resistance, and biocompatibility. Notably, these Mg alloys perform better mechanically, resist corrosion in a better way, and are more biocompatible when the calcium content is less than 1% [18–20, 61–63].

### 1.2.2  Mg-Zn Alloys

Zinc is generally considered as one the vital nutritional and trace elements in the human body owing to its nature as a cofactor for enzymatic action in different bones/ cartilages. Along with various orthopedic applications, Mg-Zn alloys possess potential biomedical applications for the repair of bile and intestinal tracts. Inclusion of zinc for the development of Mg-Zn alloys is known to enhance tensile strength besides solid solution strengthening and precipitation strengthening. Moreover, the elongation percentage was also reduced when the content of zinc in such alloys was over 5%. Mg-Zn alloys also exhibit improved corrosion resistance over pure magnesium while undergoing electrochemical investigation. Excellent biocompatible nature of zinc with improved properties make zinc a potential candidate for the development of Mg-Zn alloys.

Various studies proved that optimum concentration of zinc in Mg-Zn biomedical alloys should be 4%, above which properties start deteriorating. Hence, it should be doped with other elements as well with a view to achieve better properties of alloys. Furthermore, addition of zinc in Mg alloys is also known to enhance the tolerance limits of impurities such as copper, nickel, and iron, which, in turn, reduces the chances of possible galvanic corrosion rates [20, 54, 62, 64]. The following are the examples of commonly used biomedical Mg-Zn alloys:

- Mg-1Zn alloy
- Mg-5Zn alloy
- Mg-7Zn alloy
- Mg-1.8Zn-0.2 Gd alloy
- Mg-0.96Zn-0.21 Zr-0.3 REE alloy

### 1.2.3  Mg-Si Alloys

Human body requires vital elements, including Si. It is generally added with other elements to enhance the characteristics of Mg alloys [63].

### 1.2.4  Mg-Al Alloys

Aluminum when used for the advancement of biomedical Mg-Al alloys can enhance ultimate tensile strength along with ductility when its content is below 6%. Such alloys have orthopedic applications in general and development of screws in particular. Moreover, such alloys can cause toxicity in nerves and even excess concentration of $Al^{3+}$ ions in human brain can lead to Alzheimer's disease. This is the major limitation in the usage of Mg-Al-based alloys. Studies have found that the optimal concentration of Al in Mg-Al alloys is between 2% and 9%. The various advantages of utilizing Mg-Al-based alloys are increased corrosion resistance (due to the formation of insoluble $Al_2O_3$ layer in place of $Mg(OH)_2$, which gets soluble in chloride solution) and improved strength due to both precipitation strengthening and solid solution strengthening. Such alloys also exhibit excellent castability properties [20, 54, 77, 78]. The following are the examples of commonly used biomedical Mg-Al alloys:

- AZ-31 alloy
- AZ-61 alloy
- AZ-91 alloy, etc.

### 1.2.5 Mg-Sr ALLOYS

One of the body's trace elements is strontium. The bones are where almost all of the Sr is found. Salts of strontium can encourage the growth of bones. Sr, Mg, and Ca all perform chemically similarly (Table 1.4). Sr can efficiently refine grains and enhance all-around properties in Mg alloys. As a result, in recent years, Sr elements are frequently added to Mg-based alloys for bone implants applications. Additionally, Mg-Sr-based alloys have better biocompatibility. For example, it was found that rabbit bone tissue with new bone tissue fuses better with Mg-Zr-based alloy with Sr addition [20, 62–64].

### 1.2.6 Mg-Nd ALLOYS

Mg-Nd alloys are also in practice as biomedical alloys. They are known to increase tensile strength in addition to creep resistance owing to the growth of intermetallic compounds of $Mg_{12}Nd$, where Nd concentration is below 6%. Such alloys are known to promote healing of bone and have good compatibility with tissues. They are generally used for the development of stents and screws [20, 84, 85]. Example of such biomedical alloy is Mg-Nd-Zn-Zr alloy. Despite Mg bone fixation device's cyclical degradation and desired mechanical strength, sufficient mechanical support is evident at the preliminary stage, especially for this particular device. Compared to this, bone tissue at the site of fracture gradually increases its load-bearing capacity. The rapid collection of hydrogen hastens the degradation of the magnesium plate. Mg-Al-Mn alloy was primarily applied to screws, bolts, and plates [86].

## 1.3 CHALLENGES AND OPPORTUNITIES

It is evident from the above discussion that the major hinderance in the usage of magnesium alloys for biomedical purposes include corrosion, degradation, and stability after some time. Such issues can be taken as challenges for future research so that maximum benefit from the utilization of magnesium-based alloys can be drawn out. Besides, magnesium-based alloys must be improved in their mechanical properties and corrosion resistance to increase their biomedical application areas. Nevertheless, a rapid deterioration rate generally causes premature disintegration in mechanical integrity and hydrogen buildup, reducing the applicability of bone restoration in living tissues. Extensive studies on evaluating electrochemical corrosion rates, minimum dissolution, and maintaining the osteo-integrity of

**TABLE 1.4**

**Research Studies on Biomedical Magnesium Alloys**

| S. No. | Magnesium Alloys | Approach Used | Key Findings | Researchers |
|---|---|---|---|---|
| 1. | Pure magnesium | Usage of Ti- coating on magnesium by ion-plating technique | • Dense and homogeneous Ti- coating was deposited on the Mg surface<br>• Polarization results revealed an improvement in the corrosion resistance of Mg by the deposition of Ti on its surface | Zhang et al. [79] |
| 2. | Mg-Zn-Mn alloys | Evaluation of microstructural, mechanical, biocompatibility, and corrosion properties | • Inclusion of zinc caused refinement in grain size of extruded Mg alloys<br>• Grain refinement caused enhancement in tensile strength<br>• Formation of passivation film was accelerated due to the presence of zinc, thereby protecting Mg alloy from different body fluids | Zhang et al. [80] |
| 3. | Various Mg alloys | Surface modification techniques in biomedical Mg alloys | • Various surface modification techniques include chemical conversion coating, chemical vapor deposition, physical vapor deposition, ion implantation, thermal spraying, usage of different polymer and biomimetic coatings | Kumar et al. [81] |
| 4. | Mg-RE-Zn alloys | Enhancing corrosion resistance of biomedical Mg alloy | • New Mg-RE-Zn alloys having long period stacking ordered (LPSO) structure exhibited slow corrosion rates<br>• Other methods to improve modifying the resistance to corrosion while fabrication Mg alloys include proper heat treatments, rapid solidification rates, etc. | Chen et al. [82] |
| 5. | Mg-based metallic glass | Evaluation of glass transition temperature and thermal stability | • Inclusion of Yb improved the stability of alloy and alloy possessed excellent crystallization resistance and thermal stability for its application in biomedical systems | Baulin et al. [83] |

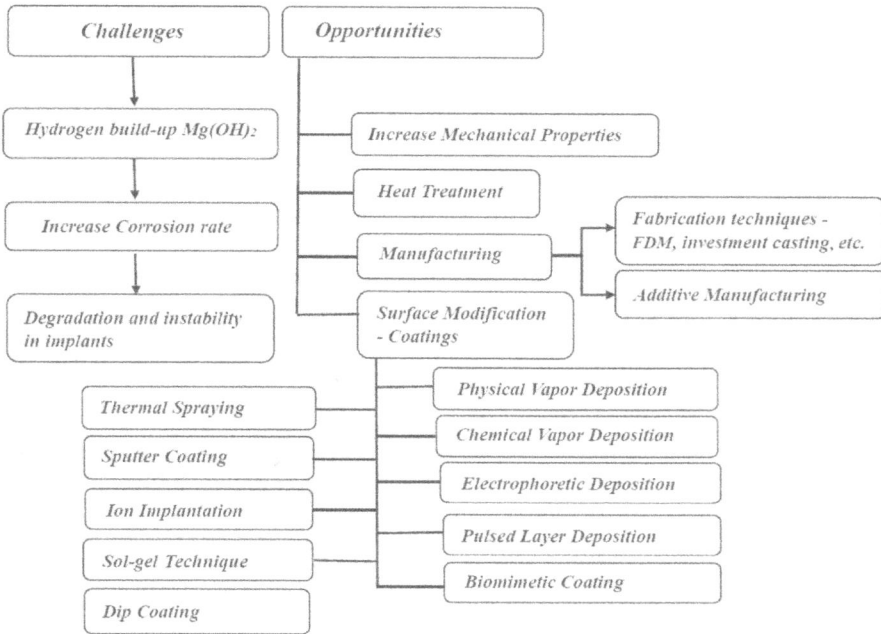

**FIGURE 1.4** The schematic diagram highlighting challenges and opportunities of Mg-based alloys in biomedical applications.

magnesium-based implants can be seen as future prospects in this area. In brief, such challenges and opportunities have been incorporated in Figure 1.4.

Development of coatings, surface modification techniques, fabrication of Mg composites, methods for improving microstructures of these alloys, etc. are the potential opportunities in this field. When the solubility of particular alloying elements differs with different factors such as temperature, surface heat treatment is employed to enhance the mechanical properties of Mg-based alloys. As compared to other processing methods, heat treatment typically modifies the microstructure of the materials rather than the form and its chemical content. Fine-grain strengthening, and second-phase strengthening are the two main methods for enhancing the mechanical properties of Mg alloys. The most widely used thermal treatments for Mg-based alloys include solid solution treatment, age treatment, and solid solution + aging treatment. Moreover, inclusion of other elements in these Mg-based alloys can also be evaluated for their performance in improving patient's health. Various alloying elements in biodegradable Mg-based alloys are employed to not only enhance the initial mechanical qualities but also to maintain mechanical integrity for a longer duration of time in vivo by improving the alloys' corrosion resistance. More in vitro and in vivo studies of such alloys can also be an opportunity to be considered in this field. Biocompatibility and biodegradation properties should be considered in order to enhance the mechanical properties of Mg-based alloys. The fields of biology, physics, chemistry, materials science, and cutting-edge technologies will all be

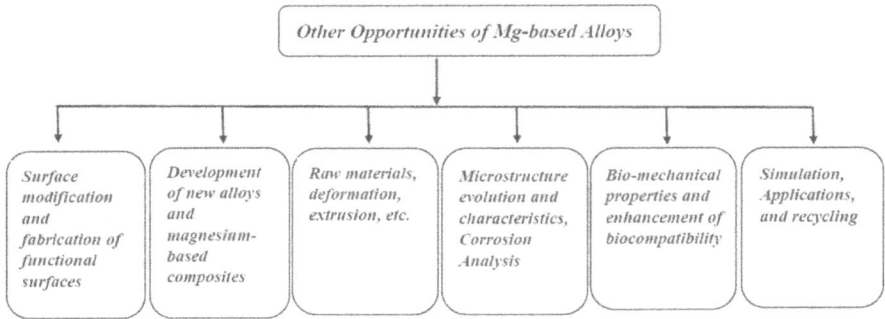

FIGURE 1.5    The schematic diagram of opportunities of magnesium alloys in biomedical applications.

covered in our discussion of magnesium and its alloy-related topics. In implant applications, there are various issues to be discussed in the future for the enhancement of biomaterials, as shown in Figure 1.5.

## 1.4    CONCLUSIONS

This chapter presents state-of-the-art work in the formation and advancement of biomedical magnesium-based alloys. This chapter has the potential to serve as a directory for various researchers/scientists working in this crucial field of development and characterization of biomedical Mg-based alloys in the case of orthopedical and cardiovascular implants. Various Mg-based alloys, their scope, challenges, and opportunities are well presented in this chapter. These alloys are known to enhance the load-bearing capacity and reduce the deterioration rates in implant applications.

## REFERENCES

1. Enderle, John, and Joseph Bronzino, eds. *Introduction to biomedical engineering.* Academic Press, 2012.
2. Berthiaume, François, and Martin L. Yarmush. *Encyclopedia of physical science and technology.* Academic Press, 2004.
3. Furth, Mark E., and Anthony Atala. "Tissue engineering: future perspectives." In *Principles of tissue engineering*, pp. 83–123. Academic Press, 2014.
4. Amini, Ami R., Cato T. Laurencin, and Syam P. Nukavarapu. "Bone tissue engineering: recent advances and challenges." *Critical Reviews™ in Biomedical Engineering* 40, no. 5 (2012): 363–408.
5. Laurencin, Cato T., Archel M. A. Ambrosio, Mark. D. Borden, and James. A. Cooper, Jr. "Tissue engineering: orthopedic applications." *Annual Review of Biomedical Engineering* 1, no. 1 (1999): 19–46.
6. Griffith, Linda G., and Gail Naughton. "Tissue engineering: current challenges and expanding opportunities." *Science* 295, no. 5557 (2002): 1009–1014.
7. Olson, Jennifer L., Anthony Atala, and James J. Yoo. "Tissue engineering: current strategies and future directions." *Chonnam Medical Journal* 47, no. 1 (2011): 1–13.
8. Atala, A., R. Lanza, and R.P. Lanza eds. *Methods of tissue engineering.* Gulf Professional Publishing, 2001.

9. Arslan-Yildiz, Ahu, Rami El Assal, Pu Chen, Sinan Guven, Fatih Inci, and Utkan Demirci. "Towards artificial tissue models: past, present, and future of 3D bioprinting." *Biofabrication* 8, no. 1 (2016): 014103.
10. O'brien, Fergal J. "Biomaterials & scaffolds for tissue engineering." *Materials Today* 14, no. 3 (2011): 88–95.
11. Kumar, Deepak, Jayant Jain, and Nitya Nand Gosvami. "Macroscale to nanoscale tribology of magnesium-based alloys: a review." *Tribology Letters* 70, no. 1 (2022): 27.
12. Berthiaume, François, Timothy J. Maguire, and Martin L. Yarmush. "Tissue engineering and regenerative medicine: history, progress, and challenges." *Annual Review of Chemical and Biomolecular Engineering* 2 (2011): 403–430.
13. Meyer, Ulrich, Thomas Meyer, Jörg Handschel, and Hans Peter Wiesmann, eds. *Fundamentals of tissue engineering and regenerative medicine.* Springer, 2009.
14. Fisher, Matthew B., and Robert L. Mauck. "Tissue engineering and regenerative medicine: recent innovations and the transition to translation." *Tissue Engineering Part B: Reviews* 19, no. 1 (2013): 1–13.
15. Pina, Sandra, Joaquim M. Oliveira, and Rui L. Reis. "Natural-based nanocomposites for bone tissue engineering and regenerative medicine: a review." *Advanced Materials* 27, no. 7 (2015): 1143–1169.
16. Lee, Esther J., F. Kurtis Kasper, and Antonios G. Mikos. "Biomaterials for tissue engineering." *Annals of Biomedical Engineering* 42 (2014): 323–337.
17. Peron, Mirco, Jan Torgersen, and Filippo Berto. "Mg and its alloys for biomedical applications: exploring corrosion and its interplay with mechanical failure." *Metals* 7, no. 7 (2017): 252.
18. Williams, David F. "On the nature of biomaterials." *Biomaterials* 30, no. 30 (2009): 5897–5909.
19. Kumar, Deepak, Nitya Nand Gosvami, and Jayant Jain. "Influence of temperature on crystallographic orientation induced anisotropy of microscopic wear in an AZ91 Mg alloy." *Tribology International* 163 (2021): 107159.
20. Chen, Junxiu, Lili Tan, Xiaoming Yu, Iniobong P. Etim, Muhammad Ibrahim, and Ke Yang. "Mechanical properties of magnesium alloys for medical application: a review." *Journal of the Mechanical Behavior of Biomedical Materials* 87 (2018): 68–79.
21. Davis, J. R. "Overview of biomaterials and their use in medical devices." In *Handbook of materials for medical devices*, pp. 1–11. ASM International, 2003.
22. Singh, Daljinder, Rupinder Singh, K. S. Boparai, Ilenia Farina, Luciano Feo, and Anita Kamra Verma. "In-vitro studies of SS 316 l biomedical implants prepared by FDM, vapor smoothing and investment casting." *Composites Part B: Engineering* 132 (2018): 107–114.
23. Kumar, D. Dinesh, and Gobi Saravanan Kaliaraj. "Multifunctional zirconium nitride/copper multilayer coatings on medical grade 316L SS and titanium substrates for biomedical applications." *Journal of the Mechanical Behavior of Biomedical Materials* 77 (2018): 106–115.
24. dos Santos, Venina, Rosmary Nichele Brandalise, Michele Savaris, Venina dos Santos, Rosmary Nichele Brandalise, and Michele Savaris. "Biomaterials: characteristics and properties." In Engineering of biomaterials, pp. 5–15. Springer, 2017.
25. Manivasagam, Geetha, Durgalakshmi Dhinasekaran, and Asokamani Rajamanickam. "Biomedical implants: corrosion and its prevention: a review." *Recent Patents on Corrosion Science* 2, no. 1 (2010): 40–54.
26. Prakash, Chander, Harmesh K. Kansal, B. S. Pabla, Sanjeev Puri, and Aditya Aggarwal. "Electric discharge machining: a potential choice for surface modification of metallic implants for orthopedic applications: a review." *Proceedings of the Institution of Mechanical Engineers, Part B: Journal of Engineering Manufacture* 230, no. 2 (2016): 331–353.

27. Nasr Azadani, Meysam, Abolfazl Zahedi, Oluwole Kingsley Bowoto, and Bankole Ibrahim Oladapo. "A review of current challenges and prospects of magnesium and its alloy for bone implant applications." *Progress in Biomaterials* 11, no. 1 (2022): 1–26.

28. Sáenz, Alejandro, E. Rivera, Witold Brostow, and Victor M. Castaño. "Ceramic biomaterials: an introductory overview." *Journal of Materials Education* 21, no. 5/6 (1999): 267–276.

29. Kumar, Deepak, Nitya Nand Gosvami, and Jayant Jain. "Influence of crystallographic orientation on nanoscale friction and wear mechanisms of the AZ91 alloy." *Tribology Letters* 68 (2020): 1–10.

30. dos Santos, Givanildo. "The importance of metallic materials as biomaterials." *Advances in Tissue Engineering & Regenerative Medicine: Open Access* 3, no. 1 (2017): 300–302.

31. Niinomi, Mitsuo. "Recent metallic materials for biomedical applications." *Metallurgical and Materials Transactions A* 33 (2002): 477–486.

32. Minnath, Mehar Al. "Metals and alloys for biomedical applications." In *Fundamental biomaterials: metals*, pp. 167–174. Woodhead Publishing, 2018.

33. Love, Brian J. *Biomaterials: a systems approach to engineering concepts.* Academic Press, 2017.

34. Dutta, Subhadeep. "Polymeric Biomaterials for Biomedical Applications Related to Human Health." PhD diss., Arizona State University, 2022.

35. Chen, Hong. "Development of multi-functional polymeric biomaterials." PhD diss., University of Akron, 2017.

36. Punj, Shivani, Jashandeep Singh, and Kulvir P. Singh. "Ceramic biomaterials: properties, state of the art and future prospectives." *Ceramics International* 47, no. 20 (2021): 28059–28074.

37. Moshiri, Ali, Neda Tekyieh Maroof, and Ali Mohammad Sharifi. "Role of organic and ceramic biomaterials on bone healing and regeneration: an experimental study with significant value in translational tissue engineering and regenerative medicine." *Iranian Journal of Basic Medical Sciences* 23, no. 11 (2020): 1426.

38. Migonney, Véronique, ed. *Biomaterials.* John Wiley & Sons, Inc., 2014.

39. Lourenço, Mariana Luna, Giovana Collombaro Cardoso, Karolyne dos Santos Jorge Sousa, Tatiani Ayako Goto Donato, Fenelon Martinho Lima Pontes, and Carlos Roberto Grandini. "Development of novel Ti-Mo-Mn alloys for biomedical applications." *Scientific Reports* 10, no. 1 (2020): 6298.

40. Chen, Qizhi, and George A. Thouas. "Metallic implant biomaterials." *Materials Science and Engineering: R: Reports* 87 (2015): 1–57.

41. Kumar, Deepak, Saurav Goel, Nitya Nand Gosvami, and Jayant Jain. "Towards an improved understanding of plasticity, friction and wear mechanisms in precipitate containing AZ91 Mg alloy." *Materialia* 10 (2020): 100640.

42. Park, Joon B., and Roderic S. Lakes. "Hard tissue replacement – II: joints and teeth." In *Biomaterials*, pp. 395–458. Springer, 2007.

43. Wong, Joyce Y., and Joseph D. Bronzino. *Biomaterials.* Taylor & Francis Group, 2007.

44. Prasad, Karthika, Olha Bazaka, Ming Chua, Madison Rochford, Liam Fedrick, Jordan Spoor, and Richard Symes et al. "Metallic biomaterials: current challenges and opportunities." *Materials* 10, no. 8 (2017): 884.

45. Hermawan, Hendra, Dadan Ramdan, and Joy R.P. Djuansjah. "Metals for biomedical applications." *Biomedical Engineering: from Theory to Applications* 1 (2011): 411–430.

46. Gupta, Vivudh, Balbir Singh, and R. K. Mishra. "Machining of titanium and titanium alloys by electric discharge machining process: a review." *International Journal of Machining and Machinability of Materials* 22, no. 2 (2020): 99–121.

47. Stadlinger, Bernd, Stephen J. Ferguson, Uwe Eckelt, Roland Mai, Anna Theresa Lode, Richard Loukota, and Falko Schlottig. "Biomechanical evaluation of a titanium implant surface conditioned by a hydroxide ion solution." *British Journal of Oral and Maxillofacial Surgery* 50, no. 1 (2012): 74–79.

48. Subramani, Karthikeyan, Reji T. Mathew, and Preeti Pachauri. "Titanium surface modification techniques for dental implants: from microscale to nanoscale." Emerging nanotechnologies in dentistry, pp. 99–124. Elsevier, 2018

49. Dvorský, Drahomír, Jiří Kubásek, and Dalibor Vojtěch. "AZ31 and WE43 alloys for biomedical applications." In *Solid state phenomena*, vol. 270, pp. 205–211. Trans Tech Publications Ltd, 2017.

50. Aherwar, Amit, Amit Kumar Singh, and Amar Patnaik. "Cobalt based alloy: a better choice biomaterial for hip implants." *Trends in Biomaterials & Artificial Organs* 30, no. 1 (2016): 50–55.

51. Kamrani, Sepideh, and Claudia Fleck. "Biodegradable magnesium alloys as temporary orthopaedic implants: a review." *Biometals* 32 (2019): 185–193.

52. Yang, Jingxin, Gerry L. Koons, Guang Cheng, Linhui Zhao, Antonios G. Mikos, and Fuzhai Cui. "A review on the exploitation of biodegradable magnesium-based composites for medical applications." *Biomedical Materials* 13, no. 2 (2018): 022001.

53. Kumar, Deepak, Basant Lal, M. F. Wani, Jibin T. Philip, and Basil Kuriachen. "Dry sliding wear behaviour of Ti-6Al-4V pin against SS316L disc in vacuum condition at high temperature." *Tribology: Materials, Surfaces & Interfaces* 13, no. 3 (2019): 182–189.

54. Amukarimi, Shukufe, and Masoud Mozafari. "Biodegradable magnesium-based biomaterials: an overview of challenges and opportunities." *MedComm* 2, no. 2 (2021): 123–144.

55. Maier, Petra, and Norbert Hort. "Magnesium alloys for biomedical applications." *Metals* 10, no. 10 (2020): 1328.

56. Thasleem, P., Deepak Kumar, M. L. Joy, and Basil Kuriachen. "Effect of heat treatment and electric discharge alloying on the lubricated tribology of Al-Si alloy fabricated by selective laser melting." *Wear* 494 (2022): 204244.

57. Ramalingam, Vaira Vignesh, Padmanaban Ramasamy, Mohan Das Kovukkal, and Govindaraju Myilsamy. "Research and development in magnesium alloys for industrial and biomedical applications: a review." *Metals and Materials International* 26 (2020): 409–430.

58. Lijesh, K. P., Deepak Kumar, and Harish Hirani. "Synthesis and field dependent shear stress evaluation of stable MR fluid for brake application." *Industrial Lubrication and Tribology* 69, no. 5 (2017): 655–665.

59. Liu, Chen, Zheng Ren, Yongdong Xu, Song Pang, Xinbing Zhao, and Ying Zhao. "Biodegradable magnesium alloys developed as bone repair materials: a review." *Scanning* 2018 (2018): 9216314.

60. Jamel, Murtatha M., Mostafa M. Jamel, and Hugo F. Lopez. "Designing advanced biomedical biodegradable Mg alloys: a review." *Metals* 12, no. 1 (2022): 85.

61. Gawlik, Marcjanna Maria, Björn Wiese, Valérie Desharnais, Thomas Ebel, and Regine Willumeit-Römer. "The effect of surface treatments on the degradation of biomedical Mg alloys a review paper." *Materials* 11, no. 12 (2018): 2561.

62. Thasleem, P., Basil Kuriachen, Deepak Kumar, Afzaal Ahmed, and M. L. Joy. "Effect of heat treatment and electric discharge alloying on the tribological performance of selective laser melted AlSi$_{10}$Mg." *Journal of Tribology* 143, no. 5 (2021): 051111.

63. Wang, Liqiang, Lechun Xie, and Daixiu Wei. "Metallic alloys in medical applications." *Frontiers in Bioengineering and Biotechnology* 10 (2022): 1041295.

64. Seitz, Jan-Marten, Dennis Utermöhlen, Eric Wulf, Christian Klose, and Friedrich-Wilhelm Bach. "The manufacture of resorbable suture material from magnesium – drawing and stranding of thin wires." *Advanced Engineering Materials* 13, no. 12 (2011): 1087–1095.

65. Zheng, Y. F., X. N. Gu, Y. L. Xi, and D. L. Chai. "In vitro degradation and cytotoxicity of Mg/Ca composites produced by powder metallurgy." *Acta Biomaterialia* 6, no. 5 (2010): 1783–1791.

66. Jähn, Katharina, Hiroaki Saito, Hanna Taipaleenmäki, Andreas Gasser, Norbert Hort, Frank Feyerabend, and Hartmut Schlüter et al. "Intramedullary $Mg_2Ag$ nails augment callus formation during fracture healing in mice." *Acta Biomaterialia* 36 (2016): 350–360.

67. Mohamed, Aya, Ahmed M. El-Aziz, and Hans-Georg Breitinger. "Study of the degradation behavior and the biocompatibility of Mg-0.8 Ca alloy for orthopedic implant applications." *Journal of Magnesium and Alloys* 7, no. 2 (2019): 249–257.

68. Agarwal, Sankalp, James Curtin, Brendan Duffy, and Swarna Jaiswal. "Biodegradable magnesium alloys for orthopaedic applications: a review on corrosion, biocompatibility and surface modifications." *Materials Science and Engineering: C* 68 (2016): 948–963.

69. Mirza, Ambreen, Andrew King, Claire Troakes, and Christopher Exley. "Aluminium in brain tissue in familial Alzheimer's disease." *Journal of Trace Elements in Medicine and Biology* 40 (2017): 30–36.

70. Dong, Jianhui, Tao Lin, Huiping Shao, Hao Wang, Xueting Wang, Ke Song, and Qianghua Li. "Advances in degradation behavior of biomedical magnesium alloys: a review." *Journal of Alloys and Compounds* (2022): 164600.

71. Yang, Youwen, Chongxian He, E. Dianyu, Wenjing Yang, Fangwei Qi, Deqiao Xie, Lida Shen, Shuping Peng, and Cijun Shuai. "Mg bone implant: features, developments and perspectives." *Materials & Design* 185 (2020): 108259.

72. Philip, Jibin T., Deepak Kumar, Jose Mathew, and Basil Kuriachen. "Tribological investigations of wear resistant layers developed through EDA and WEDA techniques on $Ti_6Al_4V$ surfaces: Part I – ambient temperature." *Wear* 458 (2020): 203409.

73. Becerra, Luis Humberto Campos, Marco Antonio Ludovic Hernández Rodríguez, Hugo Esquivel Solís, Raúl Lesso Arroyo, and Alejandro Torres Castro. "Bio-inspired biomaterial Mg-Zn-Ca: a review of the main mechanical and biological properties of Mg-based alloys." *Biomedical Physics & Engineering Express* 6, no. 4 (2020): 042001.

74. Duley, Partha, Darothi Bairagi, Lipika R. Bairi, Tapas K. Bandyopadhyay, and Sumantra Mandal. "Effect of microstructural evolution and texture change on the in-vitro bio-corrosion behaviour of hard-plate hot forged Mg-4Zn-0.5 Ca-0.16 Mn (wt%) alloy." *Corrosion Science* 192 (2021): 109860.

75. Cho, Dae Hyun, Byoung Woo Lee, Jin Young Park, Kyung Mox Cho, and Ik Min Park. "Effect of Mn addition on corrosion properties of biodegradable Mg-4Zn-0.5 Ca-$x$Mn alloys." *Journal of Alloys and Compounds* 695 (2017): 1166–1174.

76. Liu, Yang, Wei-Li Cheng, Xiong-Jie Gu, Yan-Hui Liu, Ze-Qin Cui, Li-Fei Wang, and Hong-Xia Wang. "Tailoring the microstructural characteristic and improving the corrosion resistance of extruded dilute Mg-0.5 Bi-0.5 Sn alloy by microalloying with Mn." *Journal of Magnesium and Alloys* 9, no. 5 (2021): 1656–1668.

77. Esmaily, Mohsen, Daniel B. Blücher, Jan-Erik Svensson, Mats Halvarsson, and Lars-Gunnar Johansson. "New insights into the corrosion of magnesium alloys: the role of aluminum." *Scripta Materialia* 115 (2016): 91–95.

78. Pardo, Angel I., M. Concepción Merino, Ana E. Coy, R. Arrabal, Fernando Viejo, and Endzhe Matykina. "Corrosion behaviour of magnesium/aluminium alloys in 3.5 wt.% NaCl." *Corrosion Science* 50, no. 3 (2008): 823–834.

79. Zhang, Erlin, Liping Xu, and Ke Yang. "Formation by ion plating of Ti-coating on pure Mg for biomedical applications." *Scripta Materialia* 53, no. 5 (2005): 523–527.

80. Zhang, Erlin, Dongsong Yin, Liping Xu, Lei Yang, and Ke Yang. "Microstructure, mechanical and corrosion properties and biocompatibility of Mg-Zn-Mn alloys for biomedical application." *Materials Science and Engineering: C* 29, no. 3 (2009): 987–993.

81. Kumar, Deepak, Jayant Jain, and Nitya Nand Gosvami. "Nanometer-thick base oil tribofilms with acrylamide additive as lubricants for AZ91 Mg alloy." *ACS Applied Nano Materials* 3, no. 10 (2020): 10551–10559.

82. Chen, Kai, Jianwei Dai, and Xiaobo Zhang. "Improvement of corrosion resistance of magnesium alloys for biomedical applications." *Corrosion Reviews* 33, no. 3–4 (2015): 101–117.

83. Baulin, Oriane, Damien Fabregue, Hidemi Kato, Alethea Liens, Takeshi Wada, and Jean-Marc Pelletier. "A new, toxic element-free Mg-based metallic glass for biomedical applications." *Journal of Non-Crystalline Solids* 481 (2018): 397–402.

84. Shuai, Cijun, Wenjing Yang, Shuping Peng, Chengde Gao, Wang Guo, Yuxiao Lai, and Pei Feng. "Physical stimulations and their osteogenesis-inducing mechanisms." *International Journal of Bioprinting* 4, no. 2 (2018): 138.

85. Ding, Yunfei, Cuie Wen, Peter Hodgson, and Yuncang Li. "Effects of alloying elements on the corrosion behavior and biocompatibility of biodegradable magnesium alloys: a review." *Journal of Materials Chemistry B* 2, no. 14 (2014): 1912–1933.

86. Mao, Lin, Li Shen, Jiahui Chen, Yu Wu, Minsuk Kwak, Yao Lu, and Qiong Xue et al. "Enhanced bioactivity of Mg-Nd-Zn-Zr alloy achieved with nanoscale $MgF_2$ surface for vascular stent application." *ACS Applied Materials & Interfaces* 7, no. 9 (2015): 5320–5330.

# 2 Manufacturing Methods of Mg Alloys for Biomedical Applications

*Pralhad Pesode and Shivprakash Barve*
School of Mechanical Engineering, Dr. Vishwanath Karad
MIT World Peace University, Pune, India

*Sagar V. Wankhede*
School of Mechatronics Engineering, Symbiosis Skills
and Professional University Kiwle, Pune, India

*Manoj Mugale*
Department of Mechanical Engineering,
Cleveland State University, Cleveland, USA

## 2.1 INTRODUCTION

Biomaterial implants are used to replace or repair damaged body parts. There are two types of implants: short-term implants and long-term implants. Short-term implants must be recovered after healing, whereas long-term implants are forever implanted in the body. The use of short-term implants can lead to additional surgery, increasing medical costs, treatment time, and patient pain [1]. Biodegradable or bioabsorbable materials are a new generation of biomaterials that are highly desired in medical applications because they eliminate the need for subsequent surgery by dissolving inside the body and producing bioabsorbable products following the healing process [2, 3]. These materials include ceramics or bioactive glasses, polymers, and natural polymers, including polyglycolic acid, polylactic acid, collagen, and chitin. However, these materials often have low mechanical strength and brittleness, and may not be transparent to radiation, limiting their use in applications such as bone replacements where load-bearing ability is required. On the other hand, biodegradable metals provide the necessary mechanical characteristics for artificial bone replacements, such as mechanical strength and fracture toughness for load-bearing uses.

Traditional implants fabricated from materials such as SS, Ti alloys, and Co-Cr alloys are designed to be permanent fixtures within the body after implantation [4, 5]. These materials have been found to be biocompatible, meaning they do not cause adverse reactions within the body, and they also possess mechanical properties that make them suitable for use in orthopaedic applications [6–8]. Table 2.1 shows physical and mechanical characteristics of various metallic implants and human bone.

DOI: 10.1201/9781003400462-2

**TABLE 2.1**

**Comparative Analysis of the Physical and Mechanical Characteristics of Various Metallic Implants and Human Bone**

| Properties | Density (kg/m³) | Elastic Modulus (MPa) | Compressive Yield Strength (MPa) | Fracture Toughness (MPa·m^{1/2}) |
|---|---|---|---|---|
| Natural bone | 1800–2100 | 3–20 | 130–180 | 3–6 |
| Synthetic hydroxyapatite | 3100 | 73–117 | 600 | 0.7 |
| Stainless steel | 7900–8100 | 189–205 | 170–310 | 50–200 |
| Magnesium | 1740–2000 | 41–45 | 65–100 | 15–40 |
| Co–Cr alloy | 8300–9200 | 230 | 450–1000 | NA |
| Ti alloy | 4400–4500 | 110–117 | 758–1117 | 55–115 |

*Source:* Reference [3].

The use of permanent implant materials such as stainless steel, Ti-based alloys, and CoCrMo (cobalt–chromium–molybdenum) alloys can have both biological and mechanical drawbacks. For example, stainless steel, a commonly used implant material, can suffer from pitting corrosion, which can lead to the release of harmful ions such as nickel (Ni) and chromium (Cr) into body fluids. These ions can cause inflammatory and immune reactions leading to the possibility of implant failure or other adverse effects on the body over time. Additionally, these alloys may not be suitable for certain types of applications where flexibility is important. Another issue that has been reported with some types of alloys is their tendency to undergo creep and fatigue, which can cause the implant to lose its integrity over time. This is particularly a concern for load-bearing applications such as hip replacements, where repeated loading can cause the implant to fail over time. While these alloys are widely used, researchers are constantly seeking new materials and designs to improve the performance and reduce the drawbacks of the permanent implants. Some examples of alternative materials include ceramics, polymers, and biodegradable metals [9, 10]. $Ti_6Al_4V$ is a commonly used titanium alloy in orthopaedic implants, because of its higher strength and biocompatibility. Nevertheless, it has been reported that the release of aluminium (Al) ions from this alloy can have negative effects on bone growth and may have potential links to Alzheimer's disease.

Studies have shown that Al ions can inhibit osteoblast proliferation and differentiation, which can negatively impact bone healing and growth. Additionally, there have been reports that Al ions can accumulate in the brain, which can contribute to the formation of beta-amyloid plaques, a hallmark of Alzheimer's disease. However, it is important to note that more research is needed to fully understand the potential effects of Al ion release from $Ti_6Al_4V$ on bone growth and Alzheimer's disease. It is also worth noting that other alternative materials are being researched as well, such as pure titanium, Ti-Nb alloys, and magnesium-based alloys, and they have shown promising results in terms of biocompatibility and bone healing [7]. V ion and $V_2O_5$

are toxic to cells and could pose a risk if used in vivo. CoCrMo implants are a type of metal alloy used in orthopaedic and dental surgeries. They have been found to release cobalt and chromium ions, which can have negative effects on the body, including cytotoxicity, DNA damage, metal hypersensitivity reactions, and pseudo-tumour. Above effects are triggered by the discharge of metal ions into the body after the implant is in place, which can occur over time due to wear and tear on the implant. It is important for patients and physicians to be aware of the potential risks associated with CoCrMo implants and to closely monitor patients who have received these implants. It is important to consider these potential risks before using these materials in medical applications [11].

Consequently, commonly used alloys of Al, Ni, Cr, V, etc. can contain biologically toxic elements and have mechanical compatibility issues such as stress shielding because of their high Young's modulus when comparing with human cortical bone. These issues often require invasive second surgeries for implant removal. To address these inadequacies, researchers have turned to biodegradable implants which can provide mechanical support and stability during bone reunion, degrade and disappear once bone reunion is complete, and avoid the necessity for a second surgery for implant elimination. Orthopaedic internal fixation implants made of bio-degradable polymeric materials such as polylactic acid and polylactic-*co*-glycolic have been used in the past [12]. Due to their poor strength, biodegradable polymeric implants are often employed in low loading-bearing applications. A new generation of biodegradable metal implants have been developed to provide higher strength and toughness required for orthopaedic implants. In the human body, these metallic biodegradable implants maintain the wounded tissue while corroding slowly and entirely disappear after the damaged tissue has healed.

Potential metallic materials include Ti-, Fe-, Zn-, and magnesium-based alloys, since they are non-toxic and biodegradable to varying degrees. These alloys could have a good potential for use in orthopaedic applications [13, 14]. For degradable implants, preserving mechanical integrity during the healing process is essential. Although Mg- and Fe-based implants have outstanding mechanical qualities, their usage in biodegradable implants is constrained by the low rate of disintegration of Fe-based implants. Inflammation, cell death, and other tissue-destructive processes can also be brought on by the toxic metal ions created by corrosion. Furthermore, compared to natural bone, the elastic modulus of implants made of Fe and Zn is substantially high. Due to their biocompatibility, biodegradability, and desirable Young's modulus, which really is near to that of natural bone, Mg-based alloys are one of these biodegradable metallic materials that are the subject of the most researcher for orthopaedic applications [15, 16]. Because of their ideal Young's modulus and bio-compatibility, magnesium-based alloys offer a significant amount of opportunity for application in biodegradable orthopaedic implants. However, they have a high corrosion rate in physiological environments. It was reported that a healthy adult needs 21–28 g of Mg to maintain regular functions, and 250–350 mg is recommended for daily allowance. Despite their high corrosion rate, the amount of Mg released by the implant is relatively small compared to the daily requirement and can be considered safe. Nonetheless, further research is needed to improve the corrosion resistance of Mg-based alloys before they can be widely used in orthopaedic applications [17, 18].

Mg-based alloys have potential for use in biodegradable orthopaedic implants due to their biocompatibility and required elastic modulus that matches with that of human bone. However, their high corrosion rate in physiological environments is a major drawback. Biodegradable magnesium-based alloys are intended to provide sufficient support to safeguard the fracture site from subsequent injury during the three stages of bone recovery: inflammation, repair, and reconstruction. In order to provide acceptable load-bearing capability throughout this time, Mg-based implants must have a reasonably low corrosion rate. Additionally, Mg-based alloys exhibit poor cold workability, as the dislocation slip only takes place on specific planes and directions at room temperature, which can be an issue during implant manufacturing [19]. Due to the poor cold workability of Mg-based alloys, they are typically manufactured by deformation process at higher temperatures. This is done to activate more slip systems and improve formability during manufacturing. By increasing the temperature, more slip systems are activated which allows better control over the material's shape and size during the manufacturing process. However, this can also increase the cost of production and may require special equipment [20]. This approach has the drawback of possibly oxidizing the samples, degrading the quality of the surface, and reducing processing effectiveness. Elevated temperatures can cause the Mg-based alloy samples to oxidize, which can degrade the surface quality and make it less suitable for implantation. Additionally, the increased temperature can decrease the efficiency of the manufacturing process, potentially leading to longer production times and increased costs. Therefore, it is important to consider these factors when selecting a manufacturing method for Mg-based alloys parts and balance the trade-offs between improved formability and potential downsides. There are certain optimization techniques available such as CODAS, COPRAS, GRA, and MOORA for selection of suitable materials when many options are presented [19–21].

A study by Chen et al. [21] looked into how heat treatment affected the mechanical and biodegradable characteristics of an extruded ZK60 alloy. They found that heat treatment had an impact on the mechanical characteristics of the alloy, such as strength and ductility. Additionally, heat treatment was found to affect the biodegradable properties of the alloy, such as the rate of degradation and the release of harmful ions. It was found that heat treatment can be used to tailor the mechanical and biodegradable properties of ZK60 alloy, making it more appropriate for use in orthopaedic implants. However, it is significant to note that further research is needed to understand the specific impact of heat treatments on the characteristics of this alloy, and to optimize the heat treatment parameters to achieve the desired properties. As a result of the creation of tiny, uniformly distributed MgZn phases, this study discovered that the sample that had been treated with T5 exhibited better mechanical characteristics and degrading behaviour. However, due to the creation of second phases and subsequent galvanic corrosion, the extruded specimen and the specimen treated with T6 both underwent significant corrosion.

A new extruded biomedical Mg-Zn-Ca alloy's mechanical characteristics, degradation behaviour, and cytotoxicity were investigated by Sun et al. [22]. The alloy was studied for its potential use in biomedical applications such as implants. The study aimed to understand the impact of extrusion on the mechanical characteristics, degradation, and cytotoxicity of the alloy, and to determine if it was suitable for biomedical applications. The study discovered that the extruded Mg-4.0Zn-0.2Ca alloy's peak strength, yield strength, elongation, and elastic modulus were 297 MPa, 240 MPa, 21.3%, and 45 GPa, respectively. The peak strength, yield strength, elongation, and elastic modulus were reduced to 160 MPa, 220 MPa, 8.5%, and 40 GPa, respectively, after 30 days of submersion in a simulated bodily fluid. This means that the mechanical properties of the alloy were affected by immersion in simulated body fluid, showing a decrease in strength and elongation. The influence of precipitated phases on the corrosion behaviour of Mg-5Zn alloy was studied by Song et al. [23]. The study aimed to understand how the formation of different precipitated phases in the alloy would affect its corrosion behaviour, as the corrosion resistance of Mg alloys can be significantly influenced by the presence of precipitated phases. The study focused on analysing the corrosion behaviour of the alloy under different conditions and identifying the precipitated phases that are formed and their impact on the corrosion resistance of the alloy. In summary, the T4-treated sample had the best corrosion resistance because it did not have any precipitated phases, whereas the T6-treated specimen had the poor corrosion resistance because it had precipitated phases that accelerated corrosion. Most Mg-based alloys are currently made by casting, but this method is not suitable for parts with complex shapes and the properties of the samples can be affected by the formation of thermodynamically stable phases during solidification. The distribution and morphology of precipitated phases is also difficult to control. In the work by Wei et al., the impact of Zn concentration on the corrosion resistance of Mg-$x$Zn-0.2Ca-0.1Mn alloys made by casting was investigated [24]. The study by Wei et al. found that the addition of Zn to Mg-$x$Zn-0.2Ca-0.1Mn alloys resulted in the formation of precipitated phases such as $Ca_2Mg_6Zn_3$, $Mg_2Ca$, and $Mg_4Zn_7$. The microstructure of the alloys was refined as the Zn content increased. It was shown that while the corrosion resistance of the alloys initially enhanced with the adding of Zn, it subsequently decreased. With a corrosion rate of 6.09 mm/year, the Mg-1Zn-0.1Mn-0.2Ca alloy had the maximum corrosion resistance.

Zhang et al. [25] looked into the corrosion behaviour and biocompatibility of Mg-Zn-Mn alloys made by casting for use in biomedical field. In simulated bodily fluids, they discovered that Zn can help build a passivation film that shields Mg-based alloys from corrosion damage. In addition, cell culture and haemolysis studies revealed that the Mg-based alloys had outstanding cytocompatibility. The desire for higher-quality implant materials may be satisfied by the creation of novel, high-quality Mg-based materials. The utilization of a specialized open-cell porous structure for implants would allow bone cell ingrowth and transportation channels for bodily fluids in addition to the base material. Porous implant materials such as polymeric and ceramic scaffolds have been employed, although owing to their poor mechanical strength, they cannot be used for load-bearing implant applications. Due to this, there is a desire for metallic foams with greater mechanical strength, such as Ti- and Al-based foams [26, 27]. Moreover, because Ti- and Al-based scaffold materials cannot break down in the body, they would stay there permanently. Porous bioabsorbable magnesium and magnesium alloys present fresh approaches. These substances show excellent promise for usage as bone substitutes with properties similar to bone. Host bone cells can grow inside the pores of a Mg scaffold after implantation for three to four months because the architectures of porous Mg materials and bone tissue are similar. This allows for the absorption of the implant by the body over time, reducing the risk of long-term complications associated with non-degradable materials [28, 29].

## 2.2 MANUFACTURING TECHNIQUES OF Mg ALLOY FOR BIOMEDICAL APPLICATIONS

The fundamental processes of producing and processing magnesium, including forming, casting, alloying, machining, and additive manufacturing (AM), are briefly described here.

### 2.2.1 CASTING

The variety of casting techniques has led to the categorization of these techniques, each of which is briefly explored.

#### 2.2.1.1 Gravity Casting

Despite the various benefits of casting Mg components using pressure die casting techniques, Mg products for a variety of applications are also produced via gravity casting that includes permanent and sand mould casting. The metal casting process known as "sand casting," sometimes known as "sand-moulded casting," uses sand as the mould material, while "permanent mould casting" uses metal. Both processing methods are appropriate for Mg structures that are light [30, 31].

#### 2.2.1.2 Pressure Die Casting

Pressure die casting is popular casting technique for Mg alloys and is renowned for its versatility in the design and production of intricate magnesium parts. Hot chamber die casting is a process where the metal is melted in a furnace and then poured into the die. It is called hot chamber because the metal is poured into the die from a heated chamber. Similar to hot chamber die casting, cold chamber die casting does not involve melting metal in the casting process. Instead, the metal is heated in a different furnace, moved to the die casting equipment, and then pumped under strong pressure into the die. Vacuum die casting is a variation of cold chamber die casting, where the die is placed in a vacuum chamber before the metal is injected. This process is used to eliminate the presence of gases and porosity that may be present in the metal, resulting in a better-quality casting. All of these techniques can be used to create components made of magnesium. The choice of technique will depend on the specific requirements of the component and the equipment available at the manufacturer. In each of the three forms, vacuum or pressure is used to press molten metal into a mould cavity that is sealed. However, one of the key distinctions between these approaches is the amount of pressure used [32].

#### 2.2.1.3 Stir Casting

Stir casting is another common technique used to create objects made of magnesium. This process involves heating the metal to its liquid temperature, adding reinforcing elements, and using a mechanical or ultrasonic stirrer to disseminate them throughout the molten phase. The final solid shape is subsequently provided to the molten phase once it has been cooled to room temperature. The primary issues with stir castings are the aggregated reinforced particles, their settling or floating in the molten phase, and their contact with the matrix material [33]. Cast magnesium alloys are unable to be heat-treated to increase the finished surface properties because of the inherent porosity of die casting processes, despite the fact that magnesium is known for having greater die-castability compared to other alloys such as aluminium. Using casting techniques, it seems nearly difficult, time-consuming, and expensive to produce magnesium parts with intricate shapes and exceptional attributes. In order to make complicated, net-shaped components with less time and material, there is a desire for processes that are not cost-effective [31, 34]. Adopting casting techniques depends on a number of variables, including weight, mould type, efficiency, etc. For example, gravity casting can be used to create a variety of castings made of magnesium that can weigh up to 1400 kg. Or, the HPDC method now rules the production of magnesium parts because of its increasing efficiency and the superior castability of Mg alloys. Because of its rapid cycle time (up to six components per minute), hot chamber die casting is especially economical for smaller size components [31].

## 2.2.2 FORMING

Die casting has been used to process the majority of the structural alloys made of magnesium that are used in many sectors, particularly the automotive ones. Die casting makes it possible to fabricate complex geometries, but the finished products' mechanical attributes frequently fall short of what is expected in terms of traits like endurance, strength, ductility, etc. Sheet metal forming is a dependable technique for building thinner and large-surfaced parts, such as those utilized in the vehicle body. Elements produced from sheet metal have greater mechanical qualities, such as a smoother surface with no discernible pores [30]. Therefore, using formed magnesium sheets instead of die-casted magnesium alloys can have additional benefits. Because magnesium has a hexagonal crystal structure, its alloys can be worked more easily at higher temperatures. The HCP lattice structure of Mg, which is frequently utilized, has a reduced formability at ambient temperature. A temperature of 225°C, for example, causes Mg to become more plastic. Other than the particular tooling and other methods necessary for forming Mg at high temperatures, there are no differences between the standard forming technique used for Mg and other alloys. At temperatures as high as 225°C, slip (also known as a deformation mechanism) also takes place in the hexagonal lattice structure's basal plane.

Twining is a type of shear deformation that occurs in crystals at room temperature. It involves the reflection of pieces of one crystal across a mirror or twining plane, which results in the formation of twinned crystals. This process can occur in a variety of different crystal structures and can have a noteworthy effect on the properties of the materials. Pyramidal slip planes that are triggered at high temperatures during the formation of Mg [35, 36] are where the primary portion of the twinning process takes place. As a result, temperature is very important in the formation of magnesium. According to reports, the forming temperature has a noteworthy effect on the stresses and potential strains. There is a reduction in flow stress and an increase in strain as a result of the thermally induced work softening that occurs when Mg is formed at high temperatures. Despite magnesium's low formability at low temperatures, which limits its use in cold forming to minor deformations, metal may be formed into cylinders and cones at room temperature using normal power rolls. Hot forming compared to cold forming is one of the preferred forming techniques for magnesium and its alloys. Mg alloys are typically drawn in a single step at high temperatures. Since there is no requirement for repetitive annealing and redrawing, fabrication time is reduced. Additionally, because there is less spring back in hot-formed magnesium parts compared to cold-formed ones, tighter dimensional tolerances are significantly more feasible. With one exception of pre-heating the dies and metal, the press-brake forming process for magnesium alloys is same as compared to other alloys. Hydraulic presses are preferred to mechanical presses for Mg deep drawing because they run at slower, more steady rates. Though, for the gentle draws, mechanical presses may also be employed. Manual spinning can be used to create various conical- or hemispherical-shaped parts.

Drop hammer shaping of magnesium is used to create component with shallow depths and asymmetrical shapes. When there are tiny quantities involved and a minimal amount of springback is necessary, this process is utilized. It must also be carried out at high temperatures. Lastly, near-net-shape higher quality parts are created using precision forging, a recently developed technology of die forging [36, 37].

### 2.2.3 MACHINING

The structure and qualities of Mg alloys, which make up the majority of the tonnage utilized in the various applications, rely on the casting conditions. Moreover, due to their eutectic intermetallic arrays, most of these die-cast magnesium alloys cannot be heat-treated and even cannot be age-hardened due to porosity scorching. However, compared to other materials, magnesium is more machinable, making it possible to mill Mg-based functional elements for the required function. Both dry and lubricated conditions can be used to machine magnesium. In addition to the advantages of milling magnesium, there may also be certain disadvantages, such as frequent chip ignition during dry machining or difficult chip reclamation during water/oil-based machining.

Magnesium has lower ignition point, so it is necessary to regulate the temperature of magnesium as well as the dry machining's speed and energy. At the time of machining process, the workpiece material is adhered to the cutting-edge of those materials by a process called built-up formation. Three types of build-up can be distinguished depending on the alloy being machined and the cutting speed: built-up edges, built-up layers, and flank build-up (FBU). During the machining of magnesium, these three distinct build-up patterns can be seen, but FBU is most common. FBU happens when the cutting speed surpasses its critical limit. As a result, the finishing surface degrades and the cutting force increases. Additionally, there are various machining issues related to FBU generation, such as vibrations, tolerances, and thermal expansion. Higher cutting speeds increase the possibility of chip igniting, which reduces geometrical precision, surface quality, and tool life. The friction at tool-chip and tool-workpiece also causes a rise in temperature and FBU. The accumulation of ignited chips during the dry machining of magnesium might also increase the danger of fires. Wet machining was initially developed to reduce the risks and issues associated with dry machining, although both oil- and water-based coolants have drawbacks. At high cutting speeds, oil-treatment-based machining is susceptible to deflagration [38, 39].

Additionally, because hydrogen has a low ignition point, the likelihood of hydrogen originating from water-based coolants should be taken into account. Dry machining circumstances can result in the accumulation of tiny, powder-like shards; this, in addition to creating a fire hazard, contaminates work areas and harms machine tool components. However, when the critical cutting speed is surpassed during dry machining, a high temperature might result, encouraging the adherence of the cutting tool to the workpiece as well as the FBU. Similar to wet machining, elevated process temperatures during dry machining lead to decreased workpiece surface quality, form, and dimension accuracy [38, 39]. In contrast, lubrication machining results in easy chip removal, clean machines, less tool wear, averted dust and spark production, and improved heat removal [40]. As per research, cutting magnesium alloys at extremely high or extremely low speeds and with a deeper cut increases the chance of a chip burning. Additionally, increased cutting forces may result from the development of FBU at higher cutting speeds. Furthermore, low cutting speed might result in tool wear by removing the coating from the tool because of higher cutting forces and lower cutting temperature.

Although the tool wear can be reduced and the tool's life extended by raising the cutting speed, further increases in speed, as previously indicated, bring up some other concerns, such as FBU. Additionally, the tool geometry and rake angles can be blamed for FBU. One method of avoiding the production of chips during the machining of magnesium is by adding various alloying elements. By adding more aluminium to magnesium, especially at shallower cuts and faster speeds, chips can be avoided. Additionally, yttrium and cerium can increase magnesium's oxidation resistance and keep its alloys from burning [39–41].

### 2.2.4 SEVERE PLASTIC DEFORMATION

In order to fabricate denser and heavy parts with precise structure at micro- and nanoscales for prospective usage in various industries, severe plastic deformation (SPD) methods are advantageous [42]. Although soft materials were the only ones that could be treated using SPD methods in the past, recently challenging materials like magnesium alloys have been manufactured using comparable methods. There is rising interest in using SPD methods to produce magnesium because of the metal's low ductility and formability, which are connected to its HCP crystal structure [43–45]. Naturally, it should be emphasized that each of the aforementioned techniques has a foundation from which it developed and can even be categorized under this heading. Because of discontinuous dynamic recrystallization along the grain's former boundaries, ultrafine grains of magnesium and its alloys are produced during the SPD process. During the extreme deformation of magnesium, a shear band, which is typically of a plastic nature, also forms and is regarded as the area of grain refinement. An effective parameter in grain development and refining is twinning during the SPD of Mg. Additionally, a more homogeneous microstructure is produced when the SPD of Mg is conducted at higher temperatures. The poor workability of magnesium alloys at lower temperature causes cracks at the time of processing. To prevent this cracking, SPD techniques must be used at elevated temperatures. However, increasing the process temperature might have a negative impact on the quality of the finished surface and the refinement of the grains during the SPD of Mg [46, 47]. The most significant SPDs are friction stir processing (FSP) and friction stir welding (FSW). The FSW is the basis for this process. It may concurrently homogenize and densify materials while modifying their microstructure, which improves the materials' plasticity and tensile strength. FSP alters the cast structure and makes it possible to produce Mg alloys with tiny, ultrafine, and nanoscale grains. Mg alloys' microcrystalline superplasticity is also enhanced by FSP. By swiftly displacing secondary phases, FSP improves the workability of magnesium alloys; however, this method still encounters difficulties due to the ensuing loss of alloy strength and low total and uniform elongation [48, 49].

### 2.2.5  Alloying Mg

The corrosion resistance, hardness, and grain size of Mg will be improved by alloying it with aluminium. Magnesium's tensile properties can also be enhanced by zinc, although issues with hot shortness and weldability can arise [50]. Table 2.2 displays how several alloying elements, including certain rare earth elements, affect the characteristics of magnesium. Magnesium has lately been combined with Li and Ca to make implants for the hip and knee joints lighter and more biodegradable. Another example of alloying magnesium is the development of a bone screw that uses calcium and zinc and is utilized in the femoral condyle [51].

$Mg_{17}Al_{12}$ and porosity are two phases that are thought to have an impact on the performance of commercial magnesium. Optimizing the second phase b's shape and

### TABLE 2.2
### Effect of Alloying Elements on Mg

| Elements | Alloying Element Effects |
| --- | --- |
| Cu | Strengthening while decreasing ductility |
| Zn | Improvement in corrosion resistance |
| Al | Hardness and strength increase, whereas ductility declines |
| Ce | Corrosion resistance increases, whereas yield strength decreases |
| Be and Ca | Reduced oxidation |
| Rare earth metals | Improved creep resistance, better corrosion resistance, improved strength |
| Li | Increased strength, stiffness, formability, and the transformation of magnesium from a brittle to a ductile alloy |
| Ni | Decreased ductility and corrosion resistance, increased yield and ultimate strength |
| Si | Greater resistance to corrosion |

*Sources:* References. [50, 56].

reducing porosity are the key goals of Mg alloy processing techniques. By appropriately constructing the second phase b, the toughness, formability, and texture of magnesium alloys will be enhanced, along with their fatigue and tensile strength and corrosion resistance. However, porosity is seen to be harmful and must be controlled. It manifests as voids or gas, mostly in cast Mg. However, it is manageable with the right production method selection and design [52, 53]. Another effective technique to prevent the corrosion and reactivity of Mg as well as its alloys is to coat the object, perhaps with Teflon resin coating. The coating can reduce contact corrosion as well as increase friction resistance and good lubricity while maintaining non-wetting properties [54, 55]. It appears to be difficult to create materials with characteristics that are close to their optimal theoretical strength.

The majority of techniques for creating more substantial materials are based on preventing the production of faults and slowing the movement of dislocations. These techniques do have certain drawbacks. Another method that combines the strengthening advantages of nanocrystalline materials (like magnesium) with amorphization is dual-phase nanostructuring, which results in the creation of a two-phase alloy with almost perfect strength at room temperature. The two-phase Mg-Li alloy is produced by changing the crystal structure of magnesium alloy from its HCP (a-Mg phase) to its BCC (b-Li phase). A two-phase structure (Mg-Li) will be created with Li levels ranging from 5.7 to 10.3 wt% in which the a-Mg and b-Li phases coexist in the matrix simultaneously. This alloy produces an alloy with greater ductility and formability while also covering the deficiencies of magnesium [56, 57].

## 2.2.6   AM (3D PRINTING)

Using plastic, metals, and ceramic materials, AM is a high-precision technique for creating detailed three-dimensional items directly from a computer model. Geometric freedom, a shorter design to product cycle, fewer process steps, mass customization, and material flexibility are some of AM's competitive advantages [58, 59]. AM techniques may be categorized based on their build volume, energy supply, and material feedstock. Tereolithography (SLA), developed by Charles W. Hall in 1984, is generally referred to as the predecessor of 3D printing and is recognized as the first commercially effective rapid prototyping process [60].

Powder bed fusion (PBF) and direct energy deposition (DED) systems are the two most widely utilized commercially available metallic AM technologies that first appeared in the late 1990s [61]. PBF systems melt or fuse powders using laser or electron beams as their energy source; PBF is further divided into selective laser sintering (SLS), selective laser melting (SLM), and direct metal laser sintering (DMLS), and the technique that utilizes electron beams as its source of energy is known as electron beam melting (EBM). In the PBF technique, a substrate plate is coated with metallic powder, which is then selectively melted by a laser (or electron) beam. The building platform is lowered and a new layer of powder is placed to melt additional layers after the laser scanning is finished. A levelling system, recoater blade, or any other method is employed to ensure consistent powder distribution. Until the specimens are completely constructed, this process is repeated. Inert gas is injected into the construction chamber to prevent oxidation and undesirable reactions from occurring to the metallic powder and melt [62, 63]. The type of material is a critical consideration when choosing an AM technique. For the manufacture of magnesium alloys, SLM is preferred over EBM for a number of reasons, but EBM is not always the best option. The temperature of the powder bed is high, exceeding 870 K, which causes some of the material's particles to melt. Second, the Mg and Zn elements vaporize as a result of the high concentrated energy delivered by the electron beam because of lower boiling temperatures of magnesium and Zinc. The deposition of these substances inside the construction chamber would likewise taint it. The SLM method is therefore a more effective technique for producing Mg/Zn/Al alloys [64].

## 2.3  NECESSITY FOR AM OF Mg

Through the fabrication process, the implant's microtexture can be managed and engineered. Among conventional manufacturing processes, die casting created voids and pores that had an undesirable impact on fatigue characteristics. Laser shock peening reduced stress shielding and caused the surface of magnesium alloy samples to develop micro-dents, which inhibited corrosion and increased fatigue life. The strength of die cast and hot extruded Mg specimen was also at its peak at room temperature, while ductility was more severely compromised. Although heat treatment aids in overcoming this challenge, these techniques are ineffective for producing materials with complicated shapes and functional gradients. Because of this, AM has shown to be very useful in producing the most complex geometries, which would otherwise be challenging or impossible to create using conventional machining techniques. A high degree of customization freedom offered by AM makes it possible to create tailored implants that properly match anatomical geometries. Because it avoids the lengthy, multistep processes required in traditional machining and also makes batch processing easier, the AM technology is also time- and cost-effective for implants [65].

Magnesium alloy AM is receiving a lot of interest in the community since it offers design options that conventional production cannot, as well as the capacity for the creation of biodegradable implants. The additive manufacture of Mg can be done using PBF [66, 67], wire arc [68, 69], paste extrusion deposition [70], friction stir AM [71], and jetting methods [72]. These techniques use various kinds of raw materials and process mechanics. The AM components produced by each technique have various structural characteristics.

Highly complicated parts which are challenging or difficult to manufacture with traditional machining methods can be created through these techniques. Custom implants that are better matched to anatomical geometries are made possible by AM. Furthermore, AM reduces the manufacturing time and expense for implants because multiple stages of conventional machining may be eliminated and batch manufacturing is now feasible. The development of geometrical components which will reassure cells growth, proliferation, and bone regeneration is made possible through complex internal and external geometries developed utilizing AM. In vitro toxicity of scaffolds made of WE43, a Mg alloy containing rare earth and yttrium metals, was less than 25%, and they retained their structural stiffness for four weeks [73]. Additionally, porous depositions can be created employing AM, and these might serve as ideal locations for tissue adhesion that quicken the healing process. A 3D construct's porosity can be altered by altering the print process settings, which can immediately impact corrosion rates and cell behaviour.

Current biodegradable polymer-based implants are not strong enough to serve as load-bearing orthopaedic implants. Human bone and magnesium both are quite stiff, which prevents stress shielding and makes them a perfect option for such load-carrying implants. Additionally, a comparison of Mg alloys with well-known biodegradable polylactide polymer used for non-load bearing implants showed that magnesium implants produced more bone cells [3, 74]. Throughout research, the author implanted guinea pigs with femoral implant rods made of polylactide and magnesium.

Since AM may replace some steps in traditional machining, batch processing is feasible, it can reduce the time and cost of producing implants. Magnesium produces a variety of qualities when utilized in the AM process, as opposed to other materials [75]. Geometrical characteristics that promote bone and tissue regeneration can be created by using AM to create structures with complex dimensions [76]. Samples of WE43, an in vitro magnesium alloy marked with pores as small as 600 μm and containing yttrium and rare earth elements, demonstrated a toxic impact of less than 25%.

Differences in modulus elasticity and yield strength between the as-built and as-polished samples could be insignificant. The yield strength and stress variations were shown to decrease after 1–2 days in contrast to the as-built and as-polished specimen. After 7 days, specimens usually never reach a plateau stage and even have lower stress variations [77]. Although yield strength decreases gradually over the first few days before rapidly increasing over the following few days, the Young's modulus grows in the first few days, drops dramatically in the following few days, and then practically stays unaltered until the last few days.

The researchers found that the mechanical and qualitative characteristics of the additively constructed samples were superior to those of the major component and specimens made with die casting and hot extrusion methods. Palanivel et al. [78] found that the friction stir additive manufacturing (FSAM) process generated samples based on the Mg-4Y-3ND alloy with better surface roughness under particular welding conditions. The highest hardness was 115 HV when it was manufactured, and it rose to 135 HV during ageing. Compared to the base material, welding offers up to 400 MPa more strength and 17% more ductility. One of the researchers [79] found that specimens of the magnesium alloy AZ91D produced using the SLM, PBF-based technique displayed superior tensile strength and micro hardness than die-cast Mg samples. During a stress test of 3D printed magnesium alloys, according to Yook [80], fatigue strength was unaffected by orientation, printing angle, or raster angle. Porosity was reduced by heat treatment, which also improved fatigue resistance.

## 2.4  AM OF Mg FOR BIOMEDICAL APPLICATIONS

Magnesium AM has attracted interest recently as a way to resolve problems associated with other processes and techniques; however, due to its strong reactivity and unregulated oxidation in its pure state, it has difficulties when it comes to 3D printing.

Additionally, because the raw materials for AM (such as powder, wire, or liquid resin) have a high surface energy, they are more likely to react with air oxygen and allow combustion. Figure 2.1 shows typical metal additive manufacturing (MAM)

| Design | Conversion | File Transfer | Configuration | Print |
|--------|-----------|---------------|---------------|-------|
| 3D CAD file creation. | STL file conversion. | STL uploaded to slicing software. | Parameter optimization. | Parts printed are layer by layer. |

| Handover | Inspection | Heat Treatment | Machining | Removal |
|----------|-----------|----------------|-----------|---------|
| Parts are now finalized. | Examined for defects. | Tailors properties. | Improves surfaces and tolerances. | Parts are removed from the machine. |

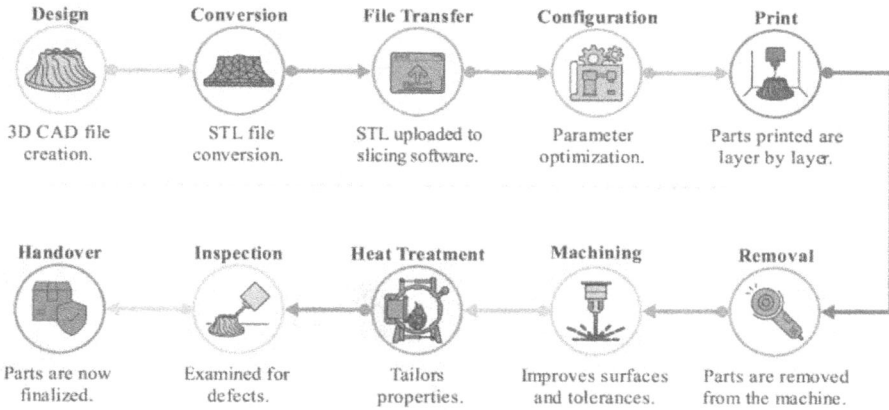

**FIGURE 2.1**    An example of a typical MAM process workflow [81].

process steps. In order to produce an environment that is inert and ensure the safety of material handling, all of these components operate as obstacles to a greater extent. Some of the Mg AM processes now in use are SLM, PBF, wire arc additive manufacturing (WAAM), paste extrusion deposition (PED), FSAM, and jetting [65, 82].

Recently, Mg alloy has been created using WAAM and SLM, two distinct AM methods. The generated metal has a well-defined grain form and few heat-affected areas because of SLM's high laser intensity, short working time, and quick cooling, which is crucial for structural integrity. The built size can vary and is influenced by the heat source. To enable maintenance or functional improvement, the DED techniques can be used for an existing object [83]. Magnesium alloys (AM) enable quick solidification to minimize coarse grains, macroscopic and microscopic composition segregation, and other defects while retaining their remarkable mechanical properties. The PBF printing process has received the greatest interest for printing magnesium alloys because of its low heat flux and ability to produce intricate internal and exterior geometries with a maximum density of 96.13% [84].

## 2.4.1  PBF

CAD design, laser processing, and system numerical control are all used in the PBF (Figure 2.2) process to create metallic components with enhanced characteristics. The following are some of the steps in the PBF technique: the system can obtain prototype segment information from three-dimensional prototypes by (i) converting them to STL files; (ii) putting a metal-powder outer film to the container used for development; (iii) using prototype data to direct the narrow light to accurately scan the powder sheet, which mop up heat and melt to make one layer; (iv) decreasing the container length by one layer while adding a new powder layer to the roller. The intended component will then be constructed by adding a new layer on top of the original layer [85].

Manufacturing component with laser additives has a number of benefits, including exact form fabrication, rapid production depending on the planned model, and

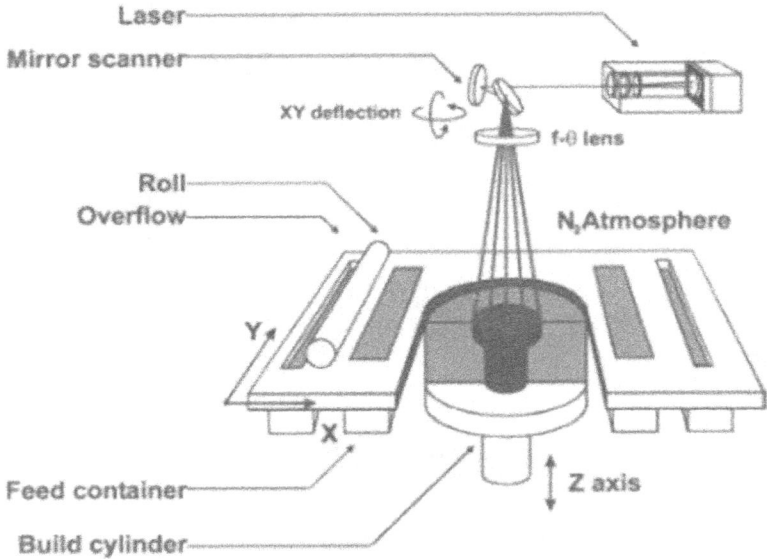

**FIGURE 2.2**   PBF system schematic diagram [65].

others [86]. The production of laser additions is compatible with a wide variety of materials, including polymers, ceramics, metals, and composites [87], thanks to the powerful laser intensity and subtle patch form [87]. In places with less load-bearing tissue, biocompatible polymers are employed as implants. Where there is a higher risk of implant materials in a body experiencing more wear and tear, ceramics are used. Implants made of metal alloys and their composites are placed in regions where they have characteristics similar to those of bone. The implant's characteristics could be better or worse than those desired for the replacement for the fractured portion. For the produced implant to work effectively in the body, it must have good biocompatibility. This processing technique is very useful for creating intricate porous materials and custom implants that may cater to specific patient requirements. A regulated rate of degradation and adequate mechanical support, particularly for the tensile modulus, have been demonstrated in recent study on the laser additive manufacture of magnesium scaffolds. After four weeks, there is a 20% reduction in the percentage of simulated fluid degradation. Similar to this, Kopp et al. [88] used laser AM to create a WE43 alloy scaffold with different pore sizes. The constructed scaffold has a bigger pore size of 1131 μm and a smaller pore size of 919 μm. The prefabricated scaffolds with minute pores had a negligible hydrogen leak and gradually lost some of their physical properties. When preparing porous structures, laser AM offers greater control over the structure than other methods. Designing bone implants for specific patients or different deficient sites is made simple with the integration of CAD and computed CT technology.

Another feature of laser AM that could assist to enhance the microstructure is rapid melting and solidification. Bär et al. [89] looked into the evolution of the WE43 microstructure throughout the manufacture of LAM. It was observed that the heat produced at different points in the molten pool influenced distinct microstructure morphologies. Besides, the particle size created by LAM was considerably smaller compared to part produced by casting technique. With lowering grain size, the fine grain strengthening method enhances the mechanical qualities of magnesium parts. Even though the findings of other researchers are inconclusive, the grain size impacts magnesium corrosion.

According to some studies, particle layers acted as a barrier against rust, slowing the pace of deterioration [90]. According to others researchers, grain boundaries function as crystallographic flaws that hasten the corrosion of magnesium [91]. It would seem that other factors that need to be considered include the type of alloy and the range of grain sizes. However, increased mechanical properties and a reduced rate of corrosion were seen in ZK60 [92] with grain refining, supporting the notion that particle layers served as degradation barriers. On the other hand, a PBF technique allows a great deal of control over the material's distribution and phase composition.

It is widely known that melting pools with strong temperature gradients generate Marangoni convection and a homogeneous alloying material dispersion as the solid–liquid boundary is swiftly crossed. At this stage in the model, the component parts of the alloy typically disintegrate. The "solvate capture effect" is another name for this phenomenon [93]. The electrochemical cell coupling between the matrix and the return leg may be minimized by the decreased precipitated phases of a wide matrix solution of alloy components, which can lower the degradation value. The application of LAM for implanted devices made of magnesium is still in its infancy when compared to metallic biomaterials such as Ti and Fe alloys. This has to deal with the physicochemical properties of magnesium. Because of its temperature ability (650°C), which is relatively close to its boiling point (1091°C), laser shaping is challenging. Ti has a higher melting and boiling point than Fe, and both materials can be manufactured utilizing a range of laser control variables [94]. However, Mg metal is easily burnt off during laser processing due to its inconsistent characteristics [95]. Furthermore, alloys need a tightly protected environment with low $O_2$ concentrations since Mg's active chemical properties make it rapidly oxidized.

One major distinction is that while magnesium bone implants made using the PBF technology are still in their infancy, this process has been used for many years to create bone implants that are made of titanium or iron. Other technologies based on AM have different constraints. Because the polymer layers on the manufactured component were not properly bonded, operations like material extrusion and vat photopolymerization reveal weaker areas. Poor calibration, incorrect printing settings, etc. are at blame for this. It is an extremely labour-intensive process that cannot be used for large production. The surface quality of the printed component is another common drawback to many AM-based methods. As a result, the manufactured part needs to be supplied for any post-processing tasks related to the selected printing medium.

If larger-sized powder particles are employed in the PBF-based processing, the component's surface polish ranges from 30 to 120 μm. Dimensional precision of the produced component is a difficult task during the binder jetting process. The AM method does not allow for custom material alloying. The composition components would remain the same regardless of the choice of raw material for printing. Size restrictions on the component being manufactured are present in all AM-based fabrication methods [96].

## 2.4.2   SLM Technology

A powerful laser light source and CAD input are used in the PBF method known as SLM to melt and fuse pre-spread powder particles layer by layer in designated regions. The term "laser" alludes to the method of handling, "melting" to the process of melting the particles, and "selective" to the treatment of only a portion of the powder [97]. SLM technique consist laser handling, a construction station, an automatic particle supply unit, monitoring software, and significant auxiliary components [98]. To regulate focus and laser beam mobility, laser diffraction unit is made of Galvano mirrors and flatter sector. To print the complete near net form part with a 99.9% relative density, the SLM process meticulously melts the powder particles layer by layer, line by line, and point by point [98, 99]. Every step of the process is managed by a production programme, including the layering mechanism, scanning, heating or cooling, and constructing.

The following phases of overall SLM processing are included: (i) Based on the thickness of each layer, CAD software-created components are divided into layers in order to construct a three-dimensional image of the component. (ii) In order to prepare for component manufacturing, a substrate is secured and levelled on the build platform. (iii) Inert gas is provided to the container to prevent surface deterioration and hydrogen absorption. (iv) A foundation sheet of exact thickness of the sliced coat should be coated with a thin layer of powder material using a powder recoater. (v) The geometry of the CAD model is used to create a layer-by-layer shape by scanning and managing powder beds in a certain way. (vi) The above two procedures must be repeated as each powder layer is produced until all necessary components are produced [96]

The first step in the SLM technique entails drawing a contour outline that emphasizes the key features of each part. The powder is subsequently melted inside the contours using correct scanning techniques [101]. SLM is a PBF-based technology that exhibits traits of various powder-based processes for component fabrication by utilizing a laser to dissolve the powder components which made up the soft beads [102, 103]. Since both powder assembly and mass approaches use the energy from the high-intensity laser, heating the powder particles is made easier [104, 105]. The powdered grains melt, clump together, and form a bowl when the energy is transformed into heat.

The boiling pool created by surface tension resembles a segmented barrel. Rapid laser contact with the powdered layer results in a solid rapid soaking effect up to 106.8°C and a transient heating range of up to 105°C [105]. Fast solidification may cause non-balance metallurgical phenomena, such as microstructural augmentation, crystalline stiffening, and the emergence of thermodynamic states, that could significantly enhance the mechanical characteristics and corrosion performance of laser materials fabrication [106]. Production of highly dense metal components is the main objective of SLM. Getting the desired result is difficult because of absence of hydraulic tension or hydrodynamics present at the time of SLM and the main driving forces are capillarity, gravitational forces, and the effects of heat. Additionally, if mechanical pressure is not applied during processing, certain components may solidify with less solubility, causing the tracks to continue to dissolve and leaving cracks, creating an uneven surface [107, 108]. Inside samples of ZK60 produced by SLM, porosity, and unmelted regions may be noticed. As a result of the materials' varying degrees of heat fluctuation, quickly solidifying laser-melting layers created during SLM produce residual tension [109].

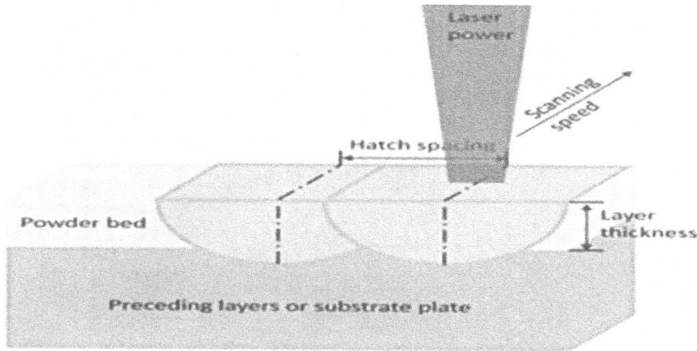

**FIGURE 2.3**   SLM process parameters [100].

Component delamination and heat blisters could result from this. Because of the quick heating and cooling that occurs during SLM, a melting pool may develop a tiny heat-affected zone (HAZ). HAZ alters material and elemental composition, which has an impact on sample characteristics and condition [97]. The transient thermal behaviour during SLM operations may be significantly controlled by processing variables such as beam strength, scan pace, hatch interval, the thickness of the border, and scan pattern.

Figure 2.3 depicts the process parameters that are typically investigated in SLM. Certain process settings are altered to permit the complete fusing of the melt vectors from the preceding layer with the subsequent melt vectors. Inadequate processing conditions could have unintended effects such as surface morphological anomalies, thermal fractures, and balling phenomena. To produce entire metal components free of cracks and fusion issues, it is crucial to link key SLM features to optimize the method's variables and ground morphology [96]. There are various restrictions related to the SLM technique in addition to the flaws with components produced using it. Some of them have incredibly sluggish processes, large power consumption, expensive beginning costs, constraints on actual size, etc.

### 2.4.3   SELECTIVE LASER SINTERING (SLS)

An alternative laser PBF-based AM method called SLS uses a laser beam to fuse powder particles into solid structures [110–113]. To aid in the sintering process, low melting temperature binder components are typically used [112, 114, 115]. Figure 2.4 shows SLS used to create metal scaffolds. Powder bed is initially heated below the melting point of material to prevent deformation and hasten the merging of the layers prior to sintering [113, 116].

Laser beam is then carefully directed to the required path of concerned layer using an optical scanning unit, sintering the particles to produce a solid structure. Lifting the feed chamber permits the powder to be dispersed evenly over the bed to obtain the required thickness. Up until the final printing of the entire item, the sintering process is repeated for the component's successive layers. Some powders may not sinter during the sintering process. A support for the portion and any overhanging

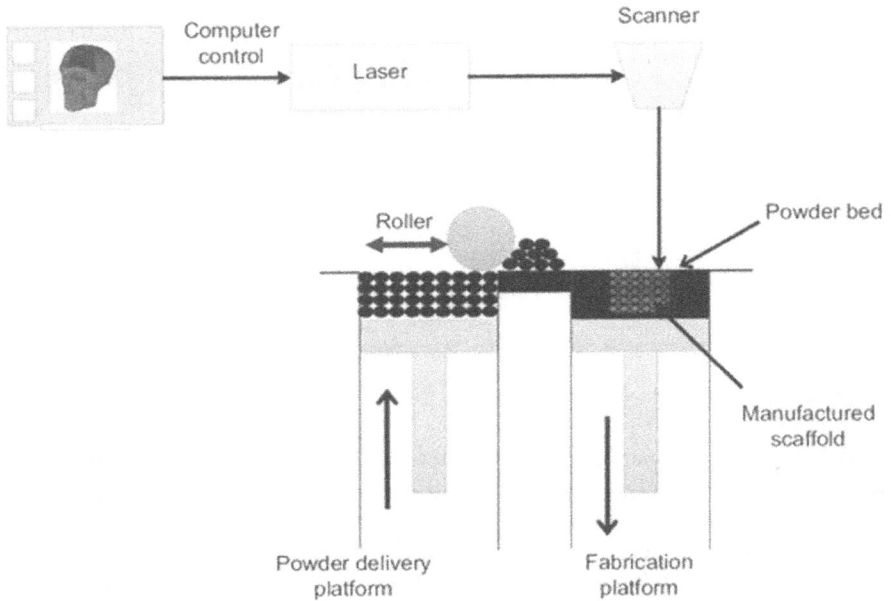

**FIGURE 2.4**  A typical setup for SLS used to create metal scaffolds [117].

features is kept on-site in the form of such powders [113, 116]. The powders were removed when the printing was finished and put to use once more. It is important to note that the SLS process only partially melts the powder particles [117]. Although SLS and SLM processes are comparable, they have some clear distinctions [112]. SLM processing is mostly used for certain metals such as Mg, Al, SS, Ti, and Co-Cr alloys; however, a variety of materials, including polymers, metals, and alloys, can be used with the SLS process [112, 115].

The laser scan used in the SLM method completely melts the powders, strengthening the connection between the particles [112]. Due to the SLS technology's focus on surface melting, powder particles are only partially melted during the laser scanning process. The scanning paths, the laser exposure length, the contouring technique, the point distance, the up-and-down-skin parameters, and the SLM technique-related variables are other elements that make up the SLS approach [112, 113, 117]. It is possible to reduce deformation and the ensuing residual stresses by altering the heat intensity distribution by optimizing the scanning paths. To achieve higher density and characteristics in the manufactured construction, however, the overall goal is to optimize all these variables [111–113].

The standard laser AM process includes the following steps [85]: (1) The shaping chamber is covered with an even layer of the desired metal powder. (2) The computer next obtains the pattern's slicing data. (3) The powder layer that absorbs heat is specifically scanned by the laser beam under computer control. The following step involves melting and solidifying this layer to create a single layer. (4) A new layer of powder is smoothed by the roller as the moulding chamber's height is reduced by one layer

[110]. After that, the subsequent layer is manufactured on top of the prior one until the designed item is created [118]. It is asserted that laser AM methods offer a wide range of advantages, including rapid manufacture, in accordance with a predetermined pattern, great process adaptability, and a higher rate of material consumption [117]. Characteristically, SLS-produced scaffolds exhibit poor formation characteristics because the melting of the particles does not occur fully, allowing formation pores to form inside the bulk metal and struts. This results in relatively low densification and poor mechanical performance for SLS-prepared implants and scaffolds, which restricts their use to load-bearing orthopaedic applications [111, 119]. Additionally, to reduce problems like oxidation and ignition, all AM process that include melting and solidification should be used in an argon-free environment [120, 121].

### 2.4.4 WAAM

Directed energy deposition (DED) in WAAM is an AM technology. Materials are melted together as they are created while using DED techniques. The metallic wire is continuously supplied into the device and then melted through an arc onto the previously deposited layers in most WAAM techniques. Tungsten inert gas (TIG) and metal inert gas are two wire-based welding processes that are essential to WAAM (MIG). In comparison to other DED methods, WAAM has the advantages of a higher deposition rate, effectiveness in terms of material consumption, and is significantly more cost-effective [65, 83].

A thin-walled AZ31 alloy component was created by Wu et al. using WAAM and the cold metal transfer (CMT) technique, which largely uses columnar dendritic structure [122]. The wire is purposefully rolled away following the short circuit in WAAM–CMT manufacturing method in order to limit the heat input during the melting and solidification stages of the metal. The anisotropic tensile properties of the produced item were found. Tensile properties of the building direction (Z-axis) specimen were identical to wrought AZ31, but those of the travel direction (X-axis) specimen were comparable to casted AZ31. The alteration in the elemental make-up of the AZ31 alloy also had an impact on the microstructure of the produced section. It is difficult to control the microstructural analysis and mechanical characteristics of the created parts since WAAM is a non-equilibrium thermal technique [123]. Greater deposition feeds and rates resulted in more refined grains being identified by TIG WAAM at arcing frequencies between 5 Hz and 10 Hz. Over and beneath this frequency range, the grain size was seen to increase [65].

### 2.4.5 Indirect Additive Manufacturing (I-AM)

The direct approach is often used in AM procedures to create functioning parts or models, i.e., the additively built part is the end result, or direct AM. However, direct AM frequently includes difficult process circumstances, such as higher temperatures and the frequent use of hazardous solvents, that could make the application of biomaterials sourced from natural sources impossible. Alternatively, the I-AM process, often known as the AM technique, can be used to build final parts or models by creating master templates, tools, or other techniques that make use of a non-AM strategy.

In the I-AM process, both traditional and cutting-edge tissue engineering techniques are integrated to create the macro- and micro-characteristics, respectively [124, 125]. The I-AM normally follows the following procedures [125]: (1) AM's creation of a negative mould; (2) using the negative mould to cast a liquid or melting biomaterial; and (3) removing the destructive/devotional mould. The negative and devotional moulds are often produced using the stereolithography or inkjet printing techniques with building components that are dissolved in non-toxic organic solvents [126, 127]. Mg-based scaffolds can easily use infiltration as an I-AM method [111]. It should be emphasized that infiltration techniques produce scaffolds with macro-scale dimensional accuracy, which might not be suitable for application in certain biomedical activities that call for open porous materials with pores that are only a few micrometers in size. Last but not least, it's important to note that the type of AM technique utilized and its parameters [111] are invariably influenced by the primary characteristics of scaffolds.

### 2.4.6 JETTING ADDITIVE MANUFACTURING

A modified two-dimensional printing technique that has been expanded to three dimensions is inkjet head 3D printing. Additionally, this approach is separated into two groups: both the binderless jetting method and binder jetting are addressed in Ref. [128]. The AM method called "binder jetting," which is based on a powder bed, particularly deposits a liquid-binding agent on the powder bed. The powder supply platform, build platform, levelling roller, and binder print head are components of a binder jetting printer [129]. Prior to putting the liquid binder over it, the platform's roller evenly spreads the powder coating over the cross-sectional area of the powder bed. Thereafter the powder bed is lowered, and an additional distance is added that is equal to the thickness of each layer. When a component is being produced, it isn't considered a green part until the desired shape is achieved; this method is carried out for each layer. Using this technique, a small batch of components can be printed. Binder jetting and sintering were used by researchers to create a 3D part while researching a semi-degradable Ti-Mg composite [130]. The printed specimen displayed enhanced interconnected pores with greater compressive strength as well as improved overall porosity. The rate of corrosion was greatly decreased. Cell proliferation increased as a result of cell–material interaction.

In a specific composition, one of the researchers employed MgP cement powder, which contains strontium carbonate ($SrCO_3$), magnesium hydroxide ($Mg(OH)_2$), and magnesium hydrogen phosphate ($MgHPO_4$). The printing variables for the binder jetting technique are influenced by the setting speed of the powdered binder system. As a result, each powder system requires a different set of printing parameters. The constructed scaffold underwent a post-hardening process that involved immersion in diammonium phosphate. $SrCO_3$ was added, and it was found to dramatically enhance microporosity while lowering the compressive strength of the MgP scaffold. Often, the powder's internal capillary forces act as a binder to bind loose powder particles altogether, and this is the basis for the binderless jetting technique's operation [131]. One of the researchers created a green body of the scaffold made of magnesium zinc and zirconium (MgeZneZr) alloy using a single-phase proprietary solvent in place of a binder solution [132]. There are no binding or solute components in this solvent. In order to prevent oxidation at high temperatures, the manufactured green portion was sintered in an inert environment furnace. The green component benefits from having all of the remaining solvent contaminations removed during sintering.

It was found that the compressive and elastic properties were greatly enhanced, and properties were closely matched with natural cortical bone. The items created with JAM technique often have higher porosity, less stiffness, and strength [110, 112]. The pieces created during the printing process must be kept in the build chamber for a few hours before outright curing. To attain the proper density and evaporate the part's binder polymers, post-thermal treatment is necessary. Due to the shrinking impact, these could lead to dimensional inaccuracies if not eliminated.

Future control over the porosity of the components manufactured may be aided by the formulation of powder characteristics and morphology. The results stated in the aforementioned publications reveal an extremely low degradation rate with a significant hydrogen evolution that strongly suggests that additional study on alloying techniques and their process parameters is required. Table 2.3 provides a summary of all the AM techniques mentioned in the chapter together with the relevant parameters and factors impacting the characteristics of the end products.

### 2.4.7   FSAM

In order to create 3D layered materials, FSAM builds on FSW [141, 142]. The spinning tool used in the FSAM process is non-consumable and has a shoulder and threaded pin. Layers are joined as a result of an intense plastic deformation brought on by the pin's movement. This heat is produced by frictional contact between the shoulder and the substrate, which causes the material to melt and fuse. Additionally, the oxidation reaction is diminished by the non-melting process and the stirring tool's rotation of the Mg surface's existing oxide layer. The $AZ_{31}$Be HA surface composite was found to have a well-defined grain matrix microstructure in the stir zone. The component matrix's density was greatly increased. However, the inclusion of HA can cause the corrosion resistance characteristic to degrade. Reduced corrosion resistance can also be a result of refined grain size. As a result of their increased reactivity, the grain boundaries are more vulnerable to corrosion. With atomized powder and rolled plate serving as filler, materials used an additive friction stir fabrication technique to create a multilayered structure out of WE43 Mg alloy [123].

Throughout this process, liquid nitrogen was used to rapidly cool the substrate's bottom in an effort to further limit the grain development. The components made using this procedure had uniform layer thickness and were free of voids or other flaws. Furthermore, it was found that the production conditions generated fully dense and fine-grained wrought microstructural parts without the requirement for an additional densification process. A rise in mechanical strength was also noted as a result of fine-grained microstructure. WE43 alloy was used to create a high-strength component by Palanivel et al. [78]. A multilayered build structure was produced using a lap joint and the successive LBL deposition process. The thickness of the sheet and the total number of assembly layers were used to calculate the joint's final thickness. Sequential building techniques and CNC machining of the welded layers were used

**TABLE 2.3**

**Benefits and Drawbacks of AM Techniques and Their Typical Applications**

| AM Techniques | Benefits | Drawbacks | Applications | References |
|---|---|---|---|---|
| WAAM | Comparatively high deposition rates, efficiency, and affordability | Geometric restrictions brought on by the nearby molten pool and surface tension | Industries related to transportation, aviation, and astronautics will certainly employ it extensively, but the medical sector is unlikely to employ it | [62, 122, 123] |
| BJ | Affordable way, swift procedure, various application materials, utilizing leftover granules, low temperatures and pressures allow for the possibility, no need for post-processing | Mechanically negative behaviour (compared to PBF methods), greater surface grit, requires post-processing, low accuracy, utilizes low-density binders | Biomedical domains, such as medication delivery, scaffolds, and implants food science, SOC, solid oxide fuel cell concrete building, storing electricity electrochemically, electronic apparatus, sand casting moulds, industrial construction | [111, 133–136] |
| SLS | High degree of mechanical precision, excellent mechanical properties decreased anisotropy, simple design changes and tweaks, good materials type flexibility, elimination of all post-curing remedies, unsintered powder can be recycled, requires no support structure | Inadequate surface quality Thermal distortion can cause warping and shrinkage to form The inability of unsintered powders to be reused, high cost of the machinery inadequate tensile strength, a poorly rough surface | Bone scaffolds and bone implants are examples of biomedical fields, automobile, military, military-related, aerospace-related, and electronics-related industries | [133, 135–138] |
| SLM | Good surface quality, good dimensional correctness, outstanding mechanical performance, outstanding repeatability, removes a few post-processing techniques, fabrication of fully dense pieces, little surface abrasion | Considerable residual tensions, higher cost, molten pool instability, responsive to corrosion | Bone implants, bone scaffolds, and cardiovascular stents are examples of biomedical areas, industries in the automotive, aerospace, and defence sectors | [111, 133, 135, 139] |

*(Continued)*

**TABLE 2.3** *(Continued)*
**Benefits and Drawbacks of AM Techniques and Their Typical Applications**

| AM Techniques | Benefits | Drawbacks | Applications | References |
|---|---|---|---|---|
| FSAM | The capacity to manufacture massive components, a number of materials can be bonded, very high repeatability, outstanding metallurgical properties in the joint area, possibility of creating flexible processes to create varied microstructures for particular applications | Tool wear happens throughout time, and the build may acquire significant residual stresses<br><br>Production scale and build speed are constrained by machine size and tool traverse speeds. The problem is clamping the material | Industries involved in rail, aerospace, automobiles, renewable energy, shipbuilding, and marine science and technology | [65, 122, 123] |
| I-AM | Superior surface quality, higher strength, and little porosity | The topological differences between as-built and as-designed scaffolds have an impact on mechanical integrity and cell ingrowth, different pore size, and strut thickness<br><br>Pores and struts are present in macro-scale and can damage biological behaviour | Clinical specialties like nasal prostheses, scaffolds, implants, and microvascular networks | [111, 136, 140] |

to make the final product. Hooking of cavities and surface were among the several defects that were observed. The cavities created were related to the existence of oxide particles and inadequate material compaction.

The most obvious flaw in the process was the cracking at the boundary between stir zone and thermomechanically impacted zone. The lingering heat tensions may have contributed to the crack's development. The significant temperature gradient across the weld nugget typically causes these problems. The grain boundaries affect how strong a structure is produced. Due to the components' exceptionally fine-grained microstructure and high density, they had a significant amount of strength and ductility. The SPD method known as FSAM produces parts with substantially smaller grain microstructures [142]. The fact that this technique has the potential to create dense, fault-free Mg alloy–based bioimplants is crucial to note. The synthesized components display high mechanical strength, while the produced bioimplants show no discernible anisotropic characteristic. Wide-ranging applications in the field of orthopaedic bioimplants have been attracted by the higher strength of the parts made using the FSAM process. FSAM has the potential to develop into an effective method for creating engineered microstructure and constructions made of various materials. It enables the addition of additional metals to magnesium to promote controlled mechanical behaviour and degradation rate of the finished product [123, 141].

## 2.5 BIOCOMPATIBILITY OF ADDITIVELY MANUFACTURED Mg ALLOYS

Biocompatibility and mechanical characteristics are crucial factors to take into account while creating new alloys [110, 143]. The capacity of a scaffold or implant to induce a proper host response after implantation is referred to as biocompatibility. In other words, biocompatibility refers to a scaffold's or implant's acceptance by the tissues around it as well as the entire human body [65, 73, 87, 144, 145]. The scaffold's biocompatibility in in vitro and/or in vivo studies is frequently ascertained to assess and describe the scaffold or implant [144, 146–148]. Factors related to biomaterials and the host/connective tissue have an impact on biocompatibility [65, 73, 87, 144, 149].

The factors that affect the 3D printed biomaterial include porosity fraction, surface features, pore shape, pore size, inclusions, chemical composition, contaminants, degradation/corrosion products, microstructure, and mechanical characteristics [65, 73, 87, 144, 149]. The biocompatibility of biodegradable Mg bioimplants and scaffolds is primarily influenced by their chemical make-up and breakdown by products [87]. It might be argued that, in light of this, attention should be paid to the chemical composition of the powders and their absolute usefulness. The acceptable limits for the degradation products must be carefully taken into account during structural design [87]. Surface treatment would increase the cells' adhesion and growth [149]. In order to encourage osteointegration, it's advisable to use both micro- and nano-textures to mimic the surface of natural bone [149]. This suggests that crystallographic texture plays a key role in the biocompatibility of Mg-based scaffolds [149]. Additionally, since they may be harmful to biocompatibility, contaminants and inclusions should be prevented from forming throughout the AM process.

Additionally, the biocompatibility of materials based on magnesium would be significantly impacted by factors associated with the burning off of elements during AM [65, 87, 120]. Human tissue has shown to be extremely biocompatible with alloys made of magnesium [149]. The human body needs to ingest 350–400 mg of magnesium on a daily basis. As a result, it is anticipated that the human immune and health systems are unaffected by the dissolution of $Mg^{2+}$ ions caused by the breakdown of a scaffold in the human body. There are no risks associated with magnesium overdose reported in the literature. The only problem with using magnesium in vivo is the excess hydrogen that is released as a result of the corrosion process occurring inside the human body [150]. By using bioactive glasses in the Mg-based alloys, it has also been demonstrated that the cytocompatibility has improved [151]. The optimal zinc concentration would increase the osteoblastic cells' ability to proliferate when added to Mg-based alloys. The cytotoxic impact, however, has been seen in vitro with increased zinc content [149]. On the other hand, 6 wt% of aluminium is the ideal amount to have in Mg alloys. This simply means that the aluminium ions generated by breakdown at such high concentrations will not be handled by the human body [149]. As a result, increasing the aluminium level to 6 wt% not only has no neurotoxic or cytotoxic effects, but also encourages the activity of osteoblastic cells. Less than 5 wt% of Zr is permitted in Mg alloys to promote biocompatibility. Bad biodegradability and biocompatibility are produced when Zr concentration is greater than 5 wt% [149, 152, 153]. Additionally, Zr and Ca components would speed up osseointegration and improve the stability of Mg-based bioimplants [149, 154].

A biomaterial is said to be biocompatible if it possesses a combination of biophysical (such as surface tension, density, wettability, etc.), biomechanical (such as Young's modulus, toughness, hardness, strength, wear behaviour, etc.), and biochemical (such as corrosion, antibacterial ability, biodegradability, cytotoxicity, etc.) properties that are same to that of the host's tissues [155]. The bioimplant and host tissue clearly play a part in this as seen by these characteristics. It should be noted that decreasing biocompatibility can cause major health issues in the body, including an unfavourable immunological response, chronic inflammation, and allergic reactions that result in host tissue rejecting the bioimplant [65, 73, 87, 144, 149]. As a result, AM can be utilized to make scaffolds that have the right amount of wettability and roughness, promoting cell adhesion, spreading, growth, and differentiation [143, 156]. Moreover, scaffolds with porous topologies and/or connected pores provide enough permeability to support cell ingrowth and the delivery of oxygen and nutrients to the cells [111]. Using the laser PBF technology, Benn et al. [157] developed the WE43 alloy for clinical uses. This method employed a laser beam with a power of 300 W, a scanning speed of 1200 mm/s, a hatching distance of 45 μm, and a layer thickness of 40 μm. The adjacent layers were exposed using a conventional zigzag laser beam exposure pattern with a 90° scanning angle. Biocompatibility behaviour demonstrated that spindle-shaped live cells (green) densely cover the control of nontoxic, whereas no live or almost live cells were observed on the control of poisonous, supporting the study [157]. Even if none of the three categories showed dead cells (red stained), alive cells with a slightly spindle and circular morphology totally cover the surfaces in comparison to the untreated sample. The treated sample specimens, however, would only contain a very small number of live cells, usually exhibiting neither a significant number of dead nor live cells on their surface [157].

## 2.6 CHALLENGES WITH MAKING MAGNESIUM-BASED ALLOYS BY AM

Despite appearing encouraging, there are still a number of challenges with AM of scaffolds manufactured from biodegradable Mg-based alloys. High chemical reactivity (oxidation) and a significant evaporation tendency characterize the powder of Mg-based alloys [111, 158–160]. Due to Mg's low boiling point, the evaporation is strong. On the other hand, Mg's rapid evaporation trend during PBF-based AM is also influenced by the fact that the gap between its melting and boiling points is less than 500 K [88, 111, 161]. A powerful exothermic reaction and explosion can occur when the magnesium powder has a high surface area similar to that employed in SLM [87, 111, 157]. In addition, difficulties with low vapour temperature, high vapour pressure, and strong inclination to oxidation can be taken into account [158]. An extraordinary amount of powder splash occurs during the manufacturing of magnesium-based alloys, which causes poor stability in AM of magnesium-based alloys. This is due to two factors: (a) the challenging preparation of Mg powder and (b) the powder splash. Magnesium has a higher vapour pressure and lower vapour temperature, which results in the powder splash. Additionally, by vapour, Mg particles along the scanning route would be removed. This could result in flaws on the subsequent scanning path and (c) cracks in the Mg alloys produced by the powder splash during AM [158].

It should be emphasized that pure magnesium and the powders of the alloys WE43 and AZ91D are easily accessible. Among all of these powders, only WE43 and pure Mg powders are being employed for biodegradable Mg-based manufacturing utilizing AM in the biomedical field. The reason AZ91D powder is not used is the biological toxicity of the aluminium element, which makes about 3–9 wt% of this alloy [158]. Due to Mg powder's lower absorption capacity, the laser beam's significant contribution would be reflected during laser AM. As a result, the Mg powder can only receive a lower intensity laser beam, which results in poor efficiency [111]. The post-process, in particular the sintering process, takes substantially longer than the primary AM technique and is therefore much more expensive [134, 144, 162]. However, it is highly desirable to create biodegradable Mg-based scaffolds whose rate of disintegration is equivalent to the pace of tissue regeneration [163–165]. Additionally, as Mg-based alloys typically have poor formability, surgeons should typically form bioimplants [166]. In order to properly realize the microstructural changes occurring during PBF-based AM, further explanation of the theory of melting and solidification is also necessary [120, 167]. Not to mention, structural shrinkage is predicted to happen during an AM sintering process in a 3D printing technology which includes a binder (like BJ) [134]. In addition to the integration and reorganization of the powders, this also relates to the disintegration of the utilized binder. The features of the 3D printed structure may change as a result of this event [134]. Homogeneous coating developed onto a porous Mg scaffolds/

implants considered as an additional post-treatment for Mg alloys produced by AM [168].

When using laser-based AM, it is challenging to produce the requisite pre-alloyed powder. However, evidence indicates that it is fine to combine elemental powder with a mixture of prealloyed powders [143]. Mechanistic investigations are still needed to understand thoroughly physical characteristics of magnesium alloys produced by AM, and more research is needed into the uniformity and blending of magnesium powder [145, 169, 170]. It is undeniable that the laser-prepared AM alloys differ from non-AM Mg alloys in a number of ways, though the physical basis for these differences is as yet unknown. Since it would also address one of the main issues with present (non-AM) Mg-alloys, there will be strong and immediate interest in the ductility that LPBF AM Mg alloys may demonstrate [171]. With magnesium and its alloys, health and safety are ongoing concerns.

Safety is always the top priority and is crucial in the production of any Mg-based goods, but in the case of AM-Mg, this also necessitates the use of least amount of powder at all times. Powder should be handled carefully and stored away from any source of ignition; precautions should be followed to handle minimally invasive and suitable testing in any non-self-extinguishing situations. Any structure that is nearby non-self-extinguishing situations should never use more powder than what is needed to put out a fire [155, 172, 173]. The reuse of used magnesium alloy powder has not yet been researched. There is currently no research on compositional alterations caused by processes. Sinter-based AM for Mg alloys is, typically, less developed than LPBF, partly because of the limited experiments carried out so far. However, the market for sinter-based AM is unique. One of the most significant AM production-ready technologies in recent years has seen significant growth is binder jetting.

Mg binder jetting could therefore advance more quickly, though it is still in its early stages. For sinter-based AM of magnesium alloy, preliminary findings indicate that more in-depth investigation is needed to completely understand the behaviour of printing and sintering, microstructural evolution, and mechanical, chemical, and electrochemical features. The post-processing of magnesium alloys created by AM has not been well studied, nor the value-adding process such as providing a homogeneous coating on Mg alloy porous scaffolds.

## 2.7    CONCLUSION AND FUTURE PROSPECTIVE

Mg alloys have excellent biocompatibility, biodegradability, and low cytotoxicity, making them very attractive materials for use in biomedicine. The creation of degradable bioimplants using various AM techniques to produce alloys based on magnesium is briefly covered in this chapter. The development of residual tension in the manufactured parts is one of the main difficulties faced by metallic bioimplant AM. By adequately heating the feedstock beforehand and homogenizing the grain structure during post-processing, the same can be further avoided. The main difficulties in 3D printing magnesium alloys come from their chemical and thermal instability, but it is also evident that the loss of mechanical properties is due to rising corrosion rates.

The evolution of the WAAM, PED, FSAM, LPBF, and jetting techniques for printing magnesium alloy tissue scaffolds is discussed. However, future research should concentrate on developed components that attain mechanical strength and controlled deterioration. When employing multiple materials with different compositions, it is preferable to combine biointegration and drug delivery capabilities (for example, metalloceramics for orthopaedic joints). The magnesium-based bioimplants may exhibit nano-surface topography, functional group attachment, surface energy alterations, among other things, as a result of plasma post-processing. One can slow down surface deterioration and enhance biointegration with host tissues by further altering the surface with beneficial MAO properties. In addition to lowering the cost of metal printing, the creation of novel materials made possible by AM methods would change the current state of many orthopaedic implants' mechanical characteristics, which could further lead to personalization of contemporary medicine. In conclusion, surface engineering by AM is a groundbreaking method for improving and evaluating the biocompatibility of novel osteoinduction and tissue-healing-supporting biodegradable metallic scaffolds with enhanced structural and degrading stability.

Mg-based alloys have recently received a lot of attention because of their potential performances in several biomedical fields. Compared to different metallic materials like SS, Ti, and Co-Cr alloys, magnesium-based alloys perform significantly better. This is because they exhibit outstanding mechanical, biodegradability, and biocompatibility properties in addition to appealing bioactivity and bioactivity traits. Mg alloys are frequently used in bone fixation devices and bone tissue scaffolds, although their breakdown rates are still unsatisfactory. The AM technique's improvements would enable the quick production of intricate and specialized porous constructions, including bone tissue scaffolds. In fact, AM techniques are routinely used to create the Mg bone tissue engineering scaffolds, as explained in this chapter. Rapid solidification and cooling during AM would result in homogenized and refined microstructures, which can enhance mechanical behaviour and corrosion/degradation resistance. AM can lead to texture development, precipitation hardening, and solid solution hardening in addition to homogenization and grain refinement. To effectively manage the properties of Mg biodegradable scaffolds, such as surface roughness, porosity, fracturing, and grain size, it is essential to accurately and appropriately select the AM process, along with its components.

The L-PBF method is a crucial step in the creation of Mg biodegradable scaffolds and implants, but evaporation must be taken into account at every stage of the process. For this, it is advised to do study utilizing the L-PBF method on how material, treatment, and microstructural change relate to one another throughout at particular temperature cycles. By doing this, it is possible to simultaneously obtain the requisite biocompatibility, cytocompatibility, biodegradability, and robust mechanical qualities. L-PBF stands out among the AM approaches because the topology can be precisely controlled, whereas EBM might be limited by the excessive Mg evaporation that affects how electron beams are distributed in a vacuum inside the built-in. The accurate and suitable selection of the AM process, together with its components, is crucial in order to properly control the characteristics of Mg biodegradable scaffolds, such as surface roughness, porosity, fracturing, and grain size.

Compared to SLS, SLM offers more functionality since Mg is completely melted and deeply infused, leaving no pores or cavities in the fabricated component with high densification. Smaller grains, homogeneous phase distribution, and increased solid solution all are benefits of SLM's rapid solidification and significant cooling rates. The mechanical and corrosive properties of Mg specimens made using SLM are therefore anticipated to be superior to those made using more traditional methods. In addition, creating structures that are near-completely dense above 99% still presents a significant problem for magnesium AM. More precise structures and specially designed implants, scaffolds, or gadgets might be produced via AM. Future advances in AM will make it simpler and better to produce Mg-based implants and scaffolds with the required shapes and characteristics for use in tissue engineering and orthopaedic surgeries. More research into the use of Mg alloys made through AM is needed since Mg-based scaffolds must exhibit the proper biological and mechanical properties in order to be implanted in the human body.

Scaffold and implant surfaces that have undergone traditional treatment, coating, or polishing may not be acceptable for use in enhancing the surface qualities of Mg alloys produced additively. The characteristics of the surfaces of the scaffolds and implants, including their wettability, roughness, and morphology, are critical to the corrosion rate and the interactions between the scaffolds and implants and cells (such as cell attachment or cellular response), which lead to bone reconstruction. Therefore, greater research on the effects of surface features and the development of surface treatment techniques are needed to further control the pace of degradation and encourage bone regeneration. These composite/hybrid constructions can be improved mechanically and biologically by future research in this field. It might be interesting to use Mg porous scaffolds in composite/hybrid manufacturing in combination with biomaterials like bioceramic, bioglass, biopolymer, and biocomposite. Innovative simulation techniques may help in fine-tuning the use of AM technology to produce desirable magnesium-based scaffolds, whereas scientists can concentrate on recreating the bone's surface using a combination of micro- and nano-textures. This research presents certain techniques, such as alloying, conversion treatment, and surface coatings, to regulate how quickly Mg-based scaffolds degrade and how resistant they are to corrosion.

In addition, new approaches or techniques must be created to successfully prevent an uncontrolled biodegradation rate. Using post-processing techniques like the hot isostatic press and heat-treatment operations, magnesium scaffolds and implants created using AM have significantly better biological and mechanical characteristics. To ascertain whether the performance of the scaffolds and implants is appropriate for implantation in human tissue, it is necessary to assess the impacts of post-processing. Additionally, it is critical to evaluate the applied surface coatings under cyclic stresses in order to boost fatigue strength because fatigue might cause the failure of Mg-based scaffolds and implants. It is also necessary to document the failure mechanism of additively manufactured Mg-based bioimplants and scaffolds. The applied loads, the AM process, the microstructure, and the surrounding environmental variables all can have an impact on the failure mechanism. It is encouraged to conduct more research to identify the failure mechanisms. The sintering performance of AM-fabricated Mg-based metals should be assessed in terms of composition, microstructural change, chemical/mechanical/degradation behaviour, and biological properties. It would be possible to create additively produced Mg-based scaffolds and bioimplants with better qualities for a range of biomedical applications by understanding and having knowledge of various failure processes, such as corrosion mechanism for controlling corrosion rate.

## DECLARATION OF COMPETING INTEREST

The authors affirm that they have no known financial or interpersonal conflicts that would have appeared to have an impact on the research presented in this study.

## REFERENCES

1. Alireza, Vahidgolpayegani, Cuie Wen, P. Hodgson, and Yuncang Li. "Production methods and characterization of porous Mg and Mg alloys for biomedical applications." In Metallic foam bone, pp. 25–82. Woodhead Publishing, 2017.
2. Pesode, Pralhad, and Shivprakash Barve. "A review: metastable β titanium alloy for biomedical applications." Journal of Engineering and Applied Science 70, no. 1 (2023): 1–36.
3. Staiger, Mark P., Alexis M. Pietak, Jerawala Huadmai, and George Dias. "Magnesium and its alloys as orthopedic biomaterials: a review." Biomaterials 27, no. 9 (2006): 1728–1734.
4. Wu, Chenliang L., Weijie J. Xie, and Hau C. Man. "Laser additive manufacturing of biodegradable Mg-based alloys for biomedical applications: a review." Journal of Magnesium and Alloys 10, no. 4 (2022): 915–937.
5. Pesode, Pralhad, and Shivprakash Barve. "Surface modification of titanium and titanium alloy by plasma electrolytic oxidation process for biomedical applications: a review." Materials Today: Proceedings 46 (2021): 594–602.
6. Vazirian, S., and A. Farzadi. "Dissimilar transient liquid phase bonding of Ti–6Al–4V and Co–Cr–Mo biomaterials using a Cu interlayer: microstructure and mechanical properties." Journal of Alloys and Compounds 829 (2020): 154510.
7. Liu, Dongni, Zhichao Ma, Hongwei Zhao, Luquan Ren, and Wei Zhang. "Nanoindentation of biomimetic artificial bone material based on porous $Ti_6Al_4V$ substrate with $Fe_{22}Co_{22}Ni_{22}Ti_{22}Al_{12}$ high entropy alloy coating." Materials Today Communications 28 (2021): 102659.
8. Wu, Yaocheng, Che Nan Kuo, T. H Wu, T. Y. Liu, Y. W. Chen, X. H. Guo, and J. C. Huang. "Empirical rule for predicting mechanical properties of Ti-6Al-4V bone implants with radial-gradient porosity bionic structures." Materials Today Communications 27 (2021): 102346.
9. Brooks, Emily K., Richard P. Brooks, and Mark T. Ehrensberger. "Effects of simulated inflammation on the corrosion of 316L stainless steel." Materials Science and Engineering: C 71 (2017): 200–205.
10. Rajasekar, Subash, Raghuram Chetty, and Lakshman Neelakantan. "Low-nickel austenitic stainless steel as an alternative to 316L bipolar plate for proton exchange membrane fuel cells." International Journal of Hydrogen Energy 40, no. 36 (2015): 12413–12423.
11. Hart, Alister J., Paul D. Quinn, Barry Sampson, Ann Sandison, Kirk D. Atkinson, John A. Skinner, Jonathan J. Powell, and J. Fred W. Mosselmans. "The chemical form of metallic debris in tissues surrounding metal-on-metal hips with unexplained failure." Acta Biomaterialia 6, no. 11 (2010): 4439–4446.

12. Adesina, Oluwagbenga Tobi, Emmanuel Rotimi Sadiku, Tamba Jamiru, Olanrewaju Seun Adesina, Olugbenga Foluso Ogunbiyi, Babatunde Abiodun Obadele, and Smith Salifu. "Polylactic acid/graphene nanocomposite consolidated by SPS technique." Journal of Materials Research and Technology 9, no. 5 (2020): 11801–11812.
13. Pesode, Pralhad A., and Shivprakash B. Barve. "Recent advances on the antibacterial coating on titanium implant by micro-Arc oxidation process." Materials Today: Proceedings 47 (2021): 5652–5662.
14. Jin, Liang, Chenxin Chen, Gaozhi Jia, Yutong Li, Jian Zhang, Hua Huang, Bin Kang, Guangyin Yuan, Hui Zeng, and Tongxin Chen. "The bioeffects of degradable products derived from a biodegradable Mg-based alloy in macrophages via heterophagy." Acta Biomaterialia 106 (2020): 428–438.
15. Jin, Shi, Dan Zhang, Xiaopeng Lu, Yang Zhang, Lili Tan, Ying Liu, and Qiang Wang. "Mechanical properties, biodegradability and cytocompatibility of biodegradable Mg-Zn-Zr-Nd/Y alloys." Journal of Materials Science & Technology 47 (2020): 190–201.
16. Zhou, Hang, Bing Liang, Haitao Jiang, Zhongliang Deng, and Kexiao Yu. "Magnesium-based biomaterials as emerging agents for bone repair and regeneration: from mechanism to application." Journal of Magnesium and Alloys 9, no. 3 (2021): 779–804.
17. Knapek, Michal, Mária Zemková, Adam Greš, Eva Jablonská, František Lukáč, Robert Král, Jan Bohlen, and Peter Minárik. "Corrosion and mechanical properties of a novel biomedical WN43 magnesium alloy prepared by spark plasma sintering." Journal of Magnesium and Alloys 9, no. 3 (2021): 853–865.
18. Singh, Gurmider, Sunpreet Singh, Chander Prakash, and Seeram Ramakrishna. "On investigating the soda-lime shot blasting of AZ31 alloy: effects on surface roughness, material removal rate, corrosion resistance, and bioactivity." Journal of Magnesium and Alloys 9, no. 4 (2021): 1272–1284.
19. Silva, Erenilton Pereira, Ricardo Henrique Buzolin, Felipe Marques, Flavio Soldera, Ulisses Alfaro, and Haroldo Cavalcanti Pinto. "Effect of Ce-base mischmetal addition on the microstructure and mechanical properties of hot-rolled ZK60 alloy." Journal of Magnesium and Alloys 9, no. 3 (2021): 995–1006.
20. Bazhenov, V. E., A. V. Li, A. A. Komissarov, A. V. Koltygin, S. A. Tavolzhanskii, V. A. Bautin, O. O. Voropaeva, A. M. Mukhametshina, and A. A. Tokar. "Microstructure and mechanical and corrosion properties of hot-extruded Mg–Zn–Ca–(Mn) biodegradable alloys." Journal of Magnesium and Alloys 9, no. 4 (2021): 1428–1442.
21. Chen, Junxiu, Lili Tan, and Ke Yang. "Effect of heat treatment on mechanical and biodegradable properties of an extruded ZK60 alloy." Bioactive Materials 2, no. 1 (2017): 19–26.
22. Sun, Yu, Baoping Zhang, Yin Wang, Lin Geng, and Xiaohui Jiao. "Preparation and characterization of a new biomedical Mg–Zn–Ca alloy." Materials & Design 34 (2012): 58–64.
23. Song, Yingwei, En-Hou Han, Dayong Shan, Chang Dong Yim, and Bong Sun You. "The role of second phases in the corrosion behavior of Mg–5Zn alloy." Corrosion Science 60 (2012): 238–245.
24. Wei, Liangyu, Jingyuan Li, Yuan Zhang, and Huiying Lai. "Effects of Zn content on microstructure, mechanical and degradation behaviors of Mg-$x$Zn-0.2 Ca-0.1 Mn alloys." Materials Chemistry and Physics 241 (2020): 122441.
25. Zhang, Erlin, Dongsong Yin, Liping Xu, Lei Yang, and Ke Yang. "Microstructure, mechanical and corrosion properties and biocompatibility of Mg–Zn–Mn alloys for biomedical application." Materials Science and Engineering: C 29, no. 3 (2009): 987–993.
26. Thakur, Bhaskar, Shivprakash Barve, and Pralhad Pesode. "Magnesium-based nanocomposites for biomedical applications." In Advanced materials for biomechanical applications, pp. 113–131. CRC Press, 2022.

27. Freyman, Toby M., Ioannis V. Yannas, and Lorna J. Gibson. "Cellular materials as porous scaffolds for tissue engineering." Progress in Materials Science 46, no. 3–4 (2001): 273–282.
28. Pesode, Pralhad, Shivprakash Barve, Yogesh Mane, Shailendra Dayane, Snehal Kolekar, and Kahtan A. Mohammed. "Recent advances on biocompatible coating on magnesium alloys by micro arc oxidation technique." Key Engineering Materials 944 (2023): 117–134.
29. Pralhad, Pesode, and Shivprakash Barve. "Magnesium alloy for biomedical applications." In Advanced materials for biomechanical applications, pp. 133–158. CRC Press, 2022.
30. Ahmadi, Mina, S. A. A. Bozorgnia Tabary, Davood Rahmatabadi, Mahmoud S. Ebrahimi, Karen Abrinia, and Ramin Hashemi. "Review of selective laser melting of magnesium alloys: advantages, microstructure and mechanical characterizations, defects, challenges, and applications." Journal of Materials Research and Technology 19 (2022): 1537–1562.
31. Pesode, Pralhad, Shivprakash Barve, Sagar V. Wankhede, and Amar Chipade. "Metal oxide coating on biodegradable magnesium alloys." 3c Empresa: Investigación y Pensamiento Crítico 12, no. 1 (2023): 392–421.
32. Michael, Nehan, and Richard Maloney. Magnesium AM60B instrument panel structure for crashworthiness FMVSS 204 and 208 compliances. No. 960419. SAE Technical Paper, 1996.
33. Kumar, Anil, SantoshChang Liu, and N. K. Mukhopadhyay. "Introduction to magnesium alloy processing technology and development of low-cost stir casting process for magnesium alloy and its composites." Journal of Magnesium and Alloys 6, no. 3 (2018): 245–254.
34. Pan, Fusheng, Mingbo Yang, and Xianhua Chen. "A review on casting magnesium alloys: modification of commercial alloys and development of new alloys." Journal of Materials Science & Technology 32, no. 12 (2016): 1211–1221.
35. Li, Ming-Zhe, Zhong-Yi Cai, Zhen Sui, and Qingguang Yan. "Multi-point forming technology for sheet metal." Journal of Materials Processing Technology 129, no. 1–3 (2002): 333–338.
36. Doege, E., and B. Behrens. "Forming of magnesium alloys." Metalworking: Sheet Forming (ASM Handbook) 14 (2006): 625–639.
37. Doege, Eckart, and K. Dröder. "Sheet metal forming of magnesium wrought alloys: formability and process technology." Journal of Materials Processing Technology 115, no. 1 (2001): 14–19.
38. Zakaria, Muhammad Syamil, Mazli Mustapha, Azwan Iskandar Azmi, Azlan Ahmad, Mohd Danish, and Saeed Rubaiee. "Machinability investigations of AZ31 magnesium alloy via submerged convective cooling in turning process." Journal of Materials Research and Technology 19 (2022): 3685–3698.
39. Tomac, Nikola, Kjell Tonnessen, and F. O. Rasch. "Formation of flank build-up in cutting magnesium alloys." CIRP Annals 40, no. 1 (1991): 79–82.
40. AKYUZ, Birol. "Machinability of magnesium and its alloys." TOJSAT 1, no. 3 (2011): 31–38.
41. Ning, Zhao, Junzhan Hou, and Shaoli Zhu. "Chip ignition in research on high-speed face milling AM50A magnesium alloy." In 2011 Second International Conference on Mechanic Automation and Control Engineering, pp. 1102–1105. IEEE, 2011.
42. Valiev, Ruslan Zafarovich, Rinat K. Islamgaliev, and Igor V. Alexandrov. "Bulk nanostructured materials from severe plastic deformation." Progress in Materials Science 45, no. 2 (2000): 103–189.
43. Rahmatabadi, Davood, Mostafa Pahlavani, Mohammad Delshad Gholami, Javad Marzbanrad, and Ramin Hashemi. "Production of Al/Mg-Li composite by the accumulative roll bonding process." Journal of Materials Research and Technology 9, no. 4 (2020): 7880–7886.

44. Yamashita, Akihiro, Zenji Horita, and Terence G. Langdon. "Improving the mechanical properties of magnesium and a magnesium alloy through severe plastic deformation." Materials Science and Engineering: A 300, no. 1–2 (2001): 142–147.
45. Xia, Xiangsheng, Qiang Chen, Zude Zhao, Minglong Ma, Xinggang Li, and Kui Zhang. "Microstructure, texture and mechanical properties of coarse-grained Mg–Gd–Y–Nd–Zr alloy processed by multidirectional forging." Journal of Alloys and Compounds 623 (2015): 62–68.
46. Mahmood, Fatemi, and Abbas Zarei-Hanzaki. "Review on ultrafined/nanostructured magnesium alloys produced through severe plastic deformation: microstructures." Journal of Ultrafine Grained and Nanostructured Materials 48, no. 2 (2015): 69–83.
47. Kim, Ho-Kyung. "The grain size dependence of flow stress in an ECAPed AZ31 Mg alloy with a constant texture." Materials Science and Engineering: A 515, no. 1–2 (2009): 66–70.
48. Ahmadi, Mina, Mostafa Pahlavani, Davood Rahmatabadi, Javad Marzbanrad, Ramin Hashemi, and Amir Afkar. "An exhaustive evaluation of fracture toughness, microstructure, and mechanical characteristics of friction stir welded Al6061 alloy and parameter model fitting using response surface methodology." Journal of Materials Engineering and Performance 31 (2022): 3418–3436.
49. Patel, Vivek, Wenya Li, Joel Andersson, and Na Li. "Enhancing grain refinement and corrosion behavior in AZ31B magnesium alloy via stationary shoulder friction stir processing." Journal of Materials Research and Technology 17 (2022): 3150–3156.
50. Kumar, D. Sameer, C. Tara Sasanka, K. Ravindra, and K. N. S. Suman. "Magnesium and its alloys in automotive applications: a review." The American Journal of Materials Science and Technology 4, no. 1 (2015): 12–30.
51. Chalisgaonkar, Rupesh. "Insight in applications, manufacturing and corrosion behaviour of magnesium and its alloys: a review." Materials Today: Proceedings 26 (2020): 1060–1071.
52. Decker, R. F., T. D. Berman, V. M. Miller, J. W. Jones, T. M. Pollock, and S. E. LeBeau. "Alloy design and processing design of magnesium alloys using 2nd phases." JOM 71 (2019): 2219–2226.
53. Jia, Guilong, Erjun Guo, Liping Wang, Yicheng Feng, and Yanhong Chen. "Evolution of phase morphologies, compositions, structures of Mg-Y-Nd system with Sm addition." Results in Physics 11 (2018): 152–157.
54. Blawert, C., N. Hort, and K. U. Kainer. "Automotive applications of magnesium and its alloys." Transactions of the Indian Institute of Metals 57, no. 4 (2004): 397–408.
55. Sharma, Asha, Sandeep Arya, Bikram Singh, Amit Tomar, Suram Singh, and Rakesh Sharma. "Sol–gel synthesis of Zn doped MgO nanoparticles and their applications." Integrated Ferroelectrics 205, no. 1 (2020): 14–25.
56. Rahmatabadi, Davood, Mina Ahmadi, Mostafa Pahlavani, and Ramin Hashemi. "DIC-based experimental study of fracture toughness through R-curve tests in a multi-layered Al-Mg (LZ91) composite fabricated by ARB." Journal of Alloys and Compounds 883 (2021): 160843.
57. Pahlavani, M., D. Rahmatabadi, M. Ahmadi, and R. Hashemi. "The role of thickness on the fracture behavior of Al/Mg–Li/Al composite processed by cold roll bonding." Materials Science and Engineering: A 824 (2021): 141851.
58. Kuai, Zezhou, Zhonghua Li, Bin Liu, Yanlei Chen, Shengyu Lu, and Peikang Bai. "Effect of heat treatment on CuCrZr alloy fabricated by selective laser melting: microstructure evolution, mechanical properties and fracture mechanism." Journal of Materials Research and Technology 23 (2023): 2658–2671.
59. Soleyman, Elyas, Mohammad Aberoumand, Davood Rahmatabadi, Kianoosh Soltan Mohammadi, I. Ghasemi, Majid Baniassadi, Karen Abrinia, and Mostafa Baghani. "Assessment of controllable shape transformation, potential applications, and tensile shape memory properties of 3D printed PETG." Journal of Materials Research and Technology 18 (2022): 4201–4215.

60. Gibson, Ian, David Rosen, Brent Stucker, Mahyar Khorasani, David Rosen, Brent Stucker, and Mahyar Khorasani. Additive manufacturing technologies, vol. 17. Cham, Switzerland: Springer, 2021.
61. Tapia, Gustavo, and Alaa Elwany. "A review on process monitoring and control in metal-based additive manufacturing." Journal of Manufacturing Science and Engineering 136, no. 6 (2014): 060801.
62. Pesode, Pralhad, and Shivprakash Barve. "Additive manufacturing of metallic biomaterials and its biocompatibility." Materials Today: Proceedings (2022). https://doi.org/10.1016/j.matpr.2022.11.248
63. Herzog, Dirk, Vanessa Seyda, Eric Wycisk, and Claus Emmelmann. "Additive manufacturing of metals." Acta Materialia 117 (2016): 371–392.
64. Konda Gokuldoss, Prashanth, Sri Kolla, and Jürgen Eckert. "Additive manufacturing processes: selective laser melting, electron beam melting and binder jetting: selection guidelines." Materials 10, no. 6 (2017): 672.
65. Karunakaran, Rakeshkumar, Sam Ortgies, Ali Tamayol, Florin Bobaru, and Michael P. Sealy. "Additive manufacturing of magnesium alloys." Bioactive Materials 5, no. 1 (2020): 44–54.
66. Niu, Xiaomiao, Hongyao Shen, and Jianzhong Fu. "Microstructure and mechanical properties of selective laser melted Mg-9 wt% Al powder mixture." Materials Letters 221 (2018): 4–7.
67. Pawlak, Andrzej, Maria Rosienkiewicz, and Edward Chlebus. "Design of experiments approach in AZ31 powder selective laser melting process optimization." Archives of Civil and Mechanical Engineering 17 (2017): 9–18.
68. Guo, Yangyang, Houhong Pan, Lingbao Ren, and Gaofeng Quan. "Microstructure and mechanical properties of wire arc additively manufactured AZ80M magnesium alloy." Materials Letters 247 (2019): 4–6.
69. Guo, Jing, Yong Zhou, Changmeng Liu, Qianru Wu, Xianping Chen, and Jiping Lu. "Wire arc additive manufacturing of AZ31 magnesium alloy: grain refinement by adjusting pulse frequency." Materials 9, no. 10 (2016): 823.
70. Farag, M. M., and Hui-Suk Yun. "Effect of gelatin addition on fabrication of magnesium phosphate-based scaffolds prepared by additive manufacturing system." Materials Letters 132 (2014): 111–115.
71. Rathee, Sandeep, Manu Srivastava, Pulak Mohan Pandey, Abhishek Mahawar, and Siddhant Shukla. "Metal additive manufacturing using friction stir engineering: a review on microstructural evolution, tooling and design strategies." CIRP Journal of Manufacturing Science and Technology 35 (2021): 560–588.
72. Salehi, Mojtaba, Saeed Maleksaeedi, Sharon Mui Ling Nai, Ganesh Kumar Meenashisundaram, Min Hao Goh, and Manoj Gupta. "A paradigm shift towards compositionally zero-sum binderless 3D printing of magnesium alloys via capillary-mediated bridging." Acta Materialia 165 (2019): 294–306.
73. Li, Yageng, Jie Zhou, Prathyusha Pavanram, M. A. Leeflang, Laura I. Fockaert, Behdad Pouran, and Nazli Tümer et al. "Additively manufactured biodegradable porous magnesium." Acta Biomaterialia 67 (2018): 378–392.
74. Witte, Frank, Volker Kaese, Heinz D. Haferkamp, Elinor N. Switzer, Andrea E. Meyer-Lindenberg, Carl J. Wirth, and Henning J. Windhagen. "In vivo corrosion of four magnesium alloys and the associated bone response." Biomaterials 26, no. 17 (2005): 3557–3563.
75. Jahangir, Md Naim, Mohammad Arif Hasan Mamun, and Michael P. Sealy. "A review of additive manufacturing of magnesium alloys." AIP Conference Proceedings 1980, no. 1 (2018): 030026.
76. Cai, Xiaoyu, Fukang Chen, Bolun Dong, Sanbao Lin, and Chunli Yang. "Microstructure and mechanical properties of GTA-based wire arc additive manufactured AZ91D magnesium alloy." Journal of Magnesium and Alloys (2022). https://doi.org/10.1016/j.jma.2022.11.018

77. Tom, Thara, Sithara P. Sreenilayam, Dermot Brabazon, Josmin P. Jose, Blessy Joseph, Kailasnath Madanan, and Sabu Thomas. "Additive manufacturing in the biomedical field: recent research developments." Results in Engineering 16 (2022): 100661.
78. Palanivel, Sivanesh, Phalgun Nelaturu, Bryan Glass, and Rajiv S. Mishra. "Friction stir additive manufacturing for high structural performance through microstructural control in an Mg based WE43 alloy." Materials & Design (1980–2015) 65 (2015): 934–952.
79. Bose, Susmita, Jens Darsell, Martha Kintner, Howard Hosick, and Amit Bandyopadhyay. "Pore size and pore volume effects on alumina and TCP ceramic scaffolds." Materials Science and Engineering: C 23, no. 4 (2003): 479–486.
80. Yook, Se-Won, Hyoun-Ee Kim, and Young-Hag Koh. "Fabrication of porous titanium scaffolds with high compressive strength using camphene-based freeze casting." Materials Letters 63, no. 17 (2009): 1502–1504.
81. Armstrong, Mark, Hamid Mehrabi, and Nida Naveed. "An overview of modern metal additive manufacturing technology." Journal of Manufacturing Processes 84 (2022): 1001–1029.
82. Allavikutty, Raja, Pallavi Gupta, Tuhin Subhra Santra, and Jayaganthan Rengaswamy. "Additive manufacturing of Mg alloys for biomedical applications: current status and challenges." Current Opinion in Biomedical Engineering 18 (2021): 100276.
83. Takagi, Hisataka, Hiroyuki Sasahara, Takeyuki Abe, Hiroki Sannomiya, Shinichiro Nishiyama, Shuichiro Ohta, and Kunimitsu Nakamura. "Material-property evaluation of magnesium alloys fabricated using wire-and-arc-based additive manufacturing." Additive Manufacturing 24 (2018): 498–507.
84. Ng, Cindy C., Monica M. Savalani, Hau Chung Man, and Ian Gibson. "Layer manufacturing of magnesium and its alloy structures for future applications." Virtual and Physical Prototyping 5, no. 1 (2010): 13–19.
85. Yang, Youwen, Chongxian He, E. Dianyu, Wenjing Yang, Fangwei Qi, Deqiao Xie, Lida Shen, Shuping Peng, and Cijun Shuai. "Mg bone implant: features, developments and perspectives." Materials & Design 185 (2020): 108259.
86. Gu, Dongdong, Yves-Christian Hagedorn, Wilhelm Meiners, Guangbin Meng, Rui João Santos Batista, Konrad Wissenbach, and Reinhart Poprawe. "Densification behavior, microstructure evolution, and wear performance of selective laser melting processed commercially pure titanium." Acta Materialia 60, no. 9 (2012): 3849–3860.
87. Qin, Yu, Peng Wen, Hui Guo, Dandan Xia, Yufeng Zheng, Lucas Jauer, Reinhart Poprawe, Maximilian Voshage, and Johannes Henrich Schleifenbaum. "Additive manufacturing of biodegradable metals: current research status and future perspectives." Acta Biomaterialia 98 (2019): 3–22.
88. Kopp, Alexander, Thomas Derra, Max Müther, Lucas Jauer, Johannes H. Schleifenbaum, Maximilian Voshage, Ole Jung, Ralf Smeets, and Nadja Kröger. "Influence of design and postprocessing parameters on the degradation behavior and mechanical properties of additively manufactured magnesium scaffolds." Acta Biomaterialia 98 (2019): 23–35.
89. Bär, Florian, Leopold Berger, Lucas Jauer, Güven Kurtuldu, Robin Schäublin, Johannes H. Schleifenbaum, and Jörg F. Löffler. "Laser additive manufacturing of biodegradable magnesium alloy WE43: a detailed microstructure analysis." Acta Biomaterialia 98 (2019): 36–49.
90. Argade, Gaurav R., Sushant K. Panigrahi, and Rajiv S. Mishra. "Effects of grain size on the corrosion resistance of wrought magnesium alloys containing neodymium." Corrosion Science 58 (2012): 145–151.
91. Zhang, Tao, Yawei Shao, Guozhe Meng, Zhongyu Cui, and Fuhui Wang. "Corrosion of hot extrusion AZ91 magnesium alloy: I-relation between the microstructure and corrosion behavior." Corrosion Science 53, no. 5 (2011): 1960–1968.

92. Shuai, Cijun, Youwen Yang, Ping Wu, Xin Lin, Yong Liu, Yuanzhuo Zhou, Pei Feng, Xinyan Liu, and Shuping Peng. "Laser rapid solidification improves corrosion behavior of Mg-Zn-Zr alloy." Journal of Alloys and Compounds 691 (2017): 961–969.

93. Shuai, Cijun, Yun Cheng, Youwen Yang, Shuping Peng, Wenjing Yang, and Fangwei Qi. "Laser additive manufacturing of Zn-2Al part for bone repair: formability, microstructure and properties." Journal of Alloys and Compounds 798 (2019): 606–615.

94. Li, Xiang, Chengtao Wang, Wenguang Zhang, and Yuanchao Li. "Fabrication and characterization of porous Ti6Al4V parts for biomedical applications using electron beam melting process." Materials Letters 63, no. 3–4 (2009): 403–405.

95. Wen, Peng, Maximilian Voshage, Lucas Jauer, Yanzhe Chen, Yu Qin, Reinhart Poprawe, and Johannes Henrich Schleifenbaum. "Laser additive manufacturing of Zn metal parts for biodegradable applications: processing, formation quality and mechanical properties." Materials & Design 155 (2018): 36–45.

96. Kaushik, V., B. Nithish Kumar, S. Sakthi Kumar, and M. Vignesh. "Magnesium role in additive manufacturing of biomedical implants: challenges and opportunities." Additive Manufacturing 55 (2022): 102802.

97. Zhang, Lai-Chang, and Hooyar Attar. "Selective laser melting of titanium alloys and titanium matrix composites for biomedical applications: a review." Advanced Engineering Materials 18, no. 4 (2016): 463–475.

98. Kruth, J-P., Peter Mercelis, J. Van Vaerenbergh, Ludo Froyen, and Marleen Rombouts. "Binding mechanisms in selective laser sintering and selective laser melting." Rapid Prototyping Journal 11, no. 1 (2005): 26–36.

99. Huang, Sheng, R. Lakshmi Narayan, Joel Heang Kuan Tan, Swee Leong Sing, and Wai Yee Yeong. "Resolving the porosity-unmelted inclusion dilemma during in-situ alloying of $Ti_{34}Nb$ via laser powder bed fusion." Acta Materialia 204 (2021): 116522.

100. Yap, Chor Yen, Chee Kai Chua, Zhi Li Dong, Zhong Hong Liu, Dan Qing Zhang, Loong Ee Loh, and Swee Leong Sing. "Review of selective laser melting: materials and applications." Applied Physics Reviews 2, no. 4 (2015): 041101.

101. Manakari, Vyasaraj, Gururaj Parande, and Manoj Gupta. "Selective laser melting of magnesium and magnesium alloy powders: a review." Metals 7, no. 1 (2016): 2.

102. Yadroitsev, Igor, and Igor Smurov. "Surface morphology in selective laser melting of metal powders." Physics Procedia 12 (2011): 264–270.

103. Riza, Syed H., Syed H. Masood, and Cuie Wen. "Laser-assisted additive manufacturing for metallic biomedical scaffolds." Comprehensive Materials Processing 10 (2014): 285–301.

104. Fischer, Pascal, Valerio Romano, Hans-Peter Weber, Nakis P. Karapatis, Eric Boillat, and Rémy Glardon. "Sintering of commercially pure titanium powder with a Nd: YAG laser source." Acta Materialia 51, no. 6 (2003): 1651–1662.

105. Li, Yali, and Dongdong Gu. "Parametric analysis of thermal behavior during selective laser melting additive manufacturing of aluminum alloy powder." Materials & Design 63 (2014): 856–867.

106. Zhang, Hongju J., Dingfei Zhang, Chunhua Ma, and Shengfeng Guo. "Improving mechanical properties and corrosion resistance of Mg6ZnMn magnesium alloy by rapid solidification." Materials Letters 92 (2013): 45–48.

107. Jean-Pierre, Kruth, Mohsen Badrossamay, Evren Yasa, Jan Deckers, Lore Thijs, and Jan Van Humbeeck. "Part and material properties in selective laser melting of metals." In Proceedings of the 16th International Symposium on Electromachining (ISEM XVI), pp. 3–14. Shanghai Jiao Tong University Press, 2010.

108. Kruth, Jean Pierre, Gideon N. Levy, Fritz Klocke, and Thomas H. C. Childs. "Consolidation phenomena in laser and powder-bed based layered manufacturing." CIRP Annals 56, no. 2 (2007): 730–759.

109. Zhang, L.-C., Hooyar Attar, Mariana Calin, and Jurgen Eckert. "Review on manufacture by selective laser melting and properties of titanium-based materials for biomedical applications." Materials Technology 31, no. 2 (2016): 66–76.
110. Badkoobeh, Farzad, Hossein Mostaan, Mahdi Rafiei, Hamid Reza Bakhsheshi-Rad, Seeram RamaKrishna, and Xiongbiao Chen. "Additive manufacturing of biodegradable magnesium-based materials: design strategies, properties, and biomedical applications." Journal of Magnesium and Alloys (2023) 9, no. 2 (2016): 392–415.
111. Sezer, Nurettin, Zafer Evis, and Muammer Koc. "Additive manufacturing of biodegradable magnesium implants and scaffolds: review of the recent advances and research trends." Journal of Magnesium and Alloys 9, no. 2 (2021): 392–415.
112. Yuan, Li, Songlin Ding, and Cuie Wen. "Additive manufacturing technology for porous metal implant applications and triple minimal surface structures: a review." Bioactive Materials 4 (2019): 56–70.
113. Charoo, Naseem A., Sogra F. Barakh Ali, Eman M. Mohamed, Mathew A. Kuttolamadom, Tanil Ozkan, Mansoor A. Khan, and Ziyaur Rahman. "Selective laser sintering 3D printing: an overview of the technology and pharmaceutical applications." Drug Development and Industrial Pharmacy 46, no. 6 (2020): 869–877.
114. Ngo, Tuan D., Alireza Kashani, Gabriele Imbalzano, Kate T. Q. Nguyen, and David Hui. "Additive manufacturing (3D printing): a review of materials, methods, applications and challenges." Composites Part B: Engineering 143 (2018): 172–196.
115. Lee, Hyub, Chin Huat Joel Lim, Mun Ji Low, Nicholas Tham, Vadakke Matham Murukeshan, and Young-Jin Kim. "Lasers in additive manufacturing: a review." International Journal of Precision Engineering and Manufacturing-Green Technology 4 (2017): 307–322.
116. Shuai, Cijun, Guofeng Liu, Youwen Yang, Fangwei Qi, Shuping Peng, Wenjing Yang, and Zheng Liu. "Construction of an electric microenvironment in piezoelectric scaffolds fabricated by selective laser sintering." Ceramics International 45, no. 16 (2019): 20234–20242.
117. Munir, Khurram Shahzad, Yuncang Li, and Cuie Wen. "Metallic scaffolds manufactured by selective laser melting for biomedical applications." In Metallic foam bone, pp. 1–23. Woodhead Publishing, 2017.
118. Kumar, Rajender, Puneet Katyal, Kamal Kumar, and Neeraj Sharma. "Investigating machining characteristics and degradation rate of biodegradable ZM21 magnesium alloy in end milling process." International Journal of Lightweight Materials and Manufacture 5, no. 1 (2022): 102–112.
119. Madrid, Ana Paula Moreno, Sonia Mariel Vrech, María Alejandra Sanchez, and Andrea Paola Rodriguez. "Advances in additive manufacturing for bone tissue engineering scaffolds." Materials Science and Engineering: C 100 (2019): 631–644.
120. Zhang, Wan-Neng, Lin-Zhi Wang, Zhong-Xue Feng, and Yu-Ming Chen. "Research progress on selective laser melting (SLM) of magnesium alloys: a review." Optik 207 (2020): 163842.
121. Aboulkhair, Nesma T., Marco Simonelli, Luke Parry, Ian Ashcroft, Christopher Tuck, and Richard Hague. "3D printing of aluminium alloys: additive manufacturing of aluminium alloys using selective laser melting." Progress in Materials Science 106 (2019): 100578.
122. Wu, Bintao, Zengxi Pan, Donghong Ding, Dominic Cuiuri, Huijun Li, Jing Xu, and John Norrish. "A review of the wire arc additive manufacturing of metals: properties, defects and quality improvement." Journal of Manufacturing Processes 35 (2018): 127–139.
123. Telang, Vicky Subhash, Rakesh Pemmada, Vinoy Thomas, Seeram Ramakrishna, Puneet Tandon, and Himansu Sekhar Nanda. "Harnessing additive manufacturing for magnesium-based metallic bioimplants: recent advances and future perspectives." Current Opinion in Biomedical Engineering 17 (2021): 100264.

124. Liu, Mie Jun Jolene, Siaw Meng Chou, Chee Kai Chua, Benjamin Chia Meng Tay, and Beng Koon Ng. "The development of silk fibroin scaffolds using an indirect rapid prototyping approach: morphological analysis and cell growth monitoring by spectral-domain optical coherence tomography." Medical Engineering & Physics 35, no. 2 (2013): 253–262.

125. Wilson, Clayton E., Clemens A. Van Blitterswijk, A. J. Verbout, W. J. A. Dhert, and Joost Dick de Bruijn. "Scaffolds with a standardized macro-architecture fabricated from several calcium phosphate ceramics using an indirect rapid prototyping technique." Journal of Materials Science: Materials in Medicine 22 (2011): 97–105.

126. Chen, Chih-Hao, Jolene Mei-Jun Liu, Chee-Kai Chua, Siaw-Meng Chou, Victor Bong-Hang Shyu, and Jyh-Ping Chen. "Cartilage tissue engineering with silk fibroin scaffolds fabricated by indirect additive manufacturing technology." Materials 7, no. 3 (2014): 2104–2119.

127. Mota, Carlos, Dario Puppi, Dinuccio Dinucci, Cesare Errico, Paulo Bártolo, and Federica Chiellini. "Dual-scale polymeric constructs as scaffolds for tissue engineering." Materials 4, no. 3 (2011): 527–542.

128. Jafari, Davoud, Tom HJ Vaneker, and Ian Gibson. "Wire and arc additive manufacturing: opportunities and challenges to control the quality and accuracy of manufactured parts." Materials & Design 202 (2021): 109471.

129. Yazdanpanah, Zahra, James D. Johnston, David ML Cooper, and Xiongbiao Chen. "3D bioprinted scaffolds for bone tissue engineering: state-of-the-art and emerging technologies." Frontiers in Bioengineering and Biotechnology 10 (2022). https://doi.org/10.3389/fbioe.2022.824156

130. Zhang, Lei, Guojing Yang, Blake N. Johnson, and Xiaofeng Jia. "Three-dimensional (3D) printed scaffold and material selection for bone repair." Acta Biomaterialia 84 (2019): 16–33.

131. Bandyopadhyay, Amit, Indranath Mitra, and Susmita Bose. "3D printing for bone regeneration." Current Osteoporosis Reports 18 (2020): 505–514.

132. Chen, Daniel X. B. Extrusion bioprinting of scaffolds for tissue engineering applications. Springer International Publishing, 2019.

133. Chua, Kaitlyn, Irfaan Khan, Raoul Malhotra, and Donghui Zhu. "Additive manufacturing and 3D printing of metallic biomaterials." Engineered Regeneration (2022). 10.1016/j.engreg.2021.11.002

134. Mostafaei, Amir, Amy M. Elliott, John E. Barnes, Fangzhou Li, Wenda Tan, Corson L. Cramer, Peeyush Nandwana, and Markus Chmielus. "Binder jet 3D printing: process parameters, materials, properties, modeling, and challenges." Progress in Materials Science 119 (2021): 100707.

135. Buj-Corral, Irene, Aitor Tejo-Otero, and Felip Fenollosa-Artés. "Development of AM technologies for metals in the sector of medical implants." Metals 10, no. 5 (2020): 686.

136. Salmi, Mika. "Additive manufacturing processes in medical applications." Materials 14, no. 1 (2021): 191.

137. Păcurar, Răzvan, Petru Berce, Anna Petrilak, Ovidiu Nemeş, Cristina Ştefana Miron Borzan, Marta Harničárová, and Ancuţa Păcurar. "Selective laser sintering of PA 2200 for hip implant applications: finite element analysis, process optimization, morphological and mechanical characterization." Materials 14, no. 15 (2021): 4240.

138. Qin, Tian, Xiaoqian Li, Hui Long, Shizhen Bin, and Yong Xu. "Bioactive tetracalcium phosphate scaffolds fabricated by selective laser sintering for bone regeneration applications." Materials 13, no. 10 (2020): 2268.

139. Ren, Zhihao, David Z. Zhang, Guang Fu, Junjie Jiang, and Miao Zhao. "High-fidelity modelling of selective laser melting copper alloy: laser reflection behavior and thermal-fluid dynamics." Materials & Design 207 (2021): 109857.

140. Aabith, Saja, Richard Caulfield, Omid Akhlaghi, Anastasia Papadopoulou, Shervanthi Homer-Vanniasinkam, and Manish K. Tiwari. "3D direct-write printing of water soluble micromoulds for high-resolution rapid prototyping." Additive Manufacturing 58 (2022): 103019.
141. Ho, Yee-Hsien, Kun Man, Sameehan S. Joshi, Mangesh V. Pantawane, Tso-Chang Wu, Yong Yang, and Narendra B. Dahotre. "In-vitro biomineralization and biocompatibility of friction stir additively manufactured AZ31B magnesium alloy-hydroxyapatite composites." Bioactive Materials 5, no. 4 (2020): 891–901.
142. Wang, Wen, Peng Han, Pai Peng, Ting Zhang, Qiang Liu, Sheng-Nan Yuan, Li-Ying Huang, Hai-Liang Yu, Ke Qiao, and Kuai-She Wang. "Friction stir processing of magnesium alloys: a review." Acta Metallurgica Sinica (English Letters) 33 (2020): 43–57.
143. Tang, Daniel, Rahul S. Tare, Liang-Yo Yang, David F. Williams, Keng-Liang Ou, and Richard OC Oreffo. "Biofabrication of bone tissue: approaches, challenges and translation for bone regeneration." Biomaterials 83 (2016): 363–382.
144. Kumar, Alok, Sourav Mandal, Srimanta Barui, Ramakrishna Vasireddi, Uwe Gbureck, Michael Gelinsky, and Bikramjit Basu. "Low temperature additive manufacturing of three-dimensional scaffolds for bone-tissue engineering applications: processing related challenges and property assessment." Materials Science and Engineering: R: Reports 103 (2016): 1–39.
145. Liu, Ruoyu, Rangan He, Jie Xiao, Meifang Tang, Hongju Zhang, and Shengfeng Guo. "Development of Fe-based bulk metallic glass composite as biodegradable metal." Materials Letters 247 (2019): 185–188.
146. Bakhsheshi-Rad, Hamid Reza, Ehsan Dayaghi, Ahmad Fauzi Ismail, Aziz Madzlan, Ali Akhavan-Farid, and Chen Xiongbiao. "Synthesis and in-vitro characterization of biodegradable porous magnesium-based scaffolds containing silver for bone tissue engineering." Transactions of Nonferrous Metals Society of China 29, no. 5 (2019): 984–996.
147. Chandorkar, Yashoda, Nitu Bhaskar, Giridhar Madras, and Bikramjit Basu. "Long-term sustained release of salicylic acid from cross-linked biodegradable polyester induces a reduced foreign body response in mice." Biomacromolecules 16, no. 2 (2015): 636–649.
148. Miramini, Saeed, Katie L. Fegan, Naomi C. Green, Daniel M. Espino, Lihai Zhang, and Lauren EJ Thomas-Seale. "The status and challenges of replicating the mechanical properties of connective tissues using additive manufacturing." Journal of the Mechanical Behavior of Biomedical Materials 103 (2020): 103544.
149. Sezer, Nurettin, Zafer Evis, Said Murat Kayhan, Aydin Tahmasebifar, and Muammer Koç. "Review of magnesium-based biomaterials and their applications." Journal of Magnesium and Alloys 6, no. 1 (2018): 23–43.
150. Witte, Frank. "The history of biodegradable magnesium implants: a review." Acta Biomaterialia 6, no. 5 (2010): 1680–1692.
151. Yin, Yong, Qianli Huang, Luxin Liang, Xiaobo Hu, Tang Liu, Yuanzhi Weng, Teng Long et al. "In vitro degradation behavior and cytocompatibility of ZK30/bioactive glass composites fabricated by selective laser melting for biomedical applications." Journal of Alloys and Compounds 785 (2019): 38–45.
152. Gu, Xuenan N., Nan Li, Yufeng F. Zheng, and Liquan Ruan. "In vitro degradation performance and biological response of a Mg–Zn–Zr alloy." Materials Science and Engineering: B 176, no. 20 (2011): 1778–1784.
153. Pesode, P., and S. Barve Surface modification of biodegradable zinc alloy for biomedical applications. BioNanoSci. (2023). https://doi.org/10.1007/s12668-023-01139-5.
154. Mushahary, Dolly, Cuie Wen, Jerald Mahesh Kumar, Jixing Lin, Nemani Harishankar, Peter Hodgson, Gopal Pande, and Yuncang Li. "Collagen type-I leads to in vivo matrix mineralization and secondary stabilization of Mg–Zr–Ca alloy implants." Colloids and Surfaces B: Biointerfaces 122 (2014): 719–728.

155. Pesode, Pralhad, and Shivprakash Barve. "Comparison and performance of α, α+β and β titanium alloy for biomedical applications." Surface Review and Letters 30, no. 12 (2023): 2330012.

156. Pesode, Pralhad, Shivprakash Barve, Sagar V. Wankhede, Dhanaji R. Jadhav, and Sumod K. Pawar. "Titanium alloy selection for biomedical application using weighted sum model methodology." Materials Today: Proceedings 72, no. 3 (2023): 724–728.

157. Benn, Felix, Nadja Kröger, Max Zinser, Kerstin van Gaalen, Ted J. Vaughan, Ming Yan, Ralf Smeets, Eric Bibiza, Savko Malinov, Fraser Buchanan, and Alexander Kopp. "Influence of surface condition on the degradation behaviour and biocompatibility of additively manufactured WE43." Materials Science and Engineering: C 124 (2021): 112016.

158. Wang, Yinchuan, Penghuai Fu, Nanqing Wang, Liming Peng, Bin Kang, Hui Zeng, Guangyin Yuan, and Wenjiang Ding. "Challenges and solutions for the additive manufacturing of biodegradable magnesium implants." Engineering 6, no. 11 (2020): 1267–1275.

159. Zumdick, Naemi A., Lucas Jauer, Lisa C. Kersting, Tatiana N. Kutz, Johannes H. Schleifenbaum, and Daniela Zander. "Additive manufactured WE43 magnesium: a comparative study of the microstructure and mechanical properties with those of powder extruded and as-cast WE43." Materials Characterization 147 (2019): 384–397.

160. Gangireddy, Sindhura, Bharat Gwalani, Kaimiao Liu, Eric J. Faierson, and Rajiv S. Mishra. "Microstructure and mechanical behavior of an additive manufactured (AM) WE43-Mg alloy." Additive Manufacturing 26 (2019): 53–64.

161. Salehi, Mojtaba, Saeed Maleksaeedi, Hamidreza Farnoush, Mui Ling Sharon Nai, Ganesh Kumar Meenashisundaram, and Manoj Gupta. "An investigation into interaction between magnesium powder and Ar gas: implications for selective laser melting of magnesium." Powder Technology 333 (2018): 252–261.

162. Li, Yageng, Holger Jahr, Jie Zhou, and Amir Abbas Zadpoor. "Additively manufactured biodegradable porous metals." Acta Biomaterialia 115 (2020): 29–50.

163. Salehi, Mojtaba, Saeed Maleksaeedi, Mui Ling Sharon Nai, and Manoj Gupta. "Towards additive manufacturing of magnesium alloys through integration of binderless 3D printing and rapid microwave sintering." Additive Manufacturing 29 (2019): 100790.

164. Thakur, Bhaskar, Shivprakash Barve, and Pralhad Pesode. "Investigation on mechanical properties of AZ31B magnesium alloy manufactured by stir casting process." Journal of the Mechanical Behavior of Biomedical Materials 138 (2023): 105641.

165. Hassan, Mohamad Nageeb, Mohammed Ahmed Yassin, Salwa Suliman, Stein Atle Lie, Harald Gjengedal, and Kamal Mustafa. "The bone regeneration capacity of 3D-printed templates in calvarial defect models: a systematic review and meta-analysis." Acta Biomaterialia 91 (2019): 1–23.

166. Badkoobeh, Farzad, Hossein Mostaan, Mahdi Rafiei, Hamid Reza Bakhsheshi-Rad, and Filippo Berto. "Friction stir welding/processing of Mg-based alloys: a critical review on advancements and challenges." Materials 14, no. 21 (2021): 6726.

167. Li, Xinzhi, Xuewei Fang, Shuaipeng Wang, Siqing Wang, Min Zha, and Ke Huang. "Selective laser melted AZ91D magnesium alloy with superior balance of strength and ductility." Journal of Magnesium and Alloys (2022). https://doi.org/10.1016/j.jma.2022.06.004

168. Zeng, Zhuoran, Mojtaba Salehi, Alexander Kopp, Shiwei Xu, Marco Esmaily, and Nick Birbilis. "Recent progress and perspectives in additive manufacturing of magnesium alloys." Journal of Magnesium and Alloys 10, no. 6 (2022): 1511–1541.

169. Wankhede, Sagar, Pralhad Pesode, Sanjay Gaikwad, Sumod Pawar, and Amar Chipade. "Implementing combinative distance base assessment (CODAS) for selection of natural fibre for long lasting composites." In Materials science forum, vol. 1081, pp. 41–48. Trans Tech Publications Ltd., 2023.

170. Wankhede, Sagar, Pralhad Pesode, Sumod Pawar, and Rayan Lobo. "Comparison study of GRA, COPRAS and MOORA for ranking of phase change material for cooling system." Materials Today: Proceedings (2023). https://doi.org/10.1016/j.matpr.2023.02.437

171. Wankhede, Sagar V., Samir L. Shinde, and Amit R. Wasnik. "Modelling of Cu-$Al_2O_3$ metal matrix composite prepared by powder metallurgy route." International Journal of Engineering and Advanced Technology 3, no. 1 (2013): 330–332.

172. Wankhede, Sagar V., and Jitendra A. Hole. "MOORA and TOPSIS based selection of input parameter in solar powered absorption refrigeration system." International Journal of Ambient Energy 43, no. 1 (2022): 3396–3401.

173. Li, Yuncang, Cuie Wen, Dolly Mushahary, Ragamouni Sravanthi, Nemani Harishankar, Gopal Pande, and Peter Hodgson. "Mg–Zr–Sr alloys as biodegradable implant materials." Acta Biomaterialia 8, no. 8 (2012): 3177–3188.

# 3 Role of Alloying Elements on Biomedical Performance of Mg Alloys

*Qazi Junaid Ashraf*
University of Kashmir, Zakura Campus, Srinagar, India
and
National Institute of Technology, Srinagar, India

*G.A. Harmain*
National Institute of Technology, Srinagar, India

## 3.1 INTRODUCTION

Magnesium alloys have gained significant attention in recent years for its potential use in biomedical applications due to their biocompatibility, mechanical properties, and biodegradability. Typical alloys used for biomedical applications, owing to their biological and mechanical performance, include cobalt–chromium alloys [1, 2], titanium and its alloys [3, 4], and stainless steel [5]. However, the extraction of the said implant materials from body after bone consolidation necessitates a second surgical procedure, which can be excruciating for the patient. Magnesium alloys can degrade in the body over time through corrosion, which is a natural process that occurs due to the interaction between the implant and the body's physiological fluids, eliminating the need for surgical removal of the implant, which is a common issue with traditional implant materials [6, 7]. Being biocompatible, they do not cause any harmful or toxic reactions when implanted in the body [8, 9]. This is due to the fact that magnesium is an essential element in the body, and it is required for several biological functions. Their low levels of ion release reduce risk of any adverse reactions. In addition, magnesium and its alloys possess mechanical properties that make them more suitable for use in biomedical applications. Magnesium has a similar density as that of bone, which reduces the risk of stress shielding, a phenomenon that can occur when the implant material is significantly denser than the surrounding bone tissue. Their high strength-to-weight ratio makes them suitable for use in load-bearing applications. However, pure magnesium has poor mechanical properties and corrosion resistance, which limits its practical application in biomedical implants. Therefore, alloying elements are added to improve the mechanical and corrosion properties of magnesium alloys (Figure 3.1).

DOI: 10.1201/9781003400462-3

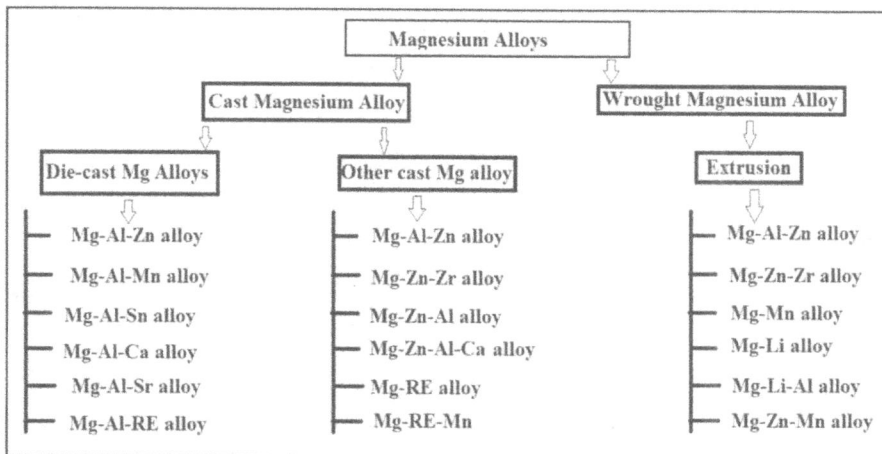

FIGURE 3.1   Various Mg alloys [9].

## 3.2   MAGNESIUM AND ITS ALLOYS

### 3.2.1   CHARACTERISTICS OF MAGNESIUM AND MAGNESIUM ALLOYS

Magnesium is a lightweight metal that possesses excellent mechanical properties and is biocompatible, making it an attractive material for use in biomedical applications. Magnesium and its alloys have been extensively studied as a potential candidate for various biomedical implants, including orthopedic implants, cardiovascular stents, and drug delivery systems [9–13].

Magnesium has several properties that make it an attractive material for biomedical applications. These properties are discussed in the following sections.

#### 3.2.1.1   Mechanical Properties

Magnesium possesses excellent mechanical properties, including high strength-to-weight ratio, good ductility, and high stiffness (Figure 3.2). These properties make it an ideal material for use in load-bearing applications. Magnesium has a low density of 1.74 $g/cm^3$, which is similar to that of bone. This makes it an ideal material for orthopedic implants as it reduces the overall weight of the implant and minimizes the load on the surrounding bone. The comparative advantage of Mg alloys over other implant materials in terms of mechanical properties has been presented in Table 3.1 [9].

#### 3.2.1.2   Biocompatibility

The biocompatibility of magnesium is one of its most attractive properties for use in biomedical applications. Magnesium ions released from the implant stimulate osteoblasts and promote the formation of new bone tissue. Magnesium is also known to possess antibacterial properties, which make it an ideal material for use in implants that are susceptible to bacterial infections. Magnesium is a biocompatible material

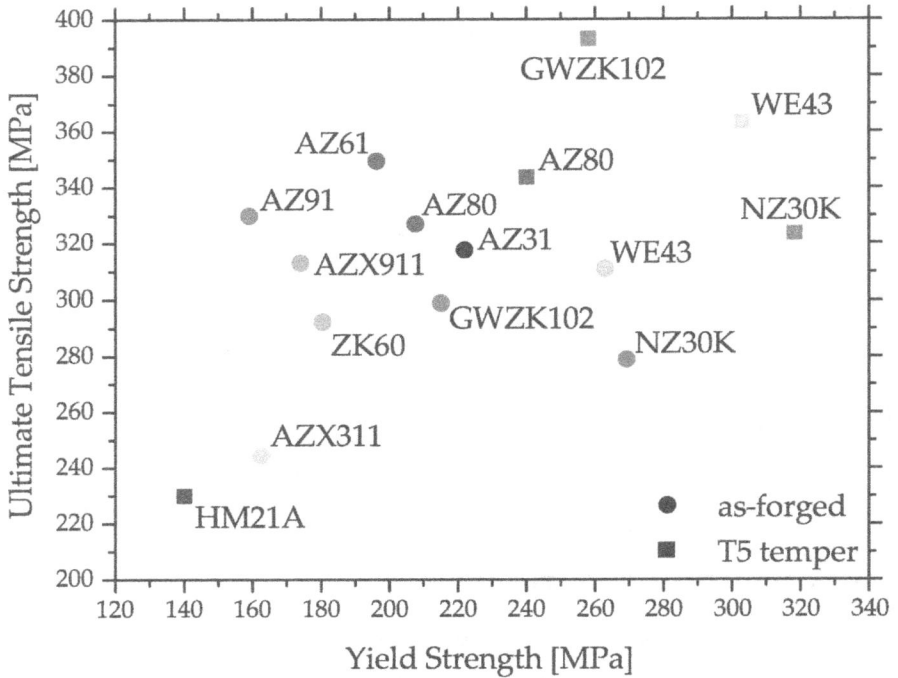

**FIGURE 3.2**  Tensile properties of various Mg alloys [13].

**TABLE 3.1**
**Mechanical Properties of Mg Alloys and Other Metallic Implants**

| S. No. | Material Property | Human Bone | Mg Alloys | Co-Cr Alloys | Ti Alloys | Stainless Steels |
|---|---|---|---|---|---|---|
| 1 | Density (g/cm³) | 1.8–2.1 | 1.74–2.00 | 8.3–9.2 | 4.4–4.5 | 7.9–8.1 |
| 2 | Tensile strength (MPa) | 70–150 | 86–280 | 655–1896 | 760–1140 | 586–1351 |
| 3 | Yield strength (MPa) | 30–114.3 | 20–200 | 448–1606 | 896–1034 | 221–1213 |
| 4 | Compressive strength (MPa) | 164–240 | 55–130 | N/A | N/A | N/A |
| 5 | Elongation (%) | 1.07–2.10 | 12–21 | N/A | 12 | N/A |
| 6 | Young's modulus (GPa) | 3–23 | 41–45 | 210–232 | 110–117 | 189–205 |
| 7 | Fracture toughness (MPa√m) | 3–7 | 15–40 | 50–200 | 55–115 | NA |

that does not cause significant immunological or inflammatory responses when implanted in the body. Furthermore, magnesium alloys have been shown to exhibit excellent biocompatibility in various in vitro and in vivo studies. For example, in vitro studies have demonstrated that magnesium alloys promote cell proliferation and differentiation, and in vivo studies indicated that the use of magnesium alloys can stimulate bone growth and enhance the process of osseointegration [14, 15].

### 3.2.1.3  Corrosion Resistance

Magnesium has excellent corrosion resistance due to the formation of a thin, protective oxide layer on its surface. However, it is also susceptible to rapid corrosion in the presence of chloride ions, which can limit its use in certain applications. The corrosion behavior of magnesium alloys can also be a challenge for their use in biomedical applications. Magnesium alloys are highly reactive in physiological environments and can corrode rapidly, leading to a reduction in mechanical properties and potential release of toxic ions. Therefore, it is important to carefully design magnesium alloys to optimize their corrosion behavior and reduce the risk of toxicity (Figure 3.3) [16, 17].

### 3.2.1.4  Thermal Conductivity

Magnesium has excellent thermal conductivity, making it suitable for use in implants that require temperature regulation, such as drug delivery systems. Several studies have investigated the thermal conductivity of magnesium alloys for biomedical

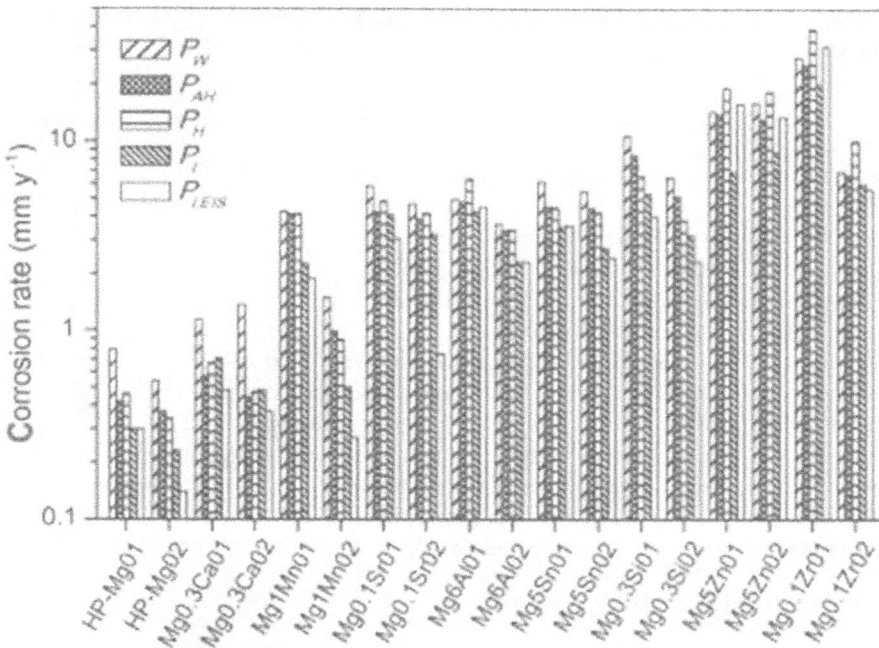

**FIGURE 3.3**  Corrosion rate of various Mg alloys [16].

applications. For example, one study found that the thermal conductivity of a magnesium alloy (AZ31) decreased with increasing porosity, which could be relevant for the design of porous implants that promote tissue ingrowth [18]. Another study investigated the thermal conductivity of magnesium alloys with different microstructures and found that grain refinement can significantly reduce the thermal conductivity, which may be useful for improving the biocompatibility of magnesium alloy implants [19].

### 3.2.2 BIOMEDICAL APPLICATIONS OF MAGNESIUM AND MAGNESIUM ALLOYS

Owing to suitable property profile (already discussed), magnesium and magnesium alloys have found a wide range of application in the field of biomedicine, including their use in orthopedics, cardiovascular medicine, and dentistry.

#### 3.2.2.1 Orthopedic Applications

Magnesium alloys are of great interest for orthopedic applications due to their high strength-to-weight ratio and biocompatibility. They are being investigated as potential materials for use in implants for bone fixation, spinal fusion, and joint replacement. The use of magnesium alloys for orthopedic applications has the potential to reduce implant-related complications, such as stress shielding and implant loosening, which can occur with traditional metallic implants [20, 21].

#### 3.2.2.2 Cardiovascular Applications

Magnesium alloys are also being studied for use in cardiovascular applications, such as stents, due to their biodegradability and ability to promote angiogenesis. Stents manufactured from magnesium alloys possess the capability to gradually dissolve inside the body, thus negating the requirement for supplementary surgery to extract them out of body. Additionally, magnesium has been shown to have a positive effect on endothelial cells, which are involved in the formation of new blood vessels, making it a promising material for promoting angiogenesis [22, 23].

#### 3.2.2.3 Dental Applications

Magnesium alloys are also being investigated for use in dental applications, such as dental implants and orthodontic wires. Dental implants made from magnesium alloys have the potential to promote bone growth and reduce implant failure rates. Additionally, orthodontic wires made from magnesium alloys have better biocompatibility and mechanical properties than traditional wires made from stainless steel. Magnesium and its alloys have also been studied for potential use in temporary dental fillings. Temporary fillings are used to restore teeth that have been damaged or decayed. Use of magnesium and its alloys in temporary fillings has the potential to lower the possibility of unfavorable reactions caused by the filling material and facilitate the development of fresh dentin, resulting in enhanced durability of the filling [22, 24].

#### 3.2.2.4 Drug Delivery Systems

Magnesium and its alloys have been studied extensively for their potential use in drug delivery systems. The unique properties of magnesium and its alloys, such as biocompatibility, biodegradability, and controlled degradation, make them attractive materials for drug delivery.

Several recent studies have explored the potential of magnesium and its alloys in drug delivery systems. For example, in Ref. [25], the use of a magnesium alloy as a drug carrier for the anticancer drug doxorubicin has been investigated. The study found that the magnesium alloy was able to deliver doxorubicin in a controlled manner, resulting in improved anticancer activity. In Ref. [26], the use of a magnesium alloy as a carrier for the antibiotic drug vancomycin has been explored. In Ref. [27], the use of magnesium-based nanocomposites for drug delivery has been investigated. One of the key advantages of using magnesium and its alloys in drug delivery systems is their ability to degrade in the body over time, which allows for controlled release of drugs.

### 3.2.2.5   Tissue Engineering Scaffolds

Magnesium and its alloys have been studied extensively for their potential use in tissue engineering scaffolds. Biocompatibility, biodegradability, and mechanical properties make them attractive materials for scaffolds. Several recent studies have explored the potential of magnesium and its alloys in tissue engineering scaffolds. For example, in Ref. [28], the use of a magnesium alloy as a scaffold for bone tissue engineering has been investigated. The study found that the magnesium alloy scaffold promoted the growth and differentiation of bone cells. In Ref. [29], the use of a magnesium alloy as a scaffold for tissue engineering has been explored. In Ref. [30], the use of a magnesium alloy as a scaffold for nerve tissue engineering has been investigated. The study found that the magnesium alloy scaffold supported the growth and differentiation of nerve cells.

### 3.2.3   Limitations of Magnesium and Magnesium Alloys

The unique combination of biocompatibility and biodegradability of magnesium and its alloys makes them a promising material for biomedical applications. However, they have several limitations that need to be addressed before they can be widely used in biomedical applications.

The high corrosion rate, poor mechanical properties, and processing challenges are some of the major limitations that need to be addressed.

The limitations of magnesium and its alloys with respect to their use in biomedical applications are discussed in the following sections.

### 3.2.3.1   Corrosion Rate

Use of magnesium in biomedical applications poses a significant obstacle due to its speedy degradation when exposed to chloride ions, which are commonly present in the human body. Moreover, the resultant corrosion products of magnesium have the potential to trigger an inflammatory response, ultimately resulting in tissue damage and implant malfunction. To overcome this challenge, several surface modification techniques have been developed, including surface coatings, surface treatments, and alloying with other elements [15, 20, 31, 32].

### 3.2.3.2   Fatigue Resistance

Magnesium alloys have poor fatigue resistance, which can limit their use in applications where cyclic loading is expected, such as orthopedic implants. The fatigue resistance can be improved through the use of surface treatments or through the addition of alloying elements [15].

### 3.2.3.3 Biocompatibility

While magnesium and its alloys are generally biocompatible, there have been reports of inflammatory reactions to magnesium implants in some patients. This can be due to the rapid corrosion rate of the implant, which can lead to the release of magnesium ions and the formation of inflammatory by-products [15, 20].

### 3.2.3.4 Processing Challenges

The processing of magnesium and its alloys can be challenging due to their low ductility and high reactivity with oxygen and moisture. Magnesium alloys are also prone to cracking during processing due to their low fracture toughness. These processing challenges can limit the production of complex shapes and geometries. In addition, magnesium and its alloys are currently more expensive than other commonly used implant materials such as titanium alloys and stainless steel. This can limit their use in certain applications where cost is a major factor [33–35].

Alloying elements play a crucial role in improving the mechanical properties, corrosion resistance, and biocompatibility of magnesium alloys for biomedical applications. The selection and optimization of alloying elements can lead to the development of novel magnesium alloys with tailored properties for specific biomedical applications. Further research is needed to identify the appropriate alloying elements with reference to a particular biomedical application and optimize the alloy composition, processing methods, and surface treatments of magnesium alloys to overcome these limitations.

## 3.3  EFFECT OF ALLOYING ELEMENTS ON MAGNESIUM ALLOYS FOR BIOMEDICAL APPLICATIONS

Pure Mg exhibits low ductility and strength due to the lack of slip systems in its HCP crystal structure. However, the addition of appropriate alloying elements can improve its properties. The composition of alloys significantly impacts the microstructure, potential difference, and surface potential between phases, ultimately influencing the mechanical performance and corrosion resistance. Among the commonly added elements to Mg, aluminum and zinc are preferred for their ability to enhance the alloy's hardness, strength, and castability. Lithium is a promising element for developing new Mg alloys due to its low density and high solid solubility. Studies suggest that adding Li can change the crystal structure from HCP to BCC, leading to better formability. Further researchers have explored the addition of various alloying elements to magnesium, including aluminum, zinc, calcium, rare earth elements (REEs), strontium, and other alloying elements, for enhancing the versatility of Mg alloys in being the candidate material for biomedical applications.

### 3.3.1  ALUMINUM

Addition of aluminum to magnesium alloys has been demonstrated to enhance their mechanical characteristics and resistance to corrosion and does not interfere significantly with compatibility with living tissue, rendering them appropriate for diverse medical implants such as orthopedic apparatus, dental implants, and cardiovascular stents. The addition of aluminum to magnesium alloys significantly improves their strength (by about 180 MPa), stiffness, and fatigue resistance [36] owing to the formation of stable precipitate phase, $Mg_{17}Al_{12}$, which enhances the strength of magnesium matrix. The precipitate phase also hinders dislocation movement, which improves the mechanical properties of the alloy (Figure 3.4). Additionally, the presence of aluminum can improve the ductility of magnesium alloys, which is important for implants that require good formability. While pure magnesium exhibits inadequate corrosion resistance, especially in biological fluids containing chloride ions, the inclusion of aluminum in magnesium alloys can enhance their corrosion resistance by producing a safeguarding oxide film on the alloy's surface [37, 38]. The oxide layer acts as a barrier to prevent the penetration of corrosive species, which slows down the corrosion rate of the alloy. Aluminum is a biocompatible element and has been used in various biomedical implants for many years. The inclusion of aluminum in magnesium alloys has a minimal impact on their biocompatibility, thereby rendering them appropriate for utilization in medical implants owing to its superior mechanical properties [39, 40]. In fact, the formation of a protective oxide layer on the surface of the alloy can reduce the degradation rate of the alloy, which is beneficial for implants that need to remain in the body for a longer period of time.

### 3.3.2  ZINC

Zinc is another commonly used alloying element in magnesium alloys for biomedical applications. The addition of zinc to magnesium alloys can significantly improve their mechanical properties, corrosion resistance, and biocompatibility, making them suitable for various biomedical implants. The incorporation of zinc

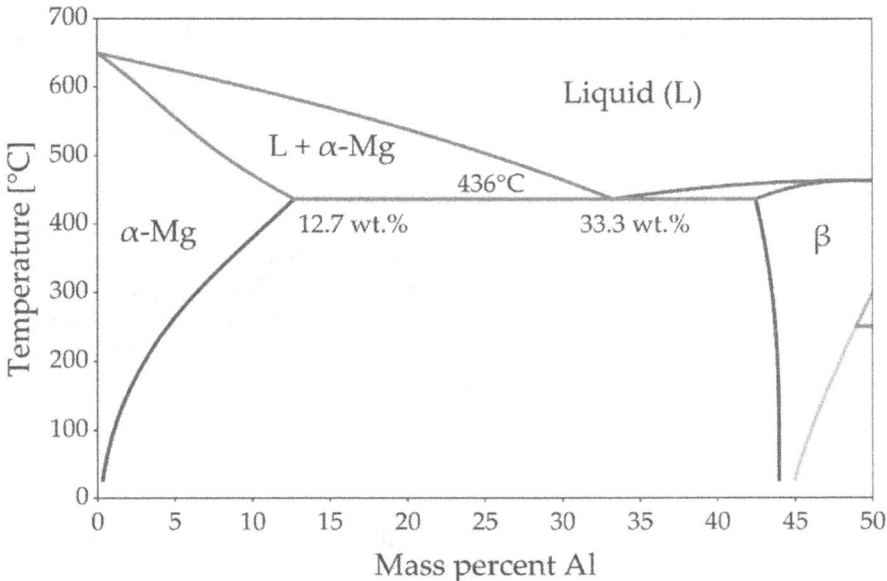

**FIGURE 3.4**  Mg-Al alloy phase diagram [40].

into magnesium alloys can enhance their processing characteristics, such as their ability to be cast and machined. Zinc's inclusion can also lead to the refinement of the magnesium alloy's grain structure, which results in improved mechanical properties and facilitates processing. It improves their corrosion resistance by forming a protective oxide layer on their surface. Zinc is a vital dietary element for human health, and its incorporation into magnesium alloys does not pose any notable health hazards. Research has revealed that the inclusion of zinc in magnesium alloys can enhance their characteristics for biomedical purposes. For example, in Ref. [41], the effect of adding different amounts of zinc to magnesium alloys on their mechanical properties and biodegradability has been investigated. The study showed that the addition of zinc improved the mechanical properties of magnesium alloys, such as their strength and ductility. The study also showed that the biodegradation rate of magnesium alloys decreased with increasing zinc content. Another study [42] investigated the effect of adding zinc to magnesium alloys on their corrosion behavior. The study showed that the incorporation of zinc enhanced the corrosion resistance of magnesium alloys by forming a protective oxide layer on their surface and that the corrosion rate significantly decreased with higher zinc content.

However, it is essential to note that the percentage limit of zinc in magnesium alloys is critical for better biomedical application. Excessive amounts of zinc can result in the formation of intermetallic phases, which can reduce the mechanical properties of magnesium alloys. Therefore, it is crucial to limit the amount of zinc in magnesium alloys for better biomedical application. In general, zinc content in magnesium alloys ranges from 0.5% to 5%. For example, the AZ31 alloy, with 3% zinc, has been used for orthopedic applications owing to its superior biocompatibility and mechanical properties. Moreover, in Ref. [43], the effect of adding different amounts of zinc to Mg-Zn alloys on their mechanical properties and biocompatibility has been investigated and it is found that a zinc content of 2% was determined to be optimal for magnesium alloys since it struck a balance between mechanical properties and biocompatibility. Similarly, in Ref, [44], the effect of zinc content on the corrosion behavior and biocompatibility of Mg-Zn-Mn alloys for biomedical applications has been investigated. The study showed that an increase in zinc content led to improved corrosion resistance but reduced biocompatibility.

A separate study [45] investigated the effects of zinc on the corrosion and bioactivity of Mg-Zn alloys specifically developed for biomedical purposes. The study showed that the addition of zinc to magnesium alloys improved their bioactivity by promoting the formation of a hydroxyapatite layer on the surface. However, the study also indicated that excessive zinc content in magnesium alloys could result in a significant decrease in the bioactivity.

### 3.3.3 CALCIUM

Calcium is a relatively new alloying element that has been explored for its potential use in magnesium alloys for biomedical applications. The addition of calcium to magnesium alloys can improve their mechanical properties and biodegradation behavior, making them promising materials for use in orthopedic implants.

By incorporating calcium into magnesium alloys, it is possible to enhance their strength, ductility, and work-hardening behavior. This improvement is primarily attributed to the development of a finely dispersed precipitate phase called $CaMg_3Zn_3$, which serves to reinforce the magnesium matrix [46]. Furthermore, the presence of calcium can refine the grain structure of the magnesium alloy, leading to an enhancement in its mechanical properties and ease of processing. Additionally, studies have shown that calcium can facilitate the formation of apatite, similar to the one found in bones, on the surface of magnesium alloys, thereby improving their biocompatibility.

One of the main advantages of magnesium alloys for biomedical applications is their ability to biodegrade in the body over time. By introducing calcium into magnesium alloys, it is possible to enhance their biodegradation properties through the regulation of both degradation rate and mechanism [47]. The deterioration of magnesium alloys within the human body primarily results from their reaction with water, which produces hydrogen gas. To address this issue, introducing calcium into the alloy can decrease the evolution of hydrogen and facilitate the creation of a calcium phosphate layer on the alloy's surface. Such a layer can bolster bone regeneration and decrease inflammation. Calcium is a vital mineral for human health, playing a critical role in several biological functions, such as bone development and upkeep. When added to magnesium alloys, calcium can improve their biocompatibility by promoting cell adhesion, proliferation, and differentiation [48]. By selecting and adjusting the calcium content in magnesium alloys, we can create tailored and innovative alloys for specific biomedical applications. However, further research is necessary to comprehend the influence of calcium on magnesium alloys' characteristics and performance in the body. The typical calcium content in magnesium alloys ranges from 0.5% to 2%. One example is the widely used Mg-1Ca alloy, which contains 1% calcium and boasts exceptional mechanical properties and biocompatibility, making it ideal for orthopedic applications. In Ref. [49], the influence of different calcium concentrations on the mechanical properties and biocompatibility of magnesium alloys has been analyzed. The study demonstrated that magnesium alloys with 1% calcium exhibited the optimal balance between mechanical properties and biocompatibility. In Refs [50, 51], the impact of calcium content on the corrosion behavior and biocompatibility of Mg-Ca alloys designed for biomedical applications has been explored. The results indicated that augmenting the calcium content led to an enhancement in the corrosion resistance and biocompatibility of magnesium alloys.

### 3.3.4 MANGANESE

Manganese is a highly promising element for improving the properties of magnesium alloys. The addition of Mn has been demonstrated to significantly enhance the mechanical properties, corrosion resistance, and biocompatibility of the resulting alloy. Mn can effectively enhance the strength, ductility, and toughness of magnesium alloys through the formation of intermetallic compounds, such as $Mg_{17}Al_{12}$ and $Mg_2Mn$. Additionally, the mechanical properties of Mn-containing magnesium alloys can be further improved by means of grain refinement and solid solution strengthening. Grain refinement can occur through the addition of Mn, which can promote the formation of finer grains and improve the mechanical properties of the alloy [52].

The addition of Mn to magnesium alloys can improve their corrosion resistance, reducing the degradation rate of the material in the body owing to the formation of a protective layer of manganese oxide on the surface of the alloy, which can inhibit further corrosion [20]. Mn-containing magnesium alloys have been shown to exhibit good biocompatibility, as they can release Mn ions that promote bone formation and have a positive effect on osteoblast cells. Mn-containing magnesium alloys can also enhance the adhesion and proliferation of osteoblast cells, leading to improved bone regeneration. Research has demonstrated that magnesium alloys containing manganese demonstrate superior performance in comparison to pure magnesium and other magnesium alloys lacking Mn. For instance, in a study [53] investigating the impact of Mn on Mg-1.0Ca alloy's mechanical and biological properties, it was discovered that the addition of Mn improved the alloy's corrosion resistance, ductility, and tensile strength. Additionally, the Mn-containing alloy demonstrated better biocompatibility, as shown by increased osteoblast cell adhesion and proliferation. Similarly, in another study [44, 45], the effect of Mn on the mechanical properties and biocompatibility of Mg-1Ca alloys was investigated, and the results revealed that the addition of Mn enhanced the alloy's strength, ductility, and corrosion resistance, while also improving its biocompatibility, as evidenced by increased osteoblast cell adhesion and proliferation.

The optimal percentage of Mn in Mg alloys for better biomedical applications varies based on the desired properties and specific application. Generally, Mn addition to Mg alloys in the range of 1–3 wt% has been observed to be effective in improving their mechanical and corrosion properties [54, 55]. Additionally, Mn addition to magnesium alloys can enhance their processing properties, including castability and machinability [53, 54, 56]. By selecting and adjusting the amount of manganese in magnesium alloys, tailored and innovative magnesium alloys for specific biomedical applications can be developed. Nevertheless, further studies are necessary to gain a complete understanding of manganese's effects on magnesium alloys' properties and their behavior in the human body.

### 3.3.5 REEs

REEs are considered potential alloying elements to enhance the mechanical properties and corrosion resistance of magnesium alloys for biomedical applications. The unique electronic configuration of REEs makes them ideal for modifying the microstructure of magnesium alloys, leading to improvements in properties such as strength, toughness, and ductility by altering crystal structure, morphology, and/ or grain size of the alloy. The strengthening mechanism is due to the formation of a fine precipitate phase that reinforces the magnesium matrix [57]. Studies have shown that cerium, lanthanum, and yttrium are the most commonly studied REEs for this purpose. For example, Ce has been found to improve the mechanical and corrosion properties of Mg alloys [58], La can enhance the corrosion and mechanical properties of Mg alloys [59], and yttrium can improve the corrosion resistance of Mg alloys [60]. The optimal percentage of REEs as alloying elements in magnesium alloys for biomedical applications may vary depending on the specific application and desired properties. However, adding 1–3 wt% of REEs to magnesium alloys has been shown to substantially improve their mechanical and biocompatibility properties. For instance, in Refs [61, 62], Mg alloys with REE has been demonstrated. Yttrium demonstrated slowed corrosion rate.

### 3.3.6 SILVER

The addition of Ag to Mg alloys can improve their mechanical properties, such as tensile strength and ductility, and enhance their corrosion resistance in physiological environments. Ag can also impart antibacterial properties to Mg alloys, making them suitable for orthopedic and dental implants. Ag ions released from Mg-Ag alloys can suppress the growth of bacteria and promote cell proliferation, leading to better tissue regeneration [63–65].

However, the incorporation of Ag in Mg alloys requires careful control of the composition and processing conditions to avoid the formation of undesirable phases and degradation of mechanical properties. Further, the use of Ag in Mg alloys is limited due to its high cost and potential toxicity at high concentrations. Several investigations have been conducted to study the impact of Ag on the characteristics of Mg alloys. One such study [66] revealed that the corrosion resistance of the Mg-3.0Nd-0.2Zn-$x$Ag-0.4Zr alloys with 0.2 wt% Ag addition is approximately that of the alloy without Ag. However, more Ag addition has a detrimental effect on corrosion resistance of the alloy. Therefore, taking corrosion resistance into account, optimum Ag addition into Mg-3.0Nd-0.2Zn-0.4Zr alloy may be about 0.2 wt%. Another study [67] demonstrated that with the Ag addition in Mg-1Zn-0.2Ca-$x$Ag, the grain size is refined due to fully dynamic recrystallization and $Ag_{17}Mg_{54}$ phase, an important strengthening phase, begins to be precipitated in the Ag-containing alloys. Due to the stronger solution strengthening and precipitation strengthening, the Mg-1Zn-0.2Ca-4Ag alloy attains the highest ultimate tensile strength.

## 3.4 PROCESSING TECHNIQUES OF MAGNESIUM ALLOYS FOR BIOMEDICAL APPLICATIONS

Magnesium alloys have gained considerable interest as implant materials due to their low density, biocompatibility, and mechanical properties. However, magnesium alloys are known to be difficult to process due to their low melting point, high reactivity, and poor formability. The processing techniques commonly used for magnesium alloys for biomedical applications include casting, extrusion, rolling, powder metallurgy, and additive manufacturing (Figure 3.5).

### 3.4.1 CASTING

Casting is a widely used processing technique for magnesium alloys due to its low cost and ability to produce complex shapes. However, it has limitations in terms of mechanical properties and surface finish. The mechanical properties of cast magnesium alloys can be improved by adding alloying elements and optimizing the casting parameters. In Refs [68, 69], the successful production of cast magnesium alloys has been reported.

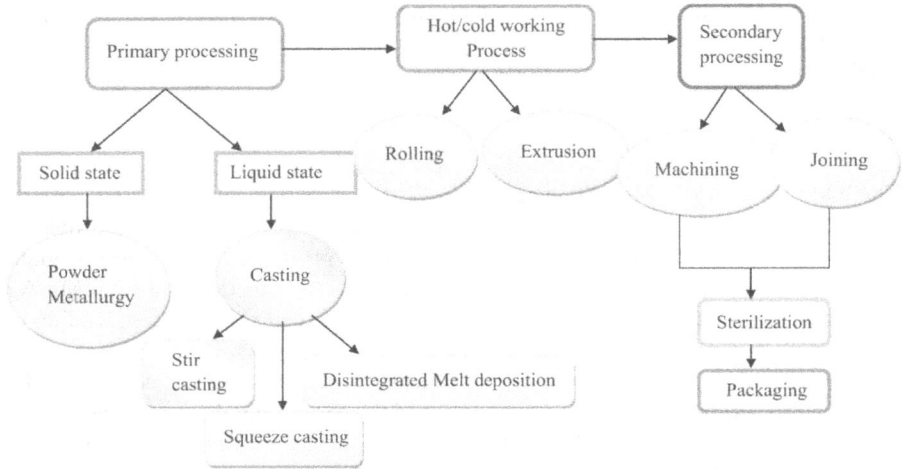

**FIGURE 3.5**   Processing steps of biodegradable Mg alloys [64].

### 3.4.2   EXTRUSION

Extrusion is a process in which a material is forced through a die to form a specific shape. It is commonly used for producing long, continuous shapes such as rods, tubes, and wires. Magnesium alloys can be extruded to improve their mechanical properties and formability [70, 71].

### 3.4.3   ROLLING

Rolling is a process in which a material is passed through a series of rollers to reduce its thickness and improve its mechanical properties. Magnesium alloys can be rolled at high temperatures to improve their strength and ductility. Rolled magnesium alloys have been used in biomedical applications, such as stents and cardiovascular implants [72–74].

### 3.4.4   POWDER METALLURGY

In powder metallurgy, Mg alloy powders are mixed with alloying elements and consolidated by cold or hot pressing to form a green compact. The compact is then sintered at high temperatures to densify the material and improve its mechanical properties. Powder metallurgy allows for the production of complex geometries with controlled microstructure and composition. However, the presence of contaminants, such as oxygen and moisture, during powder processing can have significant negative influence on corrosion resistance and biocompatibility of the final product. Surface modification and powder handling techniques can be employed to mitigate these issues [75, 76].

### 3.4.5 ADDITIVE MANUFACTURING

Additive manufacturing techniques, such as selective laser melting (SLM) and electron beam melting (EBM), allow for the production of complex geometries with precise control over composition and structure. In SLM, a laser selectively melts a layer of Mg alloy powder to create a solidified part. EBM uses an electron beam to melt the powder bed, forming a solid part through the deposition of successive layers. Additive manufacturing offers the potential for patient-specific implants with tailored mechanical properties and biocompatibility. However, the presence of residual stress and porosity in additive manufacturing Mg alloys can affect their mechanical and biological performance. Postprocessing techniques, such as hot isostatic pressing and surface finishing, can be used to reduce these issues [77–80].

## 3.5 CHALLENGES

Magnesium and its alloys have great potential for use in biomedical applications due to their excellent mechanical properties, biocompatibility, and biodegradability. However, several challenges need to be addressed for their successful clinical translation, including regulatory issues, clinical trials, standardization, and emerging technologies.

### 3.5.1 REGULATORY ISSUES

The regulatory approval process for medical devices and implants is a significant challenge for magnesium and its alloys. The regulatory agencies require extensive preclinical and clinical data to ensure the safety and efficacy of the medical devices. In the case of magnesium alloys, the high degradation rate of these materials can make it difficult to meet the regulatory requirements. Therefore, it is important to develop standard testing methods and protocols to evaluate the biocompatibility, corrosion resistance, and mechanical properties of magnesium alloys.

### 3.5.2 CLINICAL TRIALS

Clinical trials are necessary to evaluate the safety and efficacy in biomedical applications of magnesium and its alloys. Several clinical trials have been conducted to evaluate the use of magnesium alloys in orthopedic and cardiovascular applications. However, the results of these trials have been mixed, and more research is needed to understand the factors affecting the clinical outcomes of magnesium alloys.

### 3.5.3 STANDARDIZATION

Standardization of magnesium alloys is crucial for their successful clinical translation. The lack of standardized testing methods and protocols for evaluating the corrosion resistance, biocompatibility, and mechanical properties of magnesium alloys can make it difficult to compare the results from different studies. Therefore, it is important to develop standard testing methods and protocols for magnesium alloys.

### 3.5.4 Emerging Technologies

Emerging technologies, such as additive manufacturing and surface modification techniques, have the potential to improve the properties of magnesium alloys for biomedical applications. Additive manufacturing enables the creation of intricate shapes and tailored implants, whereas surface modification techniques can enhance the biocompatibility and corrosion resistance of magnesium alloys.

## 3.6 CONCLUSION AND FUTURE SCOPE

Magnesium alloys have emerged as promising materials due to their excellent mechanical properties and biocompatibility in the field of biomedical applications. However, the intrinsic properties of magnesium, like high reactivity and rapid corrosion in the physiological environment, limit their use in clinical applications. To address these issues, alloying elements have been added to magnesium to improve their mechanical and biomedical properties.

Despite the promising results, there are still challenges that need to be addressed before magnesium alloys can be widely used in biomedical applications. One of the biggest challenges is the degradation of magnesium alloys in the physiological environment, which can lead to premature failure of biomedical implants. However, recent studies have shown that the use of alloying elements can improve the corrosion resistance of magnesium alloys, making them more suitable for biomedical applications.

Another challenge is the difficulty in processing magnesium alloys due to their high reactivity and low ductility. To overcome this, several processing techniques have been developed, including casting, extrusion, and rolling. These techniques have been used to produce magnesium alloys with improved mechanical properties and biocompatibility.

In addition to these challenges, there is a lack of standardization and regulation for the use of magnesium alloys in biomedical applications. This is a significant barrier to their clinical translation, as it makes it difficult for manufacturers to comply with regulatory requirements.

The future scope of research in this field is vast and promising. One area of research is the optimization of the composition and processing techniques of magnesium alloys to improve their biocompatibility, corrosion resistance, and mechanical properties. Novel alloys and emerging technologies, such as additive manufacturing, can also provide new opportunities for the use of magnesium alloys in biomedical applications.

## REFERENCES

1. Yamanaka, Kenta, Manami Mori, and Akihiko Chiba. "Developing high strength and ductility in biomedical Co-Cr cast alloys by simultaneous doping with nitrogen and carbon." *Acta Biomaterialia* 31 (2016): 435–447.
2. Zhou, Yanan, Qi Sun, Xin Dong, Ning Li, Zhijian James Shen, Yuan Zhong, Mirva Eriksson, Jiazhen Yan, Sheng Xu, and Chenglai Xin. "Microstructure evolution and mechanical properties improvement of selective laser melted Co-Cr biomedical alloys during subsequent heat treatments." *Journal of Alloys and Compounds* 840 (2020): 155664.

3. Stráský, Josef, Dalibor Preisler, Hanuš Seiner, Lucie Bodnárová, Michaela Janovská, Tereza Košutová, and Petr Harcuba et al. "Achieving high strength and low elastic modulus in interstitial biomedical Ti-Nb-Zr-O alloys through compositional optimization." *Materials Science and Engineering: A* 839 (2022): 142833.

4. Zhang, Ting, Daixiu Wei, Eryi Lu, Wen Wang, Kuaishe Wang, Xiaoqing Li, Lai-Chang Zhang, Hidemi Kato, Weijie Lu, and Liqiang Wang. "Microstructure evolution and deformation mechanism of α + β dual-phase Ti-$x$Nb-$y$Ta-2Zr alloys with high performance." *Journal of Materials Science & Technology* 131 (2022): 68–81.

5. Du, Xiangfeng, Tong Xi, Chunguang Yang, Hanyu Zhao, and Ke Yang. "Cu addition retards the static recrystallization of cold-deformed 316L biomedical stainless steel." *Journal of Materials Research and Technology* 19 (2022): 1673–1677.

6. Zhang, Jixi, Chen Fang, and Fang Yuan. "Grain refinement of as cast Mg-Mn alloy by simultaneous addition of trace Er and Al." *International Journal of Cast Metals Research* 25, no. 6 (2012): 335–340.

7. Dong, Jianhui, Tao Lin, Huiping Shao, Hao Wang, Xueting Wang, Ke Song, and Qianghua Li. "Advances in degradation behavior of biomedical magnesium alloys: a review." *Journal of Alloys and Compounds* 908 (2022): 164600.

8. Chen, Junxiu, Lili Tan, Xiaoming Yu, Iniobong P. Etim, Muhammad Ibrahim, and Ke Yang. "Mechanical properties of magnesium alloys for medical application: a review." *Journal of the Mechanical Behavior of Biomedical Materials* 87 (2018): 68–79.

9. Sharma, Sachin Kumar, Kuldeep Kumar Saxena, Vinayak Malik, Kahtan A. Mohammed, Chander Prakash, Dharam Buddhi, and Saurav Dixit. "Significance of alloying elements on the mechanical characteristics of Mg-based materials for biomedical applications." *Crystals* 12, no. 8 (2022): 1138.

10. Zheng, Y. F., X. N. Gu, and F. Witte. "Biodegradable metals." *Materials Science and Engineering: R: Reports* 77 (2014): 1–34.

11. Li, Qing, Xiankang Zhong, Junying Hu, and Wei Kang. "Preparation and corrosion resistance studies of zirconia coating on fluorinated AZ91D magnesium alloy." *Progress in Organic Coatings* 63, no. 2 (2008): 222–227.

12. Rojaee, Ramin, Mohammadhossein Fathi, and Keyvan Raeissi. "Controlling the degradation rate of AZ91 magnesium alloy via sol–gel derived nanostructured hydroxyapatite coating." *Materials Science and Engineering: C* 33, no. 7 (2013): 3817–3825.

13. Papenberg, Nikolaus P., Stefan Gneiger, Irmgard Weißensteiner, Peter J. Uggowitzer, and Stefan Pogatscher. "Mg-alloys for forging applications: a review." *Materials* 13, no. 4 (2020): 985.

14. Witte, Frank. "The history of biodegradable magnesium implants: a review." *Acta Biomaterialia* 6, no. 5 (2010): 1680–1692.

15. Gu, Xue-Nan, and Yu-Feng Zheng. "A review on magnesium alloys as biodegradable materials." *Frontiers of Materials Science in China* 4 (2010): 111–115.

16. Feliu, Sebastián, Jr. "Electrochemical impedance spectroscopy for the measurement of the corrosion rate of magnesium alloys: brief review and challenges." *Metals* 10, no. 6 (2020): 775.

17. Kirkland, N. T., Nick Birbilis, and M. P. Staiger. "Assessing the corrosion of biodegradable magnesium implants: a critical review of current methodologies and their limitations." *Acta Biomaterialia* 8, no. 3 (2012): 925–936.

18. Lin, Tao, Xueting Wang, Liuping Jin, Wenyuan Li, Yuxuan Zhang, Aiyuan Wang, Jiang Peng, and Huiping Shao. "Manufacturing of porous magnesium scaffolds for bone tissue engineering by 3D gel-printing." *Materials & Design* 209 (2021): 109948.

19. Wang, Jing Tao, Jin Qiang Liu, Jun Tao, Yan Ling Su, and Xiang Zhao. "Effect of grain size on mechanical property of Mg-3Al-1Zn alloy." *Scripta Materialia* 59, no. 1 (2008): 63–66.

20. Witte, Frank, V. Kaese, H. Haferkamp, E. Switzer, A. Meyer-Lindenberg, C. J. Wirth, and H. Windhagen. "In vivo corrosion of four magnesium alloys and the associated bone response." *Biomaterials* 26, no. 17 (2005): 3557–3563.
21. Walker, Jemimah, Shaylin Shadanbaz, Timothy B. F. Woodfield, Mark P. Staiger, and George J. Dias. "Magnesium biomaterials for orthopedic application: a review from a biological perspective." *Journal of Biomedical Materials Research Part B: Applied Biomaterials* 102, no. 6 (2014): 1316–1331.
22. Witte, Frank, Jens Fischer, Jens Nellesen, Horst-Artur Crostack, Volker Kaese, Alexander Pisch, Felix Beckmann, and Henning Windhagen. "In vitro and in vivo corrosion measurements of magnesium alloys." *Biomaterials* 27, no. 7 (2006): 1013–1018.
23. Zhang, Ting, Wen Wang, Jia Liu, Liqiang Wang, Yujin Tang, and Kuaishe Wang. "A review on magnesium alloys for biomedical applications." *Frontiers in Bioengineering and Biotechnology* 10 (2022): 953344.
24. Li, Rachel W., Nicholas T. Kirkland, John Truong, Jian Wang, Paul N. Smith, Nick Birbilis, and David R. Nisbet. "The influence of biodegradable magnesium alloys on the osteogenic differentiation of human mesenchymal stem cells." *Journal of Biomedical Materials Research Part A* 102, no. 12 (2014): 4346–4357.
25. Vashishtha, Himanshu, Deepak Kumar, You Sub Kim, Soo Yeol Lee, E-Wen Huang, and Jayant Jain. "Effects of hot isostatic processing and hot rolling on direct energy deposited CoCrNi medium entropy alloy: microstructural heterogeneity, wear behaviour and corrosion characteristics." *Materials Characterization* 205 (2023): 113304.
26. Du, Minting, Linlin Huang, Mengke Peng, Fenyan Hu, Qiang Gao, Yashao Chen, and Peng Liu. "Preparation of vancomycin-loaded alginate hydrogel coating on magnesium alloy with enhanced anticorrosion and antibacterial properties." *Thin Solid Films* 693 (2020): 137679.
27. Saifullah, Bullo, Palanisamy Arulselvan, Sharida Fakurazi, Thomas J. Webster, Naeemullah Bullo, Mohd Zobir Hussein, and Mohamed E. El Zowalaty. "Development of a novel anti-tuberculosis nanodelivery formulation using magnesium layered hydroxide as the nanocarrier and pyrazinamide as a model drug." *Scientific Reports* 12, no. 1 (2022): 14086.
28. Parai, Rohan, and Sanchita Bandyopadhyay-Ghosh. "Engineered bio-nanocomposite magnesium scaffold for bone tissue regeneration." *Journal of the Mechanical Behavior of Biomedical Materials* 96 (2019): 45–52.
29. Yazdimamaghani, Mostafa, Mehdi Razavi, Daryoosh Vashaee, Keyvan Moharamzadeh, Aldo R. Boccaccini, and Lobat Tayebi. "Porous magnesium-based scaffolds for tissue engineering." *Materials Science and Engineering: C* 71 (2017): 1253–1266.
30. Fei, Jianjun, Xiaoxiao Wen, Xiao Lin, Weihua Wang, Olga Ren, Xinjian Chen, Lili Tan, Ke Yang, Huilin Yang, and Lei Yang. "Biocompatibility and neurotoxicity of magnesium alloys potentially used for neural repairs." *Materials Science and Engineering: C* 78 (2017): 1155–1163.
31. Song, Guang Ling, and Andrej Atrens. "Corrosion mechanisms of magnesium alloys." *Advanced Engineering Materials* 1, no. 1 (1999): 11–33.
32. Singh, Virendra Pratap, Deepak Kumar, and Basil Kuriachen. "Effect of low welding and rotational speed on microstructure and mechanical behaviour of friction stir welded AZ31-AA6061-T6." *Transactions of the Indian Institute of Metals* 76 (2023): 1–9.
33. Witte, Frank, Norbert Hort, Frank Feyerabend, and Carla Vogt. "Magnesium (Mg) corrosion: a challenging concept for degradable implants." In *Corrosion of magnesium alloys*, pp. 403–425. Woodhead Publishing, 2011.
34. Hornberger, Helga, Sannakaisa Virtanen, and Aldo R. Boccaccini. "Biomedical coatings on magnesium alloys: a review." *Acta Biomaterialia* 8, no. 7 (2012): 2442–2455.
35. Wu, Yuanzhi, Jizhao Liu, Bin Deng, Tuo Ye, Qingfen Li, Xiaotao Zhou, and Hongji Zhang. "Microstructure, texture and mechanical properties of AZ31 magnesium alloy fabricated by high strain rate biaxial forging." *Materials* 13, no. 14 (2020): 3050.

36. Vashishtha, Himanshu, Deepak Kumar, You Sub Kim, Soo Yeol Lee, E-Wen Huang, and Jayant Jain. "Role of microstructural heterogeneity on nanoscale mechanical properties and wear responses of additively manufactured CoCrNi medium entropy alloy and 316L stainless steel." *Journal of Materials Engineering and Performance* (2023): 1–10. doi: 10.1007/s11665-023-08339-w

37. Xu, Wei, Yechun Xin, Bo Zhang, and Xiuyan Li. "Stress corrosion cracking resistant nanostructured Al-Mg alloy with low angle grain boundaries." *Acta Materialia* 225 (2022): 117607.

38. Vimalanandan, Ashokanand, Asif Bashir, and Michael Rohwerder. "Zn-Mg and Zn-Mg-Al alloys for improved corrosion protection of steel: some new aspects." *Materials and Corrosion* 65, no. 4 (2014): 392–400.

39. Keim, Sigrid, Johannes G. Brunner, Ben Fabry, and Sannakaisa Virtanen. "Control of magnesium corrosion and biocompatibility with biomimetic coatings." *Journal of Biomedical Materials Research Part B: Applied Biomaterials* 96, no. 1 (2011): 84–90.

40. Predko, Pavel, Dragan Rajnovic, Maria Luisa Grilli, Bogdan O. Postolnyi, Vjaceslavs Zemcenkovs, Gints Rijkuris, Eleonora Pole, and Marks Lisnanskis. "Promising methods for corrosion protection of magnesium alloys in the case of Mg-Al, Mg-Mn-Ce and Mg-Zn-Zr: a recent progress review." *Metals* 11, no. 7 (2021): 1133.

41. Zhou, Tao, Mingbo Yang, Zhiming Zhou, Jianjun Hu, and Zhenhua Chen. "Microstructure and mechanical properties of rapidly solidified/powder metallurgy Mg-6Zn and Mg-6Zn-5Ca at room and elevated temperatures." *Journal of Alloys and Compounds* 560 (2013): 161–166.

42. Yuan, Haonan, Lin Zhang, Lihong Wu, Shijie Zhu, Yufeng Sun, and Shaokang Guan. "Significantly improved corrosion resistance of Zn layer coated Mg alloy prepared by friction stir processing." *Materials Letters* 289 (2021): 129389.

43. Kumar, Deepak, Nitya Nand Gosvami, and Jayant Jain. "Influence of temperature on crystallographic orientation induced anisotropy of microscopic wear in an AZ91 Mg alloy." *Tribology International* 163 (2021): 107159.

44. Zhang, Erlin, Dongsong Yin, Liping Xu, Lei Yang, and Ke Yang. "Microstructure, mechanical and corrosion properties and biocompatibility of Mg-Zn-Mn alloys for biomedical application." *Materials Science and Engineering: C* 29, no. 3 (2009): 987–993.

45. Vojtěch, Dalibor, Jiri Kubásek, Jan Šerák, and Pavel Novák. "Mechanical and corrosion properties of newly developed biodegradable Zn-based alloys for bone fixation." *Acta Biomaterialia* 7, no. 9 (2011): 3515–3522.

46. Zha, Min, Shi-Chao Wang, Hai-Long Jia, Yi Yang, Pin-Kui Ma, and Hui-Yuan Wang. "Effect of minor Ca addition on microstructure and mechanical properties of a low-alloyed Mg-Al-Zn-Sn alloy." *Materials Science and Engineering: A* 862 (2023): 144457.

47. Kumar, Deepak, Jayant Jain, and Nitya Nand Gosvami. Nanometer-thick base oil tribofilms with acrylamide additive as lubricants for AZ91 Mg alloy. *ACS Applied Nano Materials* 3, no. 10 (2020): 10551–10559.

48. Gao, Julia, Yingchao Su, and Yi-Xian Qin. "Calcium phosphate coatings enhance biocompatibility and degradation resistance of magnesium alloy: correlating in vitro and in vivo studies." *Bioactive Materials* 6, no. 5 (2021): 1223–1229.

49. Staiger, Mark P., Alexis M. Pietak, Jerawala Huadmai, and George Dias. "Magnesium and its alloys as orthopedic biomaterials: a review." *Biomaterials* 27, no. 9 (2006): 1728–1734.

50. Yin, Ping, Nian Feng Li, Ting Lei, Lin Liu, and Chun Ouyang. "Effects of Ca on microstructure, mechanical and corrosion properties and biocompatibility of Mg-Zn-Ca alloys." *Journal of Materials Science: Materials in Medicine* 24 (2013): 1365–1373.

51. Zhang, Baoping, Yunlong Hou, Xiaodan Wang, Yin Wang, and Lin Geng. "Mechanical properties, degradation performance and cytotoxicity of Mg-Zn-Ca biomedical alloys with different compositions." *Materials Science and Engineering: C* 31, no. 8 (2011): 1667–1673.

52. Xie, Jinshu, Jinghuai Zhang, Zihao You, Shujuan Liu, Kai Guan, Ruizhi Wu, Jun Wang, and Jing Feng. "Towards developing Mg alloys with simultaneously improved strength and corrosion resistance via RE alloying." *Journal of Magnesium and Alloys* 9, no. 1 (2021): 41–56.

53. Han, Yu Yan, Chen You, Yun Zhao, Min Fang Chen, and Liang Wang. "Effect of Mn element addition on the microstructure, mechanical properties, and corrosion properties of Mg-3Zn-0.2 Ca Alloy." *Frontiers in Materials* 6 (2019): 324.

54. Park, Sung Soo, G. T. Bae, D. H. Kang, In-Ho Jung, K. S. Shin, and Nack J. Kim. "Microstructure and tensile properties of twin-roll cast Mg-Zn-Mn-Al alloys." *Scripta Materialia* 57, no. 9 (2007): 793–796.

55. Yao, Sheng, Shuhong Liu, Guang Zeng, Xiaojing Li, Ting Lei, Yunping Li, and Yong Du. "Effect of manganese on microstructure and corrosion behavior of the Mg-3Al alloys." *Metals* 9, no. 4 (2019): 460.

56. Yu, Zhengwen, Aitao Tang, Caiyu Li, Jianguo Liu, and Fusheng Pan. "Effect of manganese on the microstructure and mechanical properties of magnesium alloys." *International Journal of Materials Research* 110, no. 11 (2019): 1016–1024.

57. Yun, B. A. I., Can-Feng Fang, H. A. O. Hai, Guo-Hong Qi, and Xing-Guo Zhang. "Effects of yttrium on microstructure and mechanical properties of Mg-Zn-Cu-Zr alloys." *Transactions of Nonferrous Metals Society of China* 20 (2010): s357–s360.

58. Dutta, Sourav, Santanu Mandal, Sanjay Gupta, and Mangal Roy. "Effects of cerium addition on the corrosion resistance and biocompatibility of Mg-2Sr-1Zr Alloy." *Journal of Materials Research* 35, no. 22 (2020): 3124–3135.

59. Kara, İsmail Hakkı, Hayrettin Ahlatçı, Yunus Türen, and Yavuz Sun. "Microstructure and corrosion properties of lanthanum-added AZ31 Mg alloys." *Arabian Journal of Geosciences* 11 (2018): 1–5.

60. Gu, Mao-Yun, Guang-Ling Wei, Jiong Zhao, Wen-Cai Liu, and Guo-Hua Wu. "Influence of yttrium addition on the corrosion behaviour of as-cast Mg-8Li-3Al-2Zn alloy." *Materials Science and Technology* 33, no. 7 (2017): 864–869.

61. Yao, Hongbin., Yi Li, and Andrew T. S. Wee. "Passivity behavior of melt-spun Mg-Y alloys." *Electrochimica Acta* 48, no. 28 (2003): 4197–4204.

62. Philip, Jibin T., Deepak Kumar, Jose Mathew, and Basil Kuriachen. "Wear characteristic evaluation of electrical discharge machined $Ti_6Al_4V$ surfaces at dry sliding conditions." *Transactions of the Indian Institute of Metals* 72 (2019): 2839–2849.

63. Jin, Shue, Jidong Li, Jian Wang, Jiaxing Jiang, Yi Zuo, Yubao Li, and Fang Yang. "Electrospun silver ion-loaded calcium phosphate/chitosan antibacterial composite fibrous membranes for guided bone regeneration." *International Journal of Nanomedicine* 13 (2018): 4591–4605.

64. Radha, Rajendran, and D. Sreekanth. "Insight of magnesium alloys and composites for orthopedic implant applications: a review." *Journal of Magnesium and Alloys* 5, no. 3 (2017): 286–312.

65. Tie, Di, Frank Feyerabend, Wolf-Dieter Mueller, Ronald Schade, Klaus Liefeith, Karl Ulrich Kainer, and Regine Willumeit. "Antibacterial biodegradable Mg-Ag alloys." *European Cells & Materials* 25 (2013): 284–298.

66. Zhang, Xiaobo, Zhixin Ba, Zhangzhong Wang, Xiancong He, Chong Shen, and Qiang Wang. "Influence of silver addition on microstructure and corrosion behavior of Mg-Nd-Zn-Zr alloys for biomedical application." *Materials Letters* 100 (2013): 188–191.

67. Ma, Yingzhong, Dexin Wang, Hongxiang Li, Fusong Yuan, Changlin Yang, and Jishan Zhang. "Microstructure, mechanical and corrosion properties of novel quaternary biodegradable extruded Mg-1Zn-0.2 Ca-xAg alloys." *Materials Research Express* 7, no. 1 (2020): 015414.

68. Kumar, Deepak, Jayant Jain, and Nitya Nand Gosvami. "Anisotropy in nanoscale friction and wear of precipitate containing AZ91 magnesium alloy." *Tribology Letters* 67 (2019): 1–8.

69. Zhang, Erlin, and Lei Yang. "Microstructure, mechanical properties and bio-corrosion properties of Mg-Zn-Mn-Ca alloy for biomedical application." *Materials Science and Engineering: A* 497, no. 1–2 (2008): 111–118.

70. Bai, Hao, Xianghui He, Pengfei Ding, Debao Liu, and Minfang Chen. "Fabrication, microstructure, and properties of a biodegradable Mg-Zn-Ca clip." *Journal of Biomedical Materials Research Part B: Applied Biomaterials* 107, no. 5 (2019): 1741–1749.

71. Tong, Libo., Mingyi Zheng, Liren Cheng, Shigeharu Kamado, and Hongjie Zhang. "Effect of extrusion ratio on microstructure, texture and mechanical properties of indirectly extruded Mg-Zn-Ca alloy." *Materials Science and Engineering: A* 569 (2013): 48–53.

72. Yuan, Yuxuan, Aibin Ma, Haoran Wu, Zheng Gao, Yaxiao Gu, and Jinghua Jiang. "Optimizing microstructure and mechanical properties of biomedical Mg-Y-Zn-Mn alloy with LPSO phases by solution treatment plus equal-channel angular pressing." *Journal of Materials Research and Technology* 16 (2022): 968–976.

73. Tong, Libo., Qingxin Zhang, Zhonghao Jiang, Jian Meng, and Hongjie Zhang. "Enhanced mechanical properties of extruded Mg-Y-Zn alloy fabricated via low-strain rolling." *Materials Science and Engineering: A* 620 (2015): 483–489.

74. Zhang, Honglin, Zhigang Xu, Sergey Yarmolenko, Laszlo J. Kecskes, and Jagannathan Sankar. "Evolution of microstructure and mechanical properties of Mg-6Al alloy processed by differential speed rolling upon post-annealing treatment." *Metals* 11, no. 6 (2021): 926.

75. Ravikanth Reddy, C., K. Satya Prasad, and B. Srinivasarao. "Microstructure and mechanical properties of Mg-Ni-Gd alloy synthesised by powder metallurgy." *Powder Metallurgy* 66 (2023): 1–8.

76. Erçetin, Ali, Kubilay Aslantas, and Özgür Özgün. "Micro-end milling of biomedical TZ54 magnesium alloy produced through powder metallurgy." *Machining Science and Technology* 24, no. 6 (2020): 924–947.

77. Zhang, Chenghang, Zhuo Li, Jikui Zhang, Haibo Tang, and Huaming Wang. "Additive manufacturing of magnesium matrix composites: comprehensive review of recent progress and research perspectives." *Journal of Magnesium and Alloys* 11 (2023): 425–461.

78. Kumar, Ashish, Virendra Pratap Singh, Akhileshwar Nirala, Ramesh Chandra Singh, Rajiv Chaudhary, Abdel Hamid I. Mourad, and Deepak Kumar. "Influence of tool rotational speed on mechanical and corrosion behaviour of friction stir processed $AZ_{31}$/$Al_2O_3$ nanocomposite." *Journal of Magnesium and Alloys* 11 (2023): 2585–2599.

79. Zeng, Zhuoran, Mojtaba Salehi, Alexander Kopp, Shiwei Xu, Marco Esmaily, and Nick Birbilis. "Recent progress and perspectives in additive manufacturing of magnesium alloys." *Journal of Magnesium and Alloys* 10, no. 6 (2022): 1511–1541.

80. Liu, Chuyi, Chengrong Ling, Cheng Chen, Dongsheng Wang, Youwen Yang, Deqiao Xie, and Cijun Shuai. "Laser additive manufacturing of magnesium alloys and its biomedical applications." *Materials Science in Additive Manufacturing* 1, no. 4 (2022): 24.

# 4 Mechanical, Chemical, Fatigue, and Biological Compatible Properties of Mg Alloys

*Aravi Muzaffar and Fatima Jalid*
National Institute of Technology, Srinagar, India

## 4.1 INTRODUCTION

Utilization in biomedical applications requires the material to have specific properties, laying enormous emphasis on strength of the implant, its load-bearing ability, and its corrosion properties. All this have acted as the continuous motivation for the development of alloys to be used as implant materials, having comparable mechanical properties as that of the bones, with optimum degradation rate so as to allow the osteoblasts to grow as the implant simultaneously degrades, as well as being nontoxic (Banerjee et al. 2019; Tan and Ramakrishna 2021). Strength of the alloys needs to match with the bones to avoid stress shielding, although various processing routes can be an alternative, e.g., creating porous materials with lower strength (to match the bone) than the bulk materials and ability to enhance osteogenesis. However, the corrosion rate could be a bigger problem. Conventional implants have extremely slow degradation rates, thereby making it difficult to use them as temporary implants. The degradation cannot be too fast for the cell growth to be inadequate, nor too slow that it needs to be removed from the body separately (Banerjee et al. 2019; Tan and Ramakrishna 2021). Some of the commonly used metal implants and their comparisons with the bone properties are given in Table 4.1. Table 4.1 also illustrates some characteristics of the common metallic implant materials.

The metals and their respective alloys commonly used for biomedical applications are broadly classified into three groups: iron, zinc, and magnesium (Zhang et al. 2009; Amukarimi and Mozafari 2021). Fe provides the highest strength and modulus to the implant, but the mechanical properties are much higher than that of the natural bones which might cause stress shielding. Also, its biodegradation is extremely slow. Zn, on the other hand, has almost ideal corrosion resistance; however, low strength ($\sigma_{UTS} \approx 30$ MPa) and poor plasticity ($\varepsilon < 0.25\%$) may hamper its prospectus of being used as a bioimplant material (Amukarimi and Mozafari 2021). Mg has similar properties to that of the bones, having a modulus of about 45 GPa that is closer to that of the bones (15–20 GPa) (Zhang et al. 2009). Also, due to its biocompatibility and accelerated corrosion in presence of chloride ions, Mg is much more

DOI: 10.1201/9781003400462-4

**TABLE 4.1**

**Properties and Characteristics of Some Common Implant Metals and Their Comparison with Natural Bone**

| Properties | Natural Bone | Mg/Mg Alloy | Ti Alloy | Co-Cr Alloy | Stainless Steel |
|---|---|---|---|---|---|
| Density (g/cc) | 1.8–2.1 | 1.74–2.0 | 4.4–4.5 | 8.3–9.2 | 7.9–8.1 |
| Elastic modulus (GPa) | 3–20 | 41–45 | 110–117 | 230 | 189–205 |
| Compressive yield strength (MPa) | 130–180 | 65–100 | 758–1117 | 450–1000 | 170–310 |
| Tensile strength (MPa) | 1.5–283 | 90–230 | 550–985 | 45–960 | 189–205 |
| Fracture toughness (MPa·m$^{1/2}$) | 3–6 | 15–40 | 55–115 | N/A | 50–200 |
| Advantages | | Biodegradable, biocompatible, trace element, mechanical properties similar to bone | High biocompatibility and corrosion resistance, fatigue strength, lightweight, low Young's modulus | High wear and corrosion resistance, fatigue strength | High wear resistance, low cost, easily available, acceptable biocompatibility |
| Disadvantages | | Low corrosion resistance, rapid loss of mechanical integrity, hydrogen evolution and alkalization during degradation | Poor tribological properties, lack of biodegradability | Biologically toxic, higher modulus than bone, expensive, lacks biodegradability | Allergic reaction, much higher modulus than bone, lack of biodegradability |

*Sources:* Staiger et al. (2006), Tan and Ramakrishna (2021), and Amukarimi and Mozafari (2021).

suited as a bioimplant (Zhang et al. 2009; Tsakiris, Tardei, and Clicinschi 2021). Thus, Mg provides one such alternative for use as potential bioimplant material due to its biodegradability, biocompatibility, lightweight, and comparable Young's modulus (Banerjee et al. 2019; Zhang et al. 2022). The strength, however, lower than the conventionally used bioimplant materials, can be improved by alloying and giving suitable thermomechanical treatments to the specified alloy (Liu et al. 2019). One of the extreme challenges with the use of Mg implants, however, is their high corrosion rates. Mg has a low standard potential of about −2.37 V because of which Mg and its alloys have low corrosion potential and are easily degradable in aqueous solutions, especially those containing chloride ions (Zhang et al. 2010). The corrosion resistance can be improved by surface modifications, coating, and alloying to make better and more efficient bioimplants (Banerjee et al. 2019).

## 4.2   BIOMEDICAL ALLOYS OF MAGNESIUM

Alloying additions like calcium, silicon, zinc, and strontium are used for the development of biocompatible Mg alloys, the properties of which can be modulated by thermomechanical means (Chen et al. 2018). Although the strength of these alloys is higher than that of unalloyed Mg, even better mechanical properties can be achieved by adding aluminum and rare earth elements (REE). The lower solubility of Ca, Si, and Sr in Mg limits their use in the biomedical industry due to noncompatible mechanical properties, although these alloys have excellent biocompatibility (Chen et al. 2018). The processing techniques for these alloys thus need to be developed further to utilize their biocompatibility benefits. Zn and RE additions, on the other hand, enhance the mechanical properties of Mg alloys; hence their use can be explored further (Chen et al. 2018). The need, thus, is to combine the use of alloying additions with better and improved processing methods to improve and expand the use of Mg alloys in biomedical applications.

The important Mg alloys for biomedical applications can be grouped broadly into five subcategories (Peron, Berto, and Torgersen 2020):

  i. Mg-Al alloys

   The Al content in Mg-Al alloys generally varies between 2 wt% and 9 wt% (Riaz, Shabib, and Haider 2019). Al is added to improve mechanical and corrosive properties as it favors solid solution and precipitation strengthening. $Al_2O_3$ layer formed in Mg-Al alloys aids in corrosion resistance (Riaz, Shabib, and Haider 2019). The most used Mg alloys in the industries belong to the AZ series (alloyed with Al and Zn) (Akyuz 2016; Bamberger and Dehm 2008). Al in Mg decreases the biodegradation of Mg in the body; however, it can be toxic (Bornapour et al. 2013). Mg-Al alloys are seen to be related to Alzheimer's disease and dementia as well as extremely harmful to osteoblasts and neurons (Zhang et al. 2010).

 ii. Mg-Zn alloys

   Zn, an essential element in the human body, helps in regulating the function of enzymes, assists in DNA synthesis, and enhances immunity. The most preferred alloying additions to Mg are Al and Zn, where Al forms the base of the alloy (Tan and Ramakrishna 2021). Zn added to Mg in quantities less than 3% decreases the grain size and when less than 5% Zn is added, corrosion resistance and mechanical properties of the alloy are enhanced (Amukarimi and Mozafari 2021; Zhang et al. 2010). Excessive Zn absorption, however, can impede the growth of bones apart from degrading the mechanical properties of the alloy (Riaz et al. 2019). Precipitation hardening as well as solid-state strengthening is accompanied by the addition of Zn, thereby improving the strength and ductility of Mg alloys (Baek et al. 2018; Riaz et al. 2019).

iii. Mg-Ca alloys

Ca is one of the important nutrients in the body, assisting in the growth of bones as well as regulating certain cell functions. The addition of Ca in Mg causes grain refinement and can result in the improvement of properties like strength, hardness, creep resistance, etc. (Baek et al. 2018; Riaz et al. 2019). It should however be noted that the Ca concentration in Mg alloys should be less than 1% as higher percentages can result in lowered corrosion resistance (Amukarimi and Mozafari 2021). Further, a higher amount of Ca can interfere with the working of the heart and other organs, can cause kidney stones, and weaken bones, etc. (Amukarimi and Mozafari 2021).

iv. Mg-RE alloys

REE are not present in quantifiable amounts inside human bodies but their addition to Mg alloys can assist in grain refinement, thereby leading to improved mechanical, corrosion, and creep properties (Riaz et al. 2019). Grain boundary pinning by the Mg-RE phase is one of the important strengthening mechanisms for these alloys (Bamberger and Dehm 2008). However, the cytotoxicity of these materials is of prime concern that needs to be worked on (Zhang et al. 2010; Amukarimi and Mozafari 2021). REE, including lanthanum (La), yttrium (Y), neodymium (Nd), cerium (Ce), scandium (Sc), and gadolinium (Gd), have been added to Mg and their influence on the mechanical and chemical properties and cytotoxicity has been studied to determine their usability as bioimplants (Liu et al. 2019). However, certain RE elements like La and Ce may cause cytotoxicity and must be carefully used as bioimplants (Liu et al. 2019).

v. Mg-Sr alloys

Sr, being a component of bone, assists in the growth of osteoblasts, prevents their resorption, and increases its strength (Bornapour et al. 2013; Riaz et al. 2019). In amounts, less than 2 wt%, Sr in Mg assists in decreasing the corrosion rate and increases the strength (Riaz et al. 2019). In higher amounts, Sr can lead to skeletal abnormalities and other defects in the body (Amukarimi and Mozafari 2021). It also acts as a grain refiner in Mg, thereby improving the strength (Bornapour et al. 2013).

Apart from these binary alloys, Mg alloys used in biomedical implants also include a combination of these elements. The combined effect of these elements further improves the properties of alloys for better utilization in the medical industry. The effect of their alloying addition on the mechanical and corrosion properties and biocompatibility is discussed in the following section.

## 4.3  MECHANICAL AND FATIGUE PROPERTIES OF
## BIOMEDICAL Mg ALLOYS

The mode of plastic deformation, i.e., the mechanical forming method to process the Mg alloys, besides the alloying addition, also affects the properties of these alloys. Extrusion, rolling, and various other severe plastic deformation (SPD) methods that include equal-channel angular processing (ECAP), high-pressure torsion (HPT), cyclic extrusion and compression (CEC), etc., are used for grain refinement and increasing the strength of the biodegradable Mg alloys (Chen et al. 2018). The aim of utilizing various processing methods as well as the alloying additions is to improve the strength by grain refinement and precipitate formation and to decrease the corrosion rate by the formation or increased protection of the corrosion protection film (Chen et al. 2018). Some alloying additions like aluminum, zinc, tin, silicon, silver, indium, and zirconium improve the yield strength (YS) and ultimate tensile strength (UTS) but manganese or yttrium do not enhance the strength (Gu et al. 2009). With Al and Zn addition, the hot-rolled Mg alloy shows significant improvement in YS and UTS, although the elongation decreases (Gu et al. 2009). These additions aim to increase the strength of the Mg alloys for their efficient utilization as a bioimplant.

Metallic biomaterial to be used as an orthopedic bioimplant must also have good fatigue characteristics, apart from compatible mechanical properties, as most of the implant failures are seen to be related to fatigue. The implants being continuously subjected to saline physiological fluid and cyclic load are susceptible to corrosion fatigue wherein the fatigue cracks are seen to originate from the localized pits created due to a corrosive environment (Antunes and De Oliveira 2012). Although the mechanical and corrosion properties of the biomedical Mg alloys are improved by alloying, there is a need to properly evaluate the effect of alloying additions and alloy processing methods of the Mg implants to prevent fatigue.

### 4.3.1  Mg-Al ALLOYS

Al is one of the most common additions in Mg with AZ91, AZ31, AE21, LAE442, and Ca-modified AZ alloys being the widely used and researched Mg alloys (Witte et al. 2008). Grain refinement and solid solution strengthening are two important phenomena occurring due to the presence of Al, thereby having direct implications on mechanical properties. Generally, the grain size decreases with the increase in Al content. Also, the hardness values increase with the increase in the Al content mainly due to decrease in the grain size (Caceres and Rovera 2001). Since Al exists as $\alpha$-Mg and $Mg_{17}Al_{12}\beta$ phase, the amounts and distribution of these phases affect the mechanical properties of the alloy (Zhang et al. 2009). It is seen that there is a decrease in the anisotropy, an improvement in ductility, and an increase in the proof stress with the increase in the Al content (Caceres and Rovera 2001). It is also seen that the maximum UTS is observed for as-cast Mg-Al alloys containing 8 wt% Al. The maximum load withstood by the alloy depends on the $Mg_{17}Al_{12}$-$\beta$ phase with the 8 wt% alloy having the optimum amount of the phase and the ductile matrix conducive for higher UTS (Cao and Wessén 2004).

Also, for the case of ternary cast Mg-Al-Zn alloy, with a minute amount of Mn as well ($\leq 0.27$ wt%), it was observed (Figure 4.1) that with the increase in the amount

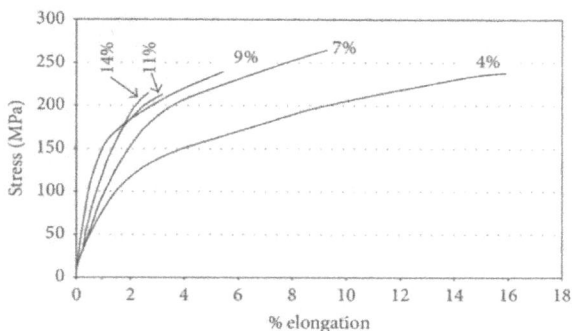

**FIGURE 4.1**    Effect of Al on tensile properties of Mg-based alloys (Abdelaziz et al. 2017).

of Al from 4 wt% to 14 wt%, the YS increased from ~120 MPa to ~153 MPa. As seen from Figure 4.1, the UTS reached a maximum at 7 wt% Al and then decreased continuously with the increase in the amount. The % elongation, however, exponentially decreased with the increase in the amount of Al. The ductile to brittle mode of fracture was observed as the Al concentration exceeds 9%. The decrease in ductility is attributed to Mg-Zn-Al as well as Mg-Al intermetallics resulting in intergranular fracture (Abdelaziz et al. 2017).

The processing conditions also influence the mechanical properties of Mg-Al (AZ91) alloy. AZ91 alloy is inherently less ductile at room temperature and has poor formability due to the presence of a high-volume fraction of the $Mg_{17}Al_{12}$ phase. The morphology of this phase and hence the resulting properties can be modified by ECAP process. It is observed that the highest YS of 289 MPa and UTS of 417 MPa are obtained after two-step ECAP with four passes at 225°C and two passes at 180°C. The elongation at failure is also seen to increase up to 8.45%. The improved mechanical properties are attributed to grain refinement and precipitation of the $Mg_{17}Al_{12}$ phase (Chen et al. 2008).

The addition of REE in Mg-Al alloys further refines the grains and improves the mechanical properties, high-temperature properties, casting characteristics, and corrosion resistance of Mg (Lü et al. 2000; Zhou et al. 2004). Some commonly used Mg-RE alloys are Mg-Al-RE (AE), Mg-Zn-RE-Zr (ZE, EZ), Mg-Ag-RE-Zr (QE), and Mg-Y-RE-Zr (WE). RE addition in AZ91 alloy as Ce-rich misch metal (MM) shows no significant change in UTS and a slight increase in YS, when tested at room temperature. The elongation, on the other hand, increases and is highest for AZ91-1RE alloy and lowest for AZ91-3RE due to coarsening of $Al_{11}RE_3$ phase. For the other alloy system, Mg-6Al, the addition of RE shows significant improvement in UTS. The UTS, YS, and elongation of Mg-6Al-1RE are highest, even higher than AZ91-RE alloy systems (Lü et al. 2000). At high temperatures, the increase in the UTS and elongation is significant for both the alloy systems. AZ91-2RE alloy has the highest UTS and elongation, much higher than AZ91 alloy without RE addition. The UTS is comparable to that of Mg-6Al-$x$RE alloys where again the property values increase due to the addition of RE elements. Even at a high temperature of 150°C, the mechanical property values for both Mg-Al-RE alloy systems are comparable to that of the room temperature (Lü et al. 2000). The

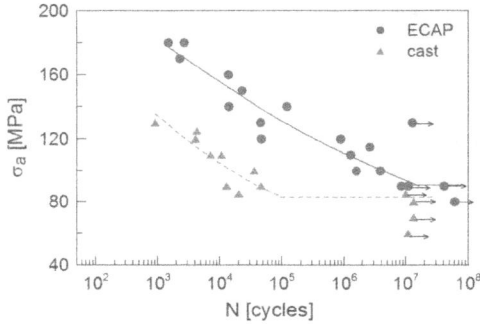

**FIGURE 4.2** *S–N* curves of as-cast AZ91 and AZ91 processed by ECAP (Fintová and Kunz 2015).

strengthening phase in AZ91 alloys is $Mg_{17}Al_{12}$ phase that softens and coarsens at a temperature of 120–130°C. The phase has a cubic structure, thus being incoherent with Mg leading to a brittle interface between the two. The addition of RE leads to the generation of $Al_{11}RE_3$ phase with high thermal stability, thereby improving the high-temperature properties (Lü et al. 2000).

Apart from the static loading, the response of dynamic loading is also seen to be a function of the alloying and processing conditions. Fatigue tests performed with the load ratio of −1 on AZ91 alloys, as shown in Figure 4.2, show that the fatigue life increased by a magnitude of two orders when the alloys were processed by ECAP. The endurance limit (based on $10^7$ cycles) of the as-cast alloy is clearly observed to be around 80 MPa, whereas for the ECAP-processed AZ91 alloy, it is around 85 MPa. It is also observed that the *S–N* curve of ECAP alloy decreases continuously with increasing number of cycles without any knee (Fintová and Kunz 2015). The cracks were seen to initiate at the cyclic slip bands. The slip bands are formed in coarse grains of ECAP processed alloys and near areas of solid solution for as-cast alloys (Fintová and Kunz 2015).

## 4.3.2 Mg-Zn Alloys

The maximum solubility of Zn in Mg is about 6.2 wt% at 325°C (Zhang et al. 2010). Mg-Zn binary alloy with 6 wt% Zn shows the tensile and compressive strength of about 279.5 ± 2.3 MPa and 433.7 ± 1.4 MPa, respectively, and the elongation of about 18.8 ± 0.8% (Zhang et al. 2010). Biological safety is ensured by the addition of Zn in Mg apart from the increase in the corrosion resistance. Strength is also increased with the addition of Zn but the amount of Zn must be toward the lower end. This increase in strength, however, leads to decrease in the corrosion rate. Hence, the optimization of strength and corrosion is to be reached, which is obtained at 4 wt%. (Jiang et al. 2019).

Further improvement in strength is obtained by the addition of Sn and the formation of $Mg_2Sn$ intermetallic compound. $Mg_2Sn$, however, acts as the site of pitting corrosion. At lower concentrations of Sn (less than 2 wt%), it decreases the corrosion rate by decreasing the amount of $Mg_2Sn$ formed and is also considered to be biologically safe (Jiang et al. 2019). The impact of Sn addition on Mg-Zn alloy can be understood by considering the increase in the amount of Sn from 1 wt% to 2 wt% and the YS and UTS increase from $133 \pm 9$ MPa and $234 \pm 12$ MPa to $147 \pm 8$ MPa and $250 \pm 11$ MPa, respectively. This is considerably higher than that of the Mg-4Zn alloy having the YS and UTS of $118 \pm 7$ MPa and $223 \pm 13$ MPa, respectively (Jiang et al. 2019). Also, these values are comparable to that of the cortical bone that has a YS of 105–114 MPa and UTS of 35–283 MPa (Jiang et al. 2019). Thus, Mg-Zn alloy can be used for orthopedic implants, and their strength can be further increased with the addition of Sn.

Apart from Sn, Mn is also added to Mg-Zn alloys for improvement in both the YS and the saltwater resistance of Mg alloys, thereby improving its corrosion resistance (Zhang et al. 2009). The YS and UTS of the extruded Mg-1Zn-1Mn alloy were observed to be 246 MPa and 280 MPa, respectively, being considerably higher than the as-cast alloy with the values of 44 MPa and 174 MPa, respectively (Zhang et al. 2009). Both these values increased with the increasing content of Zn in the alloy system, as is seen in Figure 4.3(a). This occurs due to refinement of Zn and the presence of Al-Mn and $Mg_7Zn_3$ phases (Zhang et al. 2009). As is observed in Figure 4.3(b), the elongation of the as-cast alloys increased with the Zn content; however, for the extruded alloys, the elongation drastically decreased to ~10% at 3 wt% Zn (Zhang et al. 2009).

Sr addition in Mg-Zn alloy is considered to appreciably refine the grains and promote nucleation of new osteoblasts. It is seen that as the Sr content in Mg-1Zn alloy system increased from 0.2 wt% to 1 wt%, the tensile YS increased from $89 \pm 5$ MPa to $130 \pm 10$ MPa. Similarly, the UTS and elongation increased from $187 \pm 16$ MPa and $11.0 \pm 1.4\%$ to $249 \pm 21$ MPa and $12.6 \pm 1.4\%$, respectively. Similarly, with the addition of Sr, the compressive yield strength (CYS) and ultimate compressive strength (UCS) increased from $82 \pm 7$ MPa and $241 \pm 16$ MPa to $129 \pm 11$ MPa and $278 \pm 18$ MPa, respectively. The % elongation also showed around 31% increase with 1 wt. % Sr addition (Li et al. 2014).

Apart from the static loading conditions, cyclic loading results are also seen to be affected by alloying Al and Zn in Mg. It is known that fatigue failure can be introduced by three mechanisms: cyclic deformation, the influence of the environment, and the

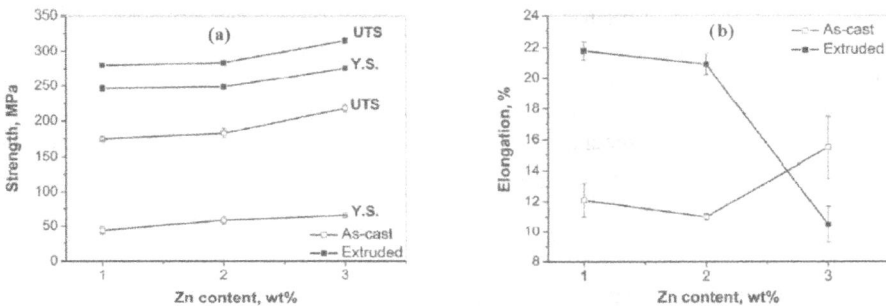

**FIGURE 4.3** Effect of Zn content (wt%) on (a) YS and UTS, and (b) % elongation of as-cast and extruded Mg-Zn-Mn alloys (Zhang et al. 2009).

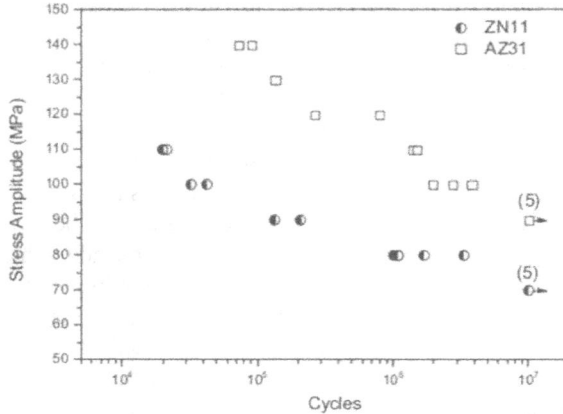

**FIGURE 4.4**   *S–N* curves of AZ31 and ZN11 alloys (Nascimento et al. 2010).

cyclic slip or deformation by mechanical twinning. The endurance limit at $10^7$ cycles, as seen in Figure 4.4, of AZ31 and ZN11 (N-Neodymium) was observed to be 90 MPa and 70 MPa, respectively. AZ31 alloy with inhomogeneous structure, strong texture responsible for $\{10\bar{1}2\}$ twinning under compressive loading and mechanical asymmetry, promotes fatigue failure. On the other hand, for ZN11 alloy, cyclic slip was the cause for fatigue failure as the initiation of crack was attributed to the hindrance of slip band movement and generation of stress concentration (Nascimento et al. 2010).

### 4.3.3   Mg-Ca Alloys

A lower density of Ca (1.55 g/cc) is a favorable factor for developing Mg-Ca alloys for biomedical implants apart from Ca being a major component of bones. This alloy system, besides giving the required strength as an implant, also assists in incorporating Ca to the bones, thereby strengthening them (Li et al. 2008). The YS and UTS as well as the elongation of as-cast Mg-Ca alloys decreased with an increase in Ca content. However, after hot rolling and extrusion, these properties increased significantly (Li et al. 2008). The UTS of the Mg-1Ca as-extruded and the as-rolled alloy was observed to be 239.63 MPa and 166.7 MPa, almost the same as that of the Mg alloys used in biomedical applications (Li et al. 2008). The ability to maneuver these properties with hot working increases their importance as optimization becomes convenient.

The low cost, good mechanical and corrosion properties, and the importance of Zn and Ca as nutrients for the human body have motivated research toward Mg-Zn-Ca alloys. Mg-Ca alloys corrode easily, hence Zn is added to improve the corrosion resistance (Baek et al. 2018). Zn in amounts of 4 wt% and Ca with less than 1 wt% have better grain structure with optimized grain refinement capabilities. The difference brought about by the addition of Ca in the mechanical properties can be considered by comparing the Mg-4Zn and Mg-4Zn-0.4Ca alloys (Hradilová et al. 2013). It was observed that the UCS of the as-cast (C), heat-treated (T4), and ECAPed (E) alloy systems of Mg-4Zn and Mg-4Zn-0.4Ca alloy systems have almost

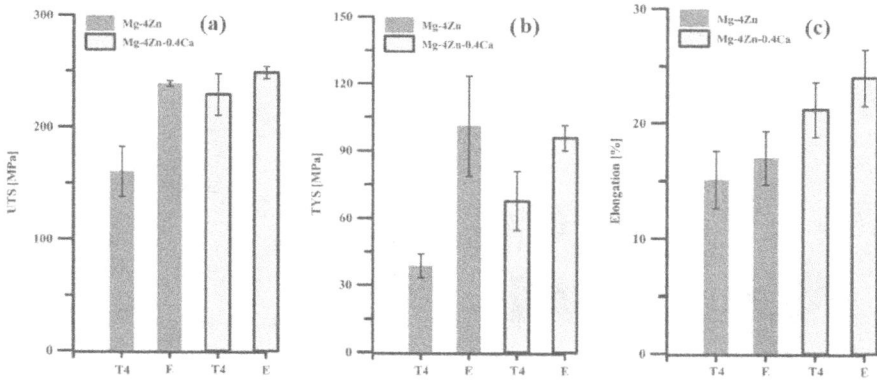

**FIGURE 4.5** Comparison of (a) UTS, (b) tensile yield strength (TYS), and (c) % elongation of Mg-4Zn and Mg-4Zn-0.4Ca alloys in the heat-treated (T4) and ECAPed (E) alloy systems (Hradilová et al. 2013).

the same value of about 350 MPa (Hradilová et al. 2013). The CYS, however, shows variation with the processing condition. The CYS of Mg-4Zn-0.4Ca alloy systems is higher than the Mg-4Zn binary alloy systems in C, T4, as well as E conditions. The dissolution of intermetallic phases decreases the values for T4 conditions, and the grain refinement by ECAP increases the values (Hradilová et al. 2013). The tensile properties of the Mg-4Zn-0.4Ca alloy system are superior to that of the binary Mg-4Zn alloy due to the formation of $Ca_2Mg_6Zn_3$ phase. It is again observed from Figure 4.5(a–c) that the ternary alloy has superior YS and UTS as well as elongation than that of the binary system. The ECAPed Mg-4Zn-0.4Ca alloy thus has better mechanical properties than the rest of the systems due to high grain refinement and removal of intradendritic intermetallic phases (Hradilová et al. 2013).

### 4.3.4 Mg-RE Alloys

Mg-RE alloys exhibit a range of mechanical properties, as shown in Figure 4.6 (a) and (b). As is seen in Figure 4.6 (a), the UTS and YS range between 76 MPa and 354 MPa and 40 MPa and 316 MPa, respectively (Liu et al. 2019). Similarly, from Figure 4.6 (b), the elongation of various Mg-RE alloys is seen to lie between 0.7% and 60% (Liu et al. 2019). For the Mg-RE binary alloys, the YS and UTS increase with the increase in RE content, although elongation decreases. For most of these binary alloys, the YS and UTS values are less than 100 MPa and 200 MPa, respectively, and the elongation is about 10% (Liu et al. 2019). Gadolinium and dysprosium have higher solubility in Mg than other RE elements and it was observed that for Mg-Gd alloys, the mechanical properties show better comparison with that of the bones. However, it was found that with the increase in implantation time, the concentration of Gd also increased in the organs of lab rats (test subject). Mg-10Dy alloy, on the other hand, showed good YS and UTS of about 83 MPa and 131 MPa, respectively. It was also observed that the grain refinement of Sc is higher than that of yttrium and Gd (Liu et al. 2019).

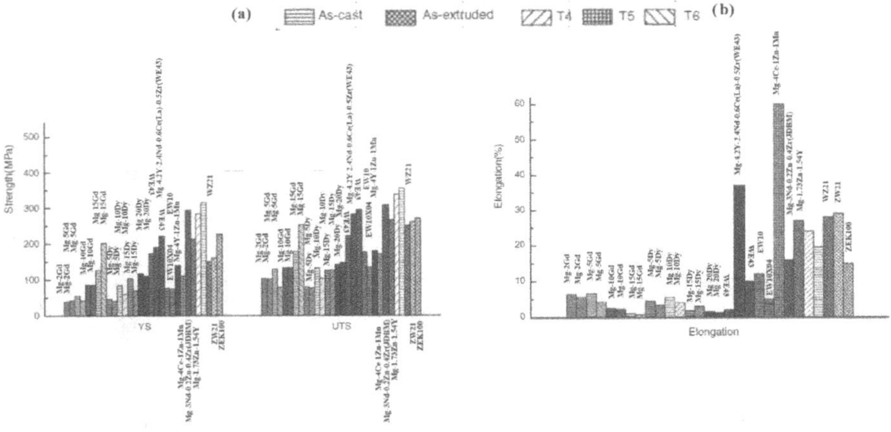

**FIGURE 4.6** (a) YS and UTS and (b) elongation of some Mg-RE alloys (Liu et al. 2019).

The ternary and quaternary Mg-RE alloys are also seen to show sufficient mechanical strength to be used in biomedical applications. Zn and Ca are the common alloying additions of Mg with RE, which are natural constituents in the body and bones. The Mg-RE alloys, in general, can be modified by appropriate heat treatment or alloying additions to better suit the properties of bones to be used as a bioimplant material (Liu et al. 2019). Mg-Zn-Y alloys showed almost similar YS and UTS to that of WE43 alloys; however, alloys like Mg-2.4Zn-0.8Gd and JDBM having strengths of 280 MPa and 310 MPa, respectively, far exceed the strength of WE43 alloys (Liu et al. 2019). The addition of Ce in Mg-Zn-Mn alloy increased the elongation up to 60%, showing the superior nature of Ce over Y (Liu et al. 2019).

Yttrium is one of the important RE elements, having good cytocompatibility (only RE) and solid solubility over a temperature range in Mg. Mg-Y alloys showed higher strength than the as-rolled Mg when tested along the rolling direction. The strength of as-rolled is seen to be higher than that of the Mg-5Y alloy due to higher solid solution strengthening. The increased ductility is attributed to weakened texture. In the annealed condition, for both alloys, the strength decreased and the ductility showed a significant increase (Ansari et al. 2021).

The cyclic deformation behavior of RE-containing Mg alloy was studied by Mirza et al. (2013). The fatigue life of Mg-10Gd-3Y-0.5Zr (GW103K) alloy was investigated and it was observed that with the increase in total strain amplitude, the stress amplitude also increased and the fatigue life decreased. Also, cyclic stabilization was observed till the strain amplitude of about 1%. The comparison of fatigue life with other alloys, as seen in Figure 4.7, shows that the cyclic hardening exponent of the GWK103K alloy is less (0.20) than that of the extruded AZ31 alloy. The fatigue life of GW103K was observed to be higher than that of RE-free Mg alloys. The tension–compression asymmetry generally observed in Mg alloys was seen to be absent in the alloy and was attributed to grain refinement, weaker texture, suppression of twinning activities, and presence of RE-containing precipitates (Mirza et al. 2013).

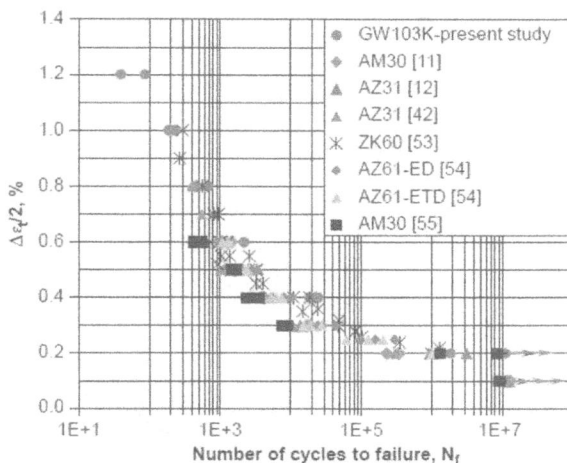

**FIGURE 4.7**    Fatigue characteristics of GW103K alloy (Mirza et al., 2013).

### 4.3.5  Mg-Sr Alloys

Sr is added to Mg for grain refinement, but it assists in stimulating bone formation and depreciates bone resorption (Brar, Wong, and Manuel 2012; Chen et al. 2020). With the increase in the Sr content, the hardness increases with the highest hardness being observed for Mg-1.5Sr alloy. In conjugation with Zn, Mg-4Zn-0.5Sr shows some age-hardening behavior as compared to Mg-2Zn-0.5Sr, which has a relatively flat hardness plot. The addition of a small quantity of Sn considerably improved the age-hardening response of Mg-6.2Zn alloy in such a way that the maximum hardness of Mg-6Zn-0.5Sr is 21 HV greater than the binary Mg-6.2Zn sample (Brar, Wong, and Manuel 2012). With the addition of Sr in Mg, both YS and UTS, as seen in Figure 4.8, increase till 2 wt% Sr and is higher than pure Mg. It is also seen that the strength starts to decrease with a further increase in the percentage of Sr. The elongation, however, decreases with the increase in Sr. The optimized mechanical properties, as seen from Figure 4.8, are observed for Mg-2Sr alloy with the values of UTS and elongation as $213.3 \pm 17.2$ MPa and $3.2 \pm 0.3\%$, respectively (Gu et al. 2012).

The solubility of Sr in Mg is about 0.11% under equilibrium conditions; thus, with the increase in the content of Sr, the grain growth is limited during solidification. This increases the strength of Mg-Sr alloy but decreases the elongation. $Mg_{17}Sr_2$ phase produced restricts the elongation in these alloys by acting as a potential crack-initiating site. Adding Sr in large quantities (3–4 wt%) increases the amount of brittle $Mg_{17}Sr_2$ phase, thereby decreasing the strength and elongation values (Gu et al. 2012).

## 4.4  CHEMICAL PROPERTIES/CORROSION RESISTANCE OF BIOMEDICAL Mg ALLOYS

Mg alloys typically corrode faster than pure Mg alloys due to micro-galvanic corrosion being accelerated by the presence of other components (Zainal Abidin et al. 2013). The processing condition apart from the alloying agent seems to determine

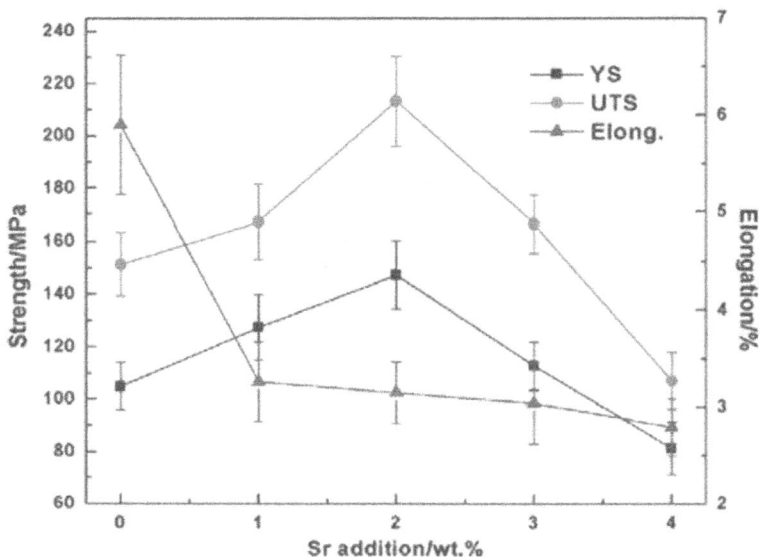

**FIGURE 4.8**   Effect of Sr content (till 4 wt%) on mechanical properties of as-rolled Mg-Sr alloys (Gu et al. 2012).

the corrosion behavior of alloys. The elements like Al, Ag, Mn, Si, and Y improve the corrosion potential of binary Mg-1X alloys. However, it is important to note that after hot rolling, the corrosion rate increases, especially of Mg-Al alloy, possibly due to precipitation of eutectic α-phase. The corrosive behavior of some of the important Mg-based biomedical alloys is described in the following sections.

## 4.4.1   Mg-Al Alloys

It is observed that the lowest hydrogen evolution rate is shown by Mg-Al and Mg-Zn alloy systems (Gu et al. 2009). Gu et al., while working on AZ31 alloys, observed that ECAP produces materials with homogenized fine grains having improved strength and superelastic properties (Gu et al. 2011). Ideally, with reduced grain size, the corrosion rate should decrease. However, it is seen that with 1–3 ECAP passes, the rate increases slightly, and after 4 passes, a reduction in the corrosion rate is observed. An initial increase in the corrosion rate may be attributed to higher stored energy, the formation of high-angle grain boundaries, and defects. After four passes, the large grains may have recrystallized, thereby releasing the strain and decreasing the dislocation density (Gu et al. 2011).

As is seen from Figure 4.9, the corrosion rates of pure Mg and AZ31 are highest at 8.008 mm/year and 8.290 mm/year, respectively, for one day. The corrosion rates of all samples decreased considerably after 8th day of immersion in m-SBF, so much so that after 24 days, the corrosion rates of pure Mg and AZ31 decreased to 1.218 mm/year and 1.997 mm/year, respectively. Sample AZ91D had the lowest corrosion

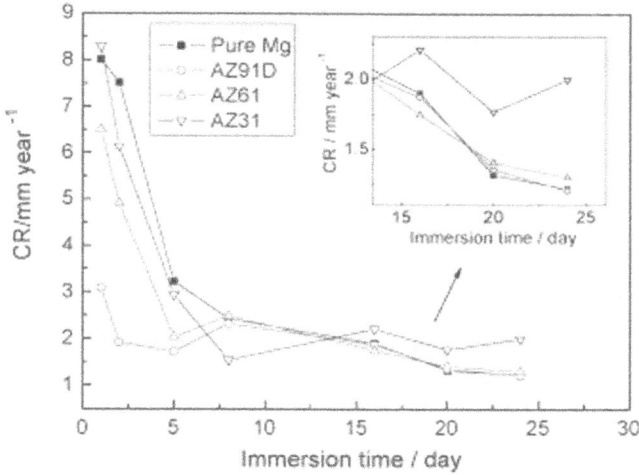

**FIGURE 4.9**  Corrosion rates of pure Mg and some Mg-Al alloys in m-SBF (Wen et al. 2009).

rate with 3.086 mm/year after 1 day of immersion and 1.206 mm/year after 24th day. The rate of pure Mg was found to be less than AZ31 and AZ61 after five days. The Al content in α-phase and the microstructure affected the corrosion rates of Mg alloys as the rates decreased with increasing Al content. For pure Mg, the corrosion was more uniform on the surface but for the alloys, the corrosion originated from the grain boundaries. AZ91D showed relatively uniform corrosion with shallow pits and in other alloys, pits were observed (Wen et al. 2009).

## 4.4.2  Mg-Zn Alloys

Zn is also seen to decrease the corrosion rate in biomedical Mg alloys so much so that Mg-6Zn alloy degrades slower than pure Mg (Zhang et al. 2009). The corrosion potential of Mg-6Zn is higher than that of pure Mg and the breakdown potential increases with the addition of Zn suggesting that the corrosion layers on Mg-6Zn are more protective than that of pure Mg (Zhang et al. 2010). Figure 4.10 shows the corrosion rates of pure Mg and Mg-Zn alloys after immersion in SBF for five days. The maximum weight loss of 0.69 mg/(cm$^2$ h) was observed for pure Mg that decreased from 0.04 mg/(cm$^2$ h) to 0.025 mg/(cm$^2$ h) to 0.063 mg/(cm$^2$ h) as the alloy composition changed to Mg-1Zn to Mg-5Zn to Mg-7Zn, respectively. The pitting corrosion was seen to be prominent in Mg-7Zn alloy leading to excessive weight loss, apart from the superficial corrosion observed in all the alloys. MgZn intermetallic formation, having cathodic potential, accelerates the localized corrosion leading to overall increase in the corrosion rate (Cai et al. 2012).

   The addition of Sn to the binary Mg-Zn is also seen to affect the corrosion behavior. The best corrosion resistance results are obtained for Mg-Zn-1.5Sn alloy, with the lowest corrosion current density ($I_{corr}$) of $1.05 \times 10^{-5}$ A/cm$^2$, the highest corrosion potential ($E_{corr}$) of $-1.51$ V, and a better pitting corrosion potential ($E_{pt}$) of $-1.47$ V, indicating better resistance against pitting corrosion. A higher percentage of Sn raises

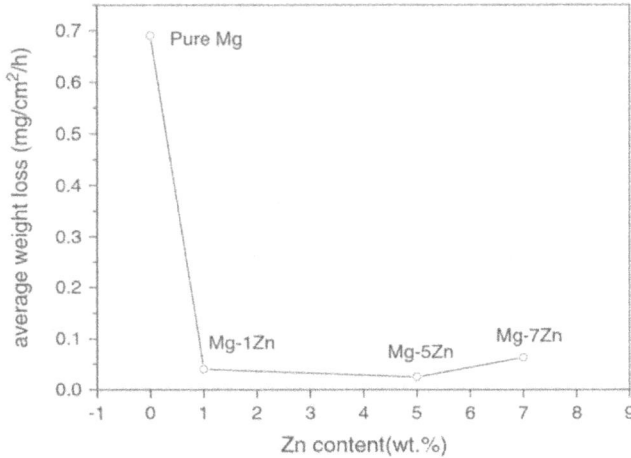

**FIGURE 4.10**   Effect of Zn addition on corrosion rates of Mg-Zn alloys (Cai et al. 2012).

$I_{corr}$ and decreases $E_{pt}$, making the composition lesser resistant to corrosion. For Mg-4Zn binary alloy, $E_{pt}$ is more negative, $I_{corr}$ is highest at $6.64 \times 10^{-5}$ A/cm², and $E_{corr}$ is lowest at $-1.58$ V. Sn assists in the formation of a protective film (as SnO and SnO$_2$) that resists the penetration of corrosive ions in the Mg matrix, when added in the composition of less than 2 wt%. An increase in the composition of Sn results in coarser Mg$_2$Sn particles that act as the initiation sites for corrosion (Jiang et al. 2019).

The corrosion rate calculated as weight loss, is highest for binary Mg-4Zn alloy and lowest for Mg-4Zn-1.5Sn alloy. The second highest corrosion rate is that of Mg-4Zn-2Sn alloy system, as was explained earlier. Mg-4Zn-1.5Sn has the lowest corrosion rate when compared with pure Mg and other Mg-Zn and Mg-Al alloys, thereby elevating the potential of Mg-Zn-Sn alloys for biomedical applications (Jiang et al. 2019).

With the addition of Mn in the system, as seen for Mg-Zn-Mn alloys, the corrosion potential decreases from $-1.47$ V for Mg-1Zn-Mn alloy to $-1.54$ V for Mg-3Zn-Mn alloy. The corrosion resistance ($R_p$) was highest for Mg-1Zn-Mn at 12.35 k$\Omega$ that decreased to 4.54 k$\Omega$ for Mg-3Zn-Mn with negligible change in pitting potential (Zhang et al. 2009). The addition of Mn in Mg-4Zn-0.5Ca alloy is seen to improve its corrosion resistance. It is observed that the $E_{corr}$ value for Mg-4Zn-0.5Ca alloy is $-1.527$ V, which increases to $-1.473$ V and $-1.414$ V with the addition of 0.4 wt% and 0.8 wt% Mn, respectively (Cho et al. 2017). The $I_{corr}$ values, however, decrease from $8.849 \times 10^{-6}$ A for Mg-4Zn-0.5Ca alloy to $2.857 \times 10^{-6}$ A for Mg-4Zn-0.5Ca-0.8Mn alloy. The corrosion rates thus show a decrease in the corrosion rate due to the addition of Mn. This is attributed to the stabilization of corrosion film (Cho et al. 2017).

## 4.4.3   Mg-Ca Alloys

Ca, an essential alloying addition to Mg, in terms of its biocompatibility is also seen to influence the corrosion behavior of Mg. The films on Mg-1Ca alloy were observed to be more protective than Mg-2Ca and Mg-3Ca alloys. The observed potential was about 320 mV for Mg-1Ca alloy, much higher than the other alloy systems having the potential of 210 mV and 170 mV, respectively. Rolling and extrusion, however, increased the potential of these alloys predicting the more protective nature of the heat-treated alloys (Li et al. 2008).

The addition of Ca in AZ alloys shifts the potential toward the positive side in the polarization curve. For the AZ91Ca alloy, with 0.4 wt% Ca addition, the shift in potential is ~140 mV, whereas for AZ91Ca with 1 wt% Ca, the shift is not significant. The insignificant shift could be because of Ca addition and Al content reduction. Further, the $I_{corr}$ values are also reduced greatly. AZ91 has the $I_{corr}$ value of 65.7 µA/cm² that decreases to 17.8 µA/cm² for AZ91Ca and to 36.5 µA/cm² for AZ61Ca alloy. It was seen that the in vitro pitting and general corrosion also reduced with the addition of Ca (Kannan and Raman 2008).

The addition of Ca in Mg-Zn alloys is interesting due to the importance of Ca and Zn inside the human body and the role played by Zn in reducing corrosion. It was seen by Abdel-Gawad and Shoeib that the lowest corrosion rate was shown by Mg-2Zn-0.6Ca alloy (Figure 4.11) with a weight loss of only 1.03 mg/cm² per day as opposed to the maximum shown by Mg-2.5Zn-1.5Ca with the weight loss of 2.6 mg/cm² per day (Abdel-Gawad and Shoeib 2019). The weight lost by pure Mg was seen to be around 2.4 mg/cm² per day. Thus, with the addition of Ca and Zn, the corrosion rate was seen to decrease mainly due to the deposition of hydroxyapatite on the surface that strengthens the corrosion barrier provided by Mg(OH)₂ layer (Abdel-Gawad and Shoeib 2019). In the same manner, for Mg-35Zn-$x$Ca ($x$ = 1–5), the highest corrosive potential of –1.26 V and –1.25 V were observed for Mg-35Zn-2Ca and Mg-35Zn-3Ca, respectively. It was observed that with Ca >3%, a large amount of Mg₂Ca phase was formed leading to the formation of dendritic structures, thereby increasing the corrosion rate (Kim et al. 2018).

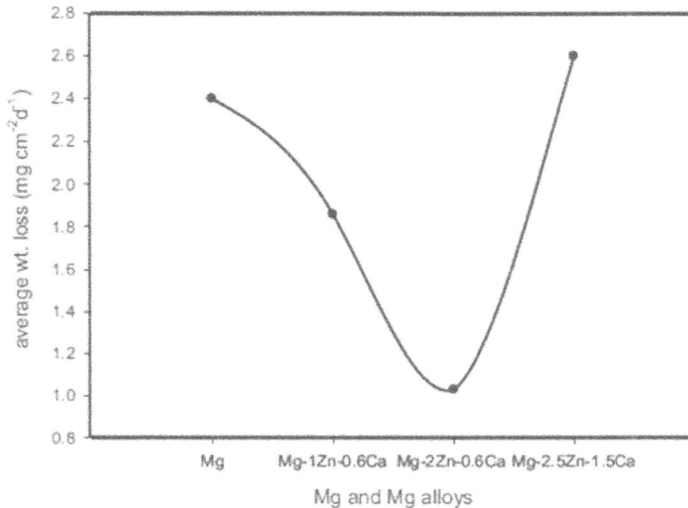

**FIGURE 4.11** Corrosion rates of some Mg-Zn-Ca alloys (Abdel-Gawad and Shoeib 2019).

### 4.4.4  Mg-RE Alloys

REE are also associated with the decreasing corrosion rates of Mg-based alloys. It is seen from Figure 4.12 that the potentiodynamic polarization curves of Mg-RE alloys are completely different from that of the pure Mg metal on NaCl solution (0.1 mol/L) (Zhao, Shi, and Xu 2013). $E_{corr}$ value of RE alloys is around 500 mV, higher than that of Mg. Also, $I_{corr}$ value is about one to two orders of magnitude higher. However, it is observed that Dy and Y show better corrosion resistance than Gd and Nd. The corrosion rate of Dy and Y is 1.2–14 mm/year and 1.9–2.4 mm/year, respectively, and is significantly less than 9.7–12.0 mm/year and 12.6–15.6 mm/year for Gd and Nd, respectively (Zhao, Shi, and Xu 2013).

Although the corrosion resistance of RE metals is significantly less than the pure Mg, it is seen that the addition of these metals in Mg increases the corrosion resistance of the alloy. This is attributed to the scavenger effect as REE form intermetallics with Fe and Ni in Mg alloys, formation of RE-rich phases with low cathodic activity, improvement in the protective film performance, and by homogenizing the microstructure (Zhao et al. 2013). The degradation behavior of Mg-RE alloys in vivo as well as in vitro shows that the lowest corrosion rates are of LAE442 and WE43 alloys. Although having better compatibility with bones in terms of mechanical properties, Gd was found with the increase in implantation time. Mg-10Dy alloy, on the other hand, showed a corrosion rate of 0.8 mm/year in 0.9% NaCl solution, which can be increased by appropriate heat treatments. Considering other alloy systems, it was seen that the addition of Y increased the corrosion resistance, being 2.17 mm/year with its addition as compared to 7.11 mm/year without the addition of Y. Mg-3Sc showed the lowest corrosion rate in Hank's solution of about 1.01 mL/cm$^2$ per day (Liu et al. 2019).

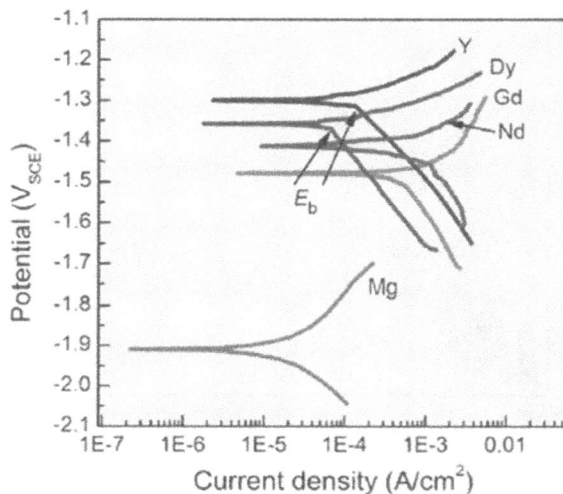

**FIGURE 4.12**  Potentiodynamic polarization curves of Mg-RE alloys in NaCl (Zhao et al. 2013).

### 4.4.5 Mg-Sr ALLOYS

Sr addition is seen to generally decrease the corrosion rate. It can be observed from Figure 4.13(a) that the corrosion rate of Mg-Sr alloys strongly depends on Sr concentration. At amounts less than 1 wt% Sr, the corrosion rate of the alloys in simulated body fluid (SBF) is less than that of pure Mg as well as that of high Sr-containing Mg alloys. It is also seen that Mg-0.5Sr has the lowest corrosion rate which is calculated to be about 2 mg/cm$^2$ per day. The polarization curves of pure Mg (as cast), compared to that of Mg-0.5Sr, show that the potential of the Mg-Sr alloy is less negative than that of pure Mg ($-1.58$ V versus $-1.6$ V) and the current density also changes from $1.259 \times 10^{-6}$ A cm$^{-2}$ for pure Mg to $5.011 \times 10^{-6}$ A cm$^{-2}$ for Mg-0.5Sr alloy, indicating better corrosion resistance of the Mg-0.5Sr alloy (Bornapour et al. 2013). With Sr addition up to 2 wt%, the corrosion rate of Mg-Sr alloy decreases and is less than that of pure Mg. As the content of Sr in Mg-Sr alloy increases to 4%, the corrosion rate increases. At low concentrations of Sr ($\leq 2\%$), the corrosion is uniform due to smaller grain size and reduced micro-shrinkage porosity. As the amount of Sr increases, corrosion becomes nonuniform leading to an increase in micropores that invariably cause increase in the exposed surface area, further accelerating the corrosion rate. Since the micropores are easily blocked by corrosion products, these pores become the sites for aggressive localized corrosion. Thus, the amount of Sr must be carefully selected due to higher corrosion rates at higher amounts of Sr (Gu et al. 2012).

To further enhance the corrosion resistance of the Mg-Sr alloys, Ca and Zn have been added to them. Their addition also refines the microstructure, thereby improving the mechanical and corrosion properties (Chen et al. 2020). The in vitro and in vivo corrosion rates of Mg-2Sr are compared with that of Mg-2Sr-Ca and Mg-2Sr-Zn alloys, as shown in Figure 4.13(b). As is seen from the figure, the in vitro corrosion rate (Hank's solution) measured by hydrogen evolution, the weight loss method, and the electrochemical test is lowest for Mg-2Sr-Zn alloy followed by Mg-2Sr-Ca alloy. The corrosion rates of these alloys were 39.6% and 65.9% of that of Mg-2Sr binary alloy, and are attributed to the refining of microstructure by the addition of Zn and Ca. The in vivo degradation rates also show the superior performance of Mg-2Sr-Zn alloy followed by Mg-2Sr-Ca alloy. The degradation rates are 0.85 mm/year and 1.10 mm/year, much slower than the Mg-2Sr alloy degrading at the rate of 1.37 mm/year (Chen et al. 2020).

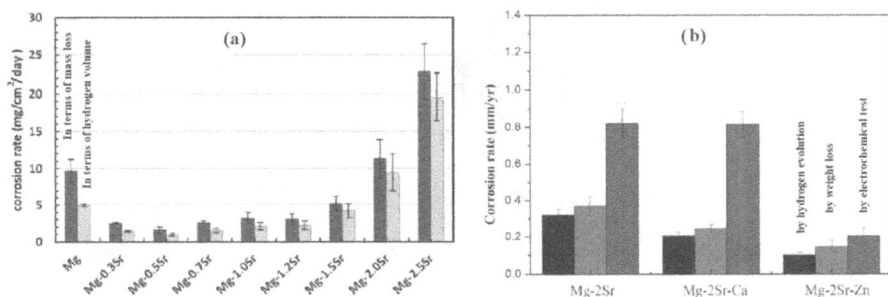

**FIGURE 4.13**  Corrosion rate of some (a) Mg-Sr biomedical alloys (Bornapour et al. 2013) and (b) Mg-Sn-Ca and Mg-Sn-Zr alloys (Chen et al. 2020).

## 4.5 BIOCOMPATIBILITY OF BIOMEDICAL Mg ALLOYS

Although biodegradation is highly essential and an advantageous trait of Mg to be used in biomedical applications, its rate, however, is a drawback. In vivo corrosion of Mg, and hence its biodegradation, can affect the utility of the implant apart from causing its failure well ahead of time. Again, alloying addition and the processing of the alloy have a more significant role in optimizing biodegradation for a better outcome and the life of the implant. Zr, Ca, Zn, Al, and Sr are considered to improve the compatibility, apart from Mg-RE alloys. The biocompatibility of these alloys, quantified as cell viability, can be observed from Figure 4.14 showing the L929 cell viability of some Mg alloys (Gu et al. 2009). The biocompatibility of the biomedical Mg alloys is discussed as follows.

### 4.5.1 Mg-Al ALLOYS

No significant cytotoxicity was observed for Mg-Al alloys considering the L-929 cell viability (Gu et al. 2009). The as-extruded and ECAPed and BP-ECAPed (back pressure ECAPed) AZ31 alloys show Grade 1 cytotoxicity concerning MG63 cells. However, the cell viability of BP-ECAP AZ31 alloy is the lowest. The alloy thereby shows Grade II level toxicity attributed to higher Al and Mg ions that cause osmolarity shock to the cells (Gu et al. 2011). When implanted in the pig femur, the mineralized bone area showed tremendous growth after 24 weeks of implanting Mg-Al alloys. When compared to the polymer group (SR-PLA96), the bone mass is seen to be higher for the Mg-Al alloys. Al stabilizes hydroxides in chloride environments, thereby stabilizing Mg. High levels of osteoblasts were observed around the implants due to the presence of magnesium ions essential for the structural biology and biochemistry of nucleic acids (Witte et al. 2005).

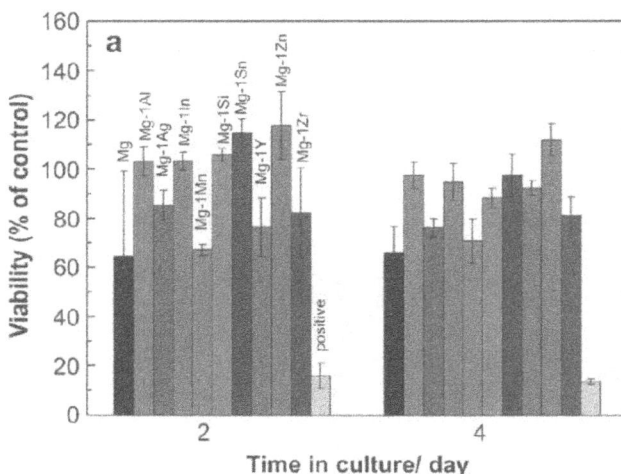

**FIGURE 4.14** L-929 cell viability of as-cast Mg-1X alloys after two and four days (Gu et al. 2009).

## 4.5.2   Mg-Zn Alloys

Mg-Zn and Mg-Ca alloys also have good biocompatibility with bones, with no observable disorders in other body organs (Zhang et al. 2010). To determine the biocompatibility of Mg-6Zn, the rods were implanted in the femoral shaft of New Zealand rabbits and no inflammation or sudden deaths were reported. It was seen that $Mg^{2+}$ serum levels were not increased nor were the lungs and kidney functions affected (Zhang et al. 2010). It was also seen that the degradation of the implants started in the first 3 weeks and after 12 weeks, the implants were not recognized clearly from the radiography tests, thereby predicting their in vivo degradation. After almost 14 weeks, the residual weight of the implant was only 13%, meaning most of the implant was decomposed. This degradation rate is higher than that of the Mg-Mn-Zn alloy, which showed ~54% degradation after 18 weeks (Zhang et al. 2010).

The cytotoxicity of Mg-6Zn observed is Grade 0–1, thereby making it suitable for cellular applications (Zhang et al. 2010). It is seen that Mg-4Zn-1Sn and Mg-4Zn-1.5Sn show cytotoxicity of level 0, with the cytocompatibility of Mg-4Zn-1.5Sn alloy being the highest (Jiang et al. 2019). Mg-1Zn-Mn with better mechanical and corrosive properties than Mg-2Zn-Mn and Mg-3Zn-Mn alloys also showed Grade 0 cytotoxicity, meaning excellent cytocompatibility (Zhang et al. 2009). The cell viability shows the same trend with the increase in incubation time, indicating a good level of cytocompatibility with Mg-Zn-Sr alloy. Also, the increment in cell viability is higher at longer exposure times, meaning cell growth is promoted by the extracted products (H. Li et al. 2014).

## 4.5.3   Mg-Sr Alloys

Sr, important for the growth and development of osteocytes, is considered beneficial as an alloying element for biomedical usage of Mg alloys. The cell viability for the cells surrounding Mg-0.5Sr alloys increases with time. Due to the initial corrosion of the alloy, the viability of the cells is less for one day of exposure, which then increases and far exceeds that of WE43 alloy after seven days. This indicates that the healthy growth of cells takes place (Bornapour et al. 2013). It was also observed that the total mass loss of Mg-0.5Sr implant, inside a dog, considered as the test subject, was 0.063 g, indicating the Sr release to be 0.015 mg/day. This release is well below the allowable limits of 4–5 mg/day (Bornapour et al. 2013). There were significantly different responses observed in terms of cytotoxicity of Mg-Sr samples. These as-rolled samples with Sr ≤2% showed higher values than Mg-3Sr and Mg-4Sr with the former showing the cytotoxicity of Grade 1 as per ISO 10993-5 (ISO 10993-5 2009). The high cytotoxicity of high Sr-containing Mg-Sr binary alloys may be attributed to higher pH levels. In vivo tests showed that Mg-2Sr alloy promoted bone mineralization and new bone formation (Gu et al. 2012).

## 4.5.4   Mg-Ca Alloys

The radiographic evaluation of the femoral implants of Mg-Ca biomaterial in rabbits showed that after three months, the implant structure was completely absorbed. Also, the growth of osteoblasts and osteocytes was observed around the Mg-Ca implants.

The L-929 cells showed better growth in Mg-1Ca alloy with the release of $Mg^{2+}$ ions increasing the cell viability. The implant constantly degraded inside the body and showed an average biocorrosion rate of $2.28 \pm 0.13$ $mg/mm^2$ per year (Li et al. 2008).

The ternary alloys of Mg-2Sr made by adding Zn and Ca show better cell viability than the binary Mg-2Sr alloy at day 1, possibly due to lower corrosion rates. With the increase in the culture period to five days, the cell viability of the ternary alloys seems comparable to that of Mg-2Sr alloy. The better bone growth was observed for Mg-2Sr-Zn and Mg-2Sr-Ca alloys as compared to that of the Mg-2Sr alloy (Chen et al. 2020).

### 4.5.5  Mg-RE Alloys

As is seen from Table 4.2, the cell viability of Mg-RE alloys matches and in some cases is better than that of the pure Mg. It is seen that Mg-1.8Zn-0.2Gd, JDBM, LAE442, and WE43 alloys show low cytotoxicity with L929. Mg-0.69La, Mg-2.13Nd, and Mg-1.27Ce showed lower cell viability with MC3T3-E1 than pure Mg, but comparable with FCV304 and VMSC. It was also seen that Mg-1.8Zn-0.2Gd, WE43, and LAE442 showed larger mineralized areas after implantation in rabbits, with eventual better growth of new bone. However, it is important to consider the cytotoxicity of the RE addition that is highest for Ce followed by La (Liu et al. 2019).

**TABLE 4.2**
**Cell Viability of Certain Mg-RE Alloy Implants**

| Materials | Formation | Cell Line | Culture Time (day) | Cell Viability (%) |
|---|---|---|---|---|
| Pure Mg | As-cast | L929 | 4 | 65.7 |
| | As-cast | MC3T3-E1 | 7 | 87.5 |
| | As-cast | ECV304 | 7 | 76.8 |
| | As-cast | VSMC | 7 | 93.6 |
| Mg-0.69La | As-cast | MC3T3-E1 | 5 | 78 |
| Mg-1.27Ce | As-cast | MC3T3-E1 | 5 | 51 |
| Mg-2.13Nd | As-cast | MC3T3-E1 | 5 | 78 |
| Mg-1.8Zn-0.2Gd | As-rolled | L929 | 5 | 82 |
| | As-rolled | MG63 | 5 | 100 |
| | As-rolled | VSMC | 5 | 90 |
| | As-rolled | ECV304 | 5 | 75 |
| Mg-1.8Zn-0.8Gd | As-rolled | L929 | 5 | 56 |
| | As-rolled | MG63 | 5 | 110 |
| | As-rolled | VSMC | 5 | 93 |
| | As-rolled | ECV304 | 5 | 65 |
| JDBM | As-extruded | L929 | 5 | 80 |
| LAE442 | ECAP | L929 | 7 | 100 |
| WE43 | Phosphating coated | L929 | 4 | 96 |

*Source:* Liu et al. (2019).

## 4.6 CONCLUSION

Mg in the body as a nutrient assisting in bone health and nucleic acid regulation is utilized by making biodegradable implants of the metal. The inherent clean degradation essential for bioimplants is controlled by alloying additions and processing methods. The strength imparted to Mg after alloying is also important for its function as an implant material. The change in mechanical properties quantified as YS and the elongation changes are shown in Figure 4.15(a). Different alloying additions like RE, Zn, Al, etc. have a tremendous effect on the strength of the alloy. From the figure, maximum improvement in YS and elongation is obtained by the addition of REE followed by Zn. The corrosive properties of Zn can be improved by controlling the amount of Zn added and by employing various processing methods, thereby making these alloys an excellent option for bioimplants (Chen et al. 2014). The amount of the metal added is seen to significantly affect the range of the property values shown by the Mg implant material. Apart from the mechanical parameters, the corrosive properties are also modulated by the addition of alloying components. Mg being highly corrosive needs alloying additions to control the degradation rate so that the implant can remain inside the body for sufficient time to promote the growth of osteoblasts. The corrosion rate of some Mg alloys is shown in Figure 4.15(b). It is seen from the figure that processing tremendously improves corrosion resistance. Also, the corrosion resistance of Mg-RE alloys is the best, especially in deformed conditions. Mg-Zn alloys also show good corrosion protection (Chen et al. 2014). Thus, alloyed Mg manufactured with proper processing routes shows significant improvement in the corrosion characteristics.

Finally, the effect of the alloying elements on biocompatibility, corrosion resistance, and mechanical properties is summarized in Table 4.3.

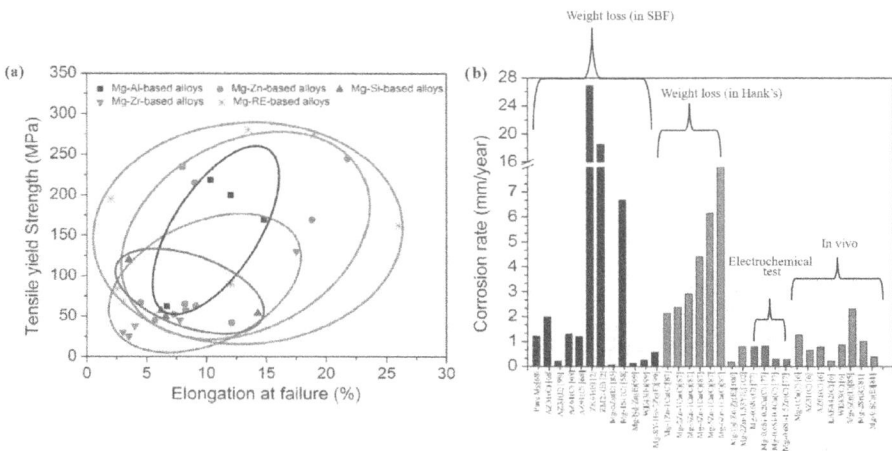

**FIGURE 4.15**  (a) YS and elongation of some typical Mg biomedical alloys, and (b) corrosion rate of typical Mg biomedical alloys (Chen et al. 2014).

**TABLE 4.3**

**Effects of Some of the Alloying Additions on Mg Alloys**

| Alloying Element | Pathophysiology/Toxicology/Biocompatibility | Corrosion Resistance | Mechanical Properties |
|---|---|---|---|
| Al | Normal blood serum level 2.1–4.8 µg/L. Neurotoxic, can cause Alzheimer's disease and muscle fiber damage, decreases osteoclast viability | • Beneficial for corrosion resistance | • Increases strength, hardness, and fluidity, while little increase in density |
| Zn | Normal blood serum level 12.4–17.4 µmol/L. Essential for the immune system, good biocompatibility, neurotoxic in higher concentration | • Improves corrosion resistance | • Assists in solid solution strengthening |
| Ca | Normal serum level 0.919–0.993 mg/L. Most abundant metal in human body, non-cytotoxic | • Corrosion resistance decreases with increasing Ca content | • Helps refine granulation, strength increases, and plasticity decreases with increasing Ca content |
| Mn | Normal blood serum level <0.8 µg/L. Influences the function of immune system, bone growth, etc., cytotoxic and neurotoxic in higher concentration | • Increases corrosion resistance in salt water for some Al-containing alloys | • Increases YS and decrease tensile strength and elongation |
| Sr | 140 mg in human body. Non-cytotoxic, promotes bone growth | • Decreases corrosion resistance with increasing Sr content | • Increases elongation resistance and reduces the incidents of fracture |
| Zr | Good biocompatibility and bone-bonding ability | • Corrosion resistance decreases with increasing Zr content | • Refines grains, increases strength and plasticity |
| Y and lanthanides | <47 g in blood serum level, compounds of drugs for treatment of cancer, basic lanthanides deposited in liver, more acidic and smaller cations are deposited on bone, Ce, La, Gd are cytotoxic, Y has good biocompatibility | • Y improves corrosion resistance<br>• Ce improves corrosion resistance when added in lower concentrations<br>• La improves corrosion resistance<br>• Gd increases corrosion resistance when added in smaller amounts | • Y improves high-temperature resistance, strength, and plasticity<br>• Ce improves strength and fatigue resistance<br>• La improves strength and creep resistance<br>• Gd improves strength due to solid solution strengthening |

*Sources*: Tsakiris, Tardei, and Clicinschi (2021) and Zhang et al. (2022).

# REFERENCES

Abdelaziz, M. H., M. Paradis, A. M. Samuel, H. W. Doty, and F. H. Samuel. 2017. "Effect of Aluminum Addition on the Microstructure, Tensile Properties, and Fractography of Cast Mg-Based Alloys." *Advances in Materials Science and Engineering* 2017. https:// doi.org/10.1155/2017/7408641

Abdel-Gawad, Soha A., and Madiha A. Shoeib. 2019. "Corrosion Studies and Microstructure of Mg-Zn-Ca Alloys for Biomedical Applications." *Surfaces and Interfaces* 14 (March): 108–16. https://doi.org/10.1016/j.surfin.2018.11.011

Akyuz, B. 2016. "A Study on Wear and Machinability of AZ Series (AZ01-AZ91) Cast Magnesium Alloys." *Metallic Materials* 52 (05): 255–62. https://doi.org/10.4149/km_2014_5_255

Amukarimi, Shukufe, and Masoud Mozafari. 2021. "Biodegradable Magnesium-based Biomaterials: An Overview of Challenges and Opportunities." *MedComm* 2 (2): 123–44. https://doi.org/10.1002/mco2.59

Ansari, Nooruddin, Soo Yeol Lee, Sudhanshu S. Singh, and Jayant Jain. 2021. "Influence of Yttrium-induced Twinning on the Recrystallization Behavior of Magnesium Alloys." *Journal of Materials Science* 56 (32): 18258–71. https://doi.org/10.1007/s10853-021-06418-8

Antunes, Renato Altobelli, and Mara Cristina Lopes De Oliveira. 2012. "Corrosion Fatigue of Biomedical Metallic Alloys: Mechanisms and Mitigation." *Acta Biomaterialia.*8 (3): 937–62. https://doi.org/10.1016/j.actbio.2011.09.012

Baek, Seung Mi, Hyung Keun Park, Jae Ik Yoon, Jaimyun Jung, Ji Hyun Moon, Seok Gyu Lee, and Jae H. Kim et al. 2018. "Effect of Secondary Phase Particles on the Tensile Behavior of Mg-Zn-Ca Alloy." *Materials Science and Engineering A* 735 (September): 288–94. https://doi.org/10.1016/j.msea.2018.08.050

Bamberger, M., and G. Dehm. 2008. "Trends in the Development of New Mg Alloys." *Annual Review of Materials Research* 38: 505–33. https://doi.org/10.1146/annurev.matsci.020408.133717

Banerjee, Parama Chakraborty, Saad Al-Saadi, Lokesh Choudhary, Shervin Eslami Harandi, and Raman Singh. 2019. "Magnesium Implants: Prospects and Challenges." *Materials.*12(1): 136. https://doi.org/10.3390/ma12010136

Bornapour, M., N. Muja, D. Shum-Tim, M. Cerruti, and M. Pekguleryuz. 2013. "Biocompatibility and Biodegradability of Mg-Sr Alloys: The Formation of Sr-Substituted Hydroxyapatite." *Acta Biomaterialia* 9 (2): 5319–30. https://doi.org/10.1016/j.actbio.2012.07.045

Brar, Harpreet S., Joey Wong, and Michele V. Manuel. 2012. "Investigation of the Mechanical and Degradation Properties of Mg-Sr and Mg-Zn-Sr Alloys for Use as Potential Biodegradable Implant Materials." *Journal of the Mechanical Behavior of Biomedical Materials* 7 (March): 87–95. https://doi.org/10.1016/j.jmbbm.2011.07.018

Caceres, C H, and D M Rovera. 2001. "Solid Solution Strengthening in Concentrated Mg-Al Alloys." *Journal of Light Metals* 1 (3): 151–56. www.elsevier.com/locate/lightmetals.

Cai, Shuhua, Ting Lei, Nianfeng Li, and Fangfang Feng. 2012. "Effects of Zn on Microstructure, Mechanical Properties and Corrosion Behavior of Mg-Zn Alloys." *Materials Science and Engineering C* 32 (8): 2570–77. https://doi.org/10.1016/j.msec.2012.07.042

Cao, H, and M Wessén. 2004. "Effect of Microstructure on Mechanical Properties of As-cast Mg-Al Alloys." *Metallurgical and Materials Transactions A* 35: 309–19.

Chen, Bin, Dong Liang Lin, Li Jin, Xiao Qin Zeng, and Chen Lu. 2008. "Equal-Channel Angular Pressing of Magnesium Alloy AZ91 and Its Effects on Microstructure and Mechanical Properties." *Materials Science and Engineering A* 483–484 (1–2 C): 113–16. https://doi.org/10.1016/j.msea.2006.10.199

Chen, Junxiu, Lili Tan, Xiaoming Yu, Iniobong P. Etim, Muhammad Ibrahim, and Ke Yang. 2018. "Mechanical Properties of Magnesium Alloys for Medical Application: A Review." *Journal of the Mechanical Behavior of Biomedical Materials* 87: 68–79. https://doi.org/10.1016/j.jmbbm.2018.07.022

Chen, Kai, Xinhui Xie, Hongyan Tang, Hui Sun, Ling Qin, Yufeng Zheng, Xuenan Gu, and Yubo Fan. 2020. "In Vitro and in Vivo Degradation Behavior of Mg-2Sr-Ca and Mg-2Sr-Zn Alloys." *Bioactive Materials* 5 (2): 275–85. https://doi.org/10.1016/j.bioactmat.2020.02.014

Chen, Yongjun, Zhigang Xu, Christopher Smith, and Jag Sankar. 2014. "Recent Advances on the Development of Magnesium Alloys for Biodegradable Implants." *Acta Biomaterialia* 10 (11): 4561–73. https://doi.org/10.1016/j.actbio.2014.07.005

Cho, Dae Hyun, Byoung Woo Lee, Jin Young Park, Kyung Mox Cho, and Ik Min Park. 2017. "Effect of Mn Addition on Corrosion Properties of Biodegradable Mg-4Zn-0.5Ca-$x$Mn Alloys." *Journal of Alloys and Compounds* 695: 1166–74. https://doi.org/10.1016/j.jallcom.2016.10.244

Fintová, Stanislava, and Ludvík Kunz. 2015. "Fatigue Properties of Magnesium Alloy AZ91 Processed by Severe Plastic Deformation." *Journal of the Mechanical Behavior of Biomedical Materials* 42 (February): 219–28. https://doi.org/10.1016/j.jmbbm.2014.11.019

Gu, X. N., N. Li, Y. F. Zheng, F. Kang, J. T. Wang, and Liquan Ruan. 2011. "In Vitro Study on Equal Channel Angular Pressing AZ31 Magnesium Alloy With and Without Back Pressure." *Materials Science and Engineering B: Solid-State Materials for Advanced Technology* 176: 1802–6. https://doi.org/10.1016/j.mseb.2011.04.003

Gu, X. N., X. H. Xie, N. Li, Y. F. Zheng, and L. Qin. 2012. "In Vitro and In Vivo Studies on a Mg-Sr Binary Alloy System Developed as a New Kind of Biodegradable Metal." *Acta Biomaterialia* 8 (6): 2360–74. https://doi.org/10.1016/j.actbio.2012.02.018

Gu, Xuenan, Yufeng Zheng, Yan Cheng, Shengping Zhong, and Tingfei Xi. 2009. "In Vitro Corrosion and Biocompatibility of Binary Magnesium Alloys." *Biomaterials* 30 (4): 484–98. https://doi.org/10.1016/j.biomaterials.2008.10.021

Hradilová, Monika, Dalibor Vojtěch, Jiří Kubásek, Jaroslav Čapek, and Martin Vlach. 2013. "Structural and Mechanical Characteristics of Mg-4Zn and Mg-4Zn-0.4Ca Alloys after Different Thermal and Mechanical Processing Routes." *Materials Science and Engineering A* 586 (December): 284–91. https://doi.org/10.1016/j.msea.2013.08.008

ISO 10993-5. 2009. "Biological Evaluation of Medical Devices Part 5 – Tests for In Vitro Cytotoxicity."

Jiang, Weiyan, Jingfeng Wang, Weikang Zhao, Qingshan Liu, Dianming Jiang, and Shengfeng Guo. 2019. "Effect of Sn Addition on the Mechanical Properties and Bio-corrosion Behavior of Cytocompatible Mg-4Zn Based Alloys." *Journal of Magnesium and Alloys* 7 (1): 15–26. https://doi.org/10.1016/j.jma.2019.02.002

Kannan, M. Bobby, and R. K. Singh Raman. 2008. "In Vitro Degradation and Mechanical Integrity of Calcium-Containing Magnesium Alloys in Modified-Simulated Body Fluid." *Biomaterials* 29 (15): 2306–14. https://doi.org/10.1016/j.biomaterials.2008.02.003

Kim, Seo Young, Yu Kyoung Kim, Yang Kwang-kyun, Kwang Bok Lee, and Min ho Lee. 2018. "Determination of Ideal Mg-35Zn-XCa Alloy Depending on Ca Concentration for Biomaterials." *Journal of Alloys and Compounds* 766 (October): 994–1002. https://doi.org/10.1016/j.jallcom.2018.06.088

Li, Zijian, Xunan Gu, Siquan Lou, and Yufeng Zheng. 2008. "The Development of Binary Mg-Ca Alloys for Use as Biodegradable Materials within Bone." *Biomaterials* 29 (10): 1329–44. https://doi.org/10.1016/j.biomaterials.2007.12.021

Li, Hui, Qiuming Peng, Xuejun Li, Kun Li, Zengsheng Han, and Daqing Fang. 2014. "Microstructures, Mechanical and Cytocompatibility of Degradable Mg-Zn Based Orthopedic Biomaterials." *Materials and Design* 58: 43–51. https://doi.org/10.1016/j.matdes.2014.01.031

Liu, Dexue, Donglin Yang, Xinling Li, and Shiwen Hu. 2019. "Mechanical Properties, Corrosion Resistance and Biocompatibilities of Degradable Mg-RE Alloys: A Review." *Journal of Materials Research and Technology* 8: 1538–49. https://doi.org/10.1016/j.jmrt.2018.08.003.

Lü, Yizhen, Qudong Wang, Xiaoqin Zeng, Wenjiang Ding, Chunquan Zhai, and Yanping Zhu. 2000. "Effects of Rare Earths on the Microstructure, Properties and Fracture Behavior of Mg-Al Alloys." *Materials Science and Engineering* 278 : 66–76. www. elsevier.com/locate/msea.

Mirza, F. A., D. L. Chen, D. J. Li, and X. Q. Zeng. 2013. "Low Cycle Fatigue of a Rare-Earth Containing Extruded Magnesium Alloy." *Materials Science and Engineering A* 575 (July): 65–73. https://doi.org/10.1016/j.msea.2013.03.041

Nascimento, L., S. Yi, J. Bohlen, L. Fuskova, D. Letzig, and K. U. Kainer. 2010. "High Cycle Fatigue Behaviour of Magnesium Alloys." *Procedia Engineering* 2: 743–50. https://doi. org/10.1016/j.proeng.2010.03.080

Peron, Mirco, Filippo Berto, and Jan Torgersen. 2020. Magnesium and *its alloys as implant materials; corrosion, mechanical and biological performances*, 1st edition. Boca Raton: CRC Press.

Riaz, Usman, Ishraq Shabib, and Waseem Haider. 2019. "The Current Trends of Mg Alloys in Biomedical Applications: A Review." *Journal of Biomedical Materials Research: Part B: Applied Biomaterials* 107 (6): 1970–96. https://doi.org/10.1002/jbm.b.34290

Staiger, Mark P., Alexis M. Pietak, Jerawala Huadmai, and George Dias. 2006. "Magnesium and Its Alloys as Orthopedic Biomaterials: A Review." *Biomaterials* 27 (9): 1728–34. https://doi.org/10.1016/j.biomaterials.2005.10.003

Tan, Jovan, and Seeram Ramakrishna. 2021. "Applications of Magnesium and Its Alloys: A Review." *Applied Sciences* 11 (15): 6861. https://doi.org/10.3390/app11156861

Tsakiris, Violeta, Christu Tardei, and Florentina Marilena Clicinschi. 2021. "Biodegradable Mg Alloys for Orthopedic Implants: A Review." *Journal of Magnesium and Alloys* 2 (3): 214–35. https://doi.org/10.1016/j.jma.2021.06.024

Wen, Zhaohui, Changjun Wu, Changsong Dai, and Feixia Yang. 2009. "Corrosion Behaviors of Mg and Its Alloys with Different Al Contents in a Modified Simulated Body Fluid." *Journal of Alloys and Compounds* 488 (1): 392–99. https://doi.org/10.1016/j. jallcom.2009.08.147

Witte, Frank, Norbert Hort, Carla Vogt, Smadar Cohen, Karl Ulrich Kainer, Regine Willumeit, and Frank Feyerabend. 2008. "Degradable Biomaterials Based on Magnesium Corrosion." *Current Opinion in Solid State and Materials Science* 12 (5–6): 63–72. https://doi.org/10.1016/j.cossms.2009.04.001

Witte, F., V. Kaese, H. Haferkamp, E. Switzer, A. Meyer-Lindenberg, C. J. Wirth, and H. Windhagen. 2005. "In Vivo Corrosion of Four Magnesium Alloys and the Associated Bone Response." *Biomaterials* 26 (17): 3557–63. https://doi.org/10.1016/j. biomaterials.2004.09.049

Zainal, Abidin, Nor Ishida, Barbara Rolfe, Helen Owen, Julian Malisano, Darren Martin, Joelle Hofstetter, Peter J. Uggowitzer, and Andrej Atrens. 2013. "The In Vivo and In Vitro Corrosion of High-Purity Magnesium and Magnesium Alloys WZ21 and AZ91." *Corrosion Science* 75 (October): 354–66. https://doi.org/10.1016/j.corsci. 2013.06.019

Zhang, L., Z. Y. Cao, Y. B. Liu, G. H. Su, and L. R. Cheng. 2009. "Effect of Al Content on the Microstructures and Mechanical Properties of Mg-Al Alloys." *Materials Science and Engineering A* 508 (1–2): 129–33. https://doi.org/10.1016/j.msea.2008.12.029

Zhang, Shaoxiang, Jianan Li, Yang Song, Changli Zhao, Xiaonong Zhang, Chaoying Xie, and Yan Zhang, Tao, Hairong, He, Yaohua, Jiang, Yao, Bian, Yujian 2009. "In Vitro Degradation, Hemolysis and MC3T3-E1 Cell Adhesion of Biodegradable Mg-Zn Alloy." *Materials Science and Engineering C* 29 (6): 1907–12. https://doi.org/10.1016/j. msec.2009.03.001

Zhang, Ting, Wen Wang, Jia Liu, Liqiang Wang, Yujin Tang, and Kuaishe Wang. 2022. "A Review on Magnesium Alloys for Biomedical Applications." *Frontiers in Bioengineering and Biotechnology* 10: 953344. https://doi.org/10.3389/fbioe.2022.953344

Zhang, Erlin, Dongsong Yin, Liping Xu, Lei Yang, and Ke Yang. 2009. "Microstructure, Mechanical and Corrosion Properties and Biocompatibility of Mg-Zn-Mn Alloys for Biomedical Application." *Materials Science and Engineering C* 29 (3): 987–93. https://doi.org/10.1016/j.msec.2008.08.024

Zhang, Shaoxiang, Xiaonong Zhang, Changli Zhao, Jianan Li, Yang Song, Chaoying Xie, and Hairong Tao, et al. 2010. "Research on an Mg-Zn Alloy as a Degradable Biomaterial." *Acta Biomaterialia* 6 (2): 626–40. https://doi.org/10.1016/j.actbio.2009.06.028

Zhao, Xu, Ling-ling Shi, and Jian Xu. 2013. "A Comparison of Corrosion Behavior in Saline Environment: Rare Earth Metals (Y, Nd, Gd, Dy) for Alloying of Biodegradable Magnesium Alloys." *Journal of Materials Science and Technology* 29 (9): 781–87. https://doi.org/10.1016/j.jmst.2013.05.017

Zhou, Haitao, Xiaoqin Zeng, Liufa Liu, Y A Zhang, and Yanping Zhu. 2004. "Effect of Cerium on Microstructures and Mechanical Properties of AZ61 Wrought Magnesium Alloy." *Journal of Materials Science* 39: 7061–66.

# 5 Surface Modification of Magnesium Alloy Employing External Coating for Biomedical Applications

*Kamlendra Vikram and Sumit Pramanik*
Department of Mechanical Engineering, College
of Engineering and Technology, SRM Institute
of Science and Technology, Chennai, India

*Viorel Paleu*
Mechanical Engineering Faculty, Gheorghe Asachi
Technical University of Iași, Iași, Romania

*Shubrajit Bhaumik*
Tribology and Interactive Surfaces Research
Laboratory (TRISUL), Department of Mechanical
Engineering, Amrita School of Engineering, Amrita
Vishwa Vidyapeetham, Chennai, India

## 5.1 INTRODUCTION

Magnesium is one of the elements that is found in high quantities in nature. Dolomite, magnesite, and kainite are examples of the types of minerals that contain this element, which accounts for 2.7% of the crust of the earth [1]. Pure Mg does not have very good mechanical properties, so alloying additives are used to improve their performance. The Mg alloys which have the most extensive application in industry are the ones in which aluminum is the primary additive and generally accounts for between 6% and 10% of the total. Both long-term implants (such as joint prostheses) and short-term implants (such as plates, bone screws), which are used in medical practice to stabilize broken bones, are produced from titanium alloys, cobalt alloys, or stainless steel. Long-term implants include joint prostheses and short-term implants include plates and bone screws. As long as protective layers – typically oxide – remain on the surface of the implant, medical professionals consider it to be inert – that is, harmless to the body – and so classify it as neutral. Eventually, corrosion and destruction to these layers allow implant components, which are often physiologically incompatible (toxic to the body), to get into the human body, where they can pose a serious risk to health and even life. Short-term orthopedic implants have traditionally been made of metal alloys, but resorbable biomaterials provide an alternative. Although many of the components that make up commercially accessible materials for industrial purposes are particularly harmful to the human body, the composition of the material under consideration is vital for biomedical applications. Hence, the material must not only possess the necessary mechanical qualities for a specific biomedical application, but it also needs to be biocompatible. Ideally, biodegradable biomedical equipment would be made from nontoxic or noncarcinogenic materials or alloys. In addition, the material must have either a dissolution rate that is adjustable or a corrosion rate that is slow enough to allow the biomedical device or implant to keep its mechanical integrity while the surrounding tissues recover and become capable of bearing the load. Once the healing process is complete, the biomedical implant load-bearing characteristics are no longer necessary, and the implant material can be allowed to disintegrate naturally. Additionally, the degradation process should produce nontoxic by-products that can be ingested, absorbed by nearby tissues, or dissolved and easily eliminated by the kidneys. Therefore, it is necessary to regulate the corrosion behavior of Mg and its alloys in the body fluid environment if they are to be used as an efficient biodegradable implant. In this chapter, we will discuss the function of magnesium within the body as well as its application in the medical field. It addresses the concept of Mg alloys, as well as prospective uses of Mg alloys, classification of Mg alloys as potential biomaterials according to the structure (amorphous, crystalline), and alloying elements of Mg alloys (rare earth elements, noble metals, etc.) in the medical field. This chapter also discusses the reasons behind the deterioration of Mg alloys and how they behave (in vitro) as a result of their structure. The effect of alloy additions (rare earth elements, noble metals), as well as protective coatings, on the process of Mg alloys degrading in vitro for use in biomedical applications has also been evaluated.

## 5.2  INFLUENCING FACTORS OF Mg ALLOYS PERFORMANCES IN BIOMEDICAL APPLICATIONS

Mg is considered a "life-sustaining" element due to its involvement in so many cellular reactions. In order for the human body to continue operating normally, homeostasis must be maintained. The average human body has 22–26 g of Mg, according to several sources [2]. Figure 5.1 depicts the influence parameters for Mg alloy corrosion. There are a number of parameters, such as (a) alloy composition, (b) surface morphology, (c) environmental medium, and (d) stress conditions, that can have an effect on the Mg alloy when it is being used in a biomedical application [3]. The most significant application of magnesium in the medical field is in the treatment of illnesses depicted in Figure 5.2 [4].

In particular, the use of suitable alloying elements can help to refine grains, optimize the type and size of the second phase, as well as optimize its distribution, which ultimately results in an increase in the corrosion resistance of Mg alloys. In addition, components have the ability to generate passive films or layers composed

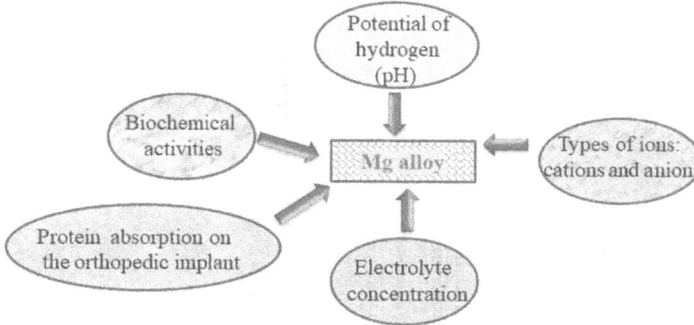

**FIGURE 5.1**   Influence parameters for magnesium alloy corrosion [3].

of corrosion products, which can stop the further spread of corrosion. Alloying elements that are often utilized nowadays include aluminum, zinc, manganese, calcium, strontium, zirconium, and neodymium. Table 5.1 illustrates how the presence of these components influences the performance of Mg alloys.

## 5.3   Mg ALLOYS IN MEDICINE: CONCEPT AND PRACTICAL APPLICATIONS

The development of both medical science and the engineering of materials lead to an increase in the number of research efforts focusing on developing novel biomaterials. In today's world, Mg alloys are seen to be prospective alternatives for use as resorbable metallic biomaterials. In addition, it is generally believed that a Mg alloy used as a resorbable biomaterial should progressively break down in the human body until the bone fuses. The use of implants developed in accordance with this approach eliminates the need for additional surgical procedures and enables the foreign substance (implant) to continue to be kept within the human body [7]. Table 5.2 provides a full explanation of the advantage and drawbacks associated with the use of Mg alloys in biomedical applications. Figure 5.3 depicts some of the possible applications of Mg alloys in the field of implantology [2].

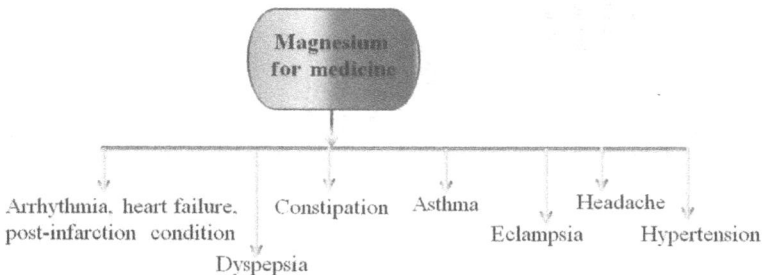

**FIGURE 5.2**   The most significant applications of magnesium in the medical field is in the treatment of illnesses.

**TABLE 5.1**

**The Influence of Alloying Element on the Properties of Mg Alloys**

| Alloying Elements | Biocompatibility | Corrosion Resistance | Mechanical Behavior |
|---|---|---|---|
| Aluminum | Due to its neurotoxicity, Al is considered of contributing to the development of Alzheimer's disease and can also generate muscle fiber damage | It has a positive impact on resistance to corrosion | The addition of Al enhances both the material's strength and its flexibility |
| Zinc | Zn is an essential nutrient that is essential for the human body; it is non-cytotoxic and has an excellent biocompatibility | It causes the corrosion resistance to decrease in proportion to the increasing amount of zinc concentration | Zn is mainly responsible for the role of strengthening the solid solution, and the strength increases with the increase in the Zn concentration |
| Manganese | The human body cannot function properly without manganese, which is a trace element. On the other hand, cytotoxicity and neurotoxicity both have been attributed to Mn | It helps to ensure that the corrosion resistance is maintained | It has a positive effect on yield strength while having a negative effect on tensile strength and elongation |
| Calcium | Ca is an essential component of human bone, and it does not have any harmful effects | The corrosion resistance will decrease in direct proportion to the amount of Ca present | Strength improves and plasticity decreases with increased Ca concentration |
| Strontium | Sr is an essential component of human bone and does not have any cytotoxic effects. It has the potential to encourage bone growth | It causes the corrosion resistance of Mg alloys to decrease in proportion to the amount of strontium present | A higher Sr concentration results in a more robust product |
| Zirconium | Zr has excellent biocompatibility and the potential to connect with bone | The corrosion resistance will decrease proportionately with the increasing Zr concentration | It improves the grain structure, resulting in greater strength and flexibility |
| Silicon | Si is a trace element that is necessary for the human body | It has a negative impact on the resistance to corrosion | A coarse $Mg_2Si$ phase is created, strength is increased, and plasticity is decreased |

*(Continued)*

**TABLE 5.1 (Continued)**
**The Influence of Alloying Element on the Properties of Mg Alloys**

| Alloying Elements | Biocompatibility | Corrosion Resistance | Mechanical Behavior |
|---|---|---|---|
| Lithium | Li might potentially lead to problems in human cardiovascular development | It reduces the material's resistance to corrosion | As the amount of Li added exceeds 5.5%, changes occur in the microstructure, the strength decreases, and the plasticity improves |
| Neodymium | At high concentrations, Nd is cytotoxic, but at low concentrations, it is somewhat biosafe | It enhances the corrosion resistance | It results in the formation of novel phases, the refinement of microstructure, and enhanced mechanical properties |
| Yttrium | Y has good biocompatibility | It enhances the resistance to corrosion | It enhances the strength and plasticity |
| Cerium | Ce is highly cytotoxic | It makes the corrosion resistance better, but a result in excessive makes the corrosion resistance worse | It makes the material stronger and less resistant to fatigue |
| Lanthanum | La is highly cytotoxic | It has an effect that makes the corrosion resistance stronger | It enhances the tensile strength as well as the creep resistance |
| Erbium | Er is cytotoxic | It has a positive effect on the resistance to corrosion | It increases both rigidity and malleability |
| Gadolinium | Gd is cytotoxic | It enhances corrosion resistance, which is something that suffers when there is a high Gd concentration | Strength is increased as a result of the strengthening of the solid solution |

*Sources*: Refs. [5, 6].

**TABLE 5.2**

**Advantages and Disadvantages of Mg Alloy for Biomedical Application**

| Advantages | Description |
|---|---|
| Low density and elastic modulus | Both the density and the elastic modulus are similar to those seen in cortical bone |
| High specific strength | Strength-to-weight ratio of around 35–260 kNm/kg should be expected |
| Stress shielding effect | Mg offers great machinability, dimensional stability, and ease of processing into complicated forms |
| Biocompatibility | Due to the fact that the elastic modulus of Mg is so similar to that of bone, the number of complications related with implant stress shielding can be drastically minimized |
| Degradability | Magnesium's biocompatibility and shown osteogenic functions make it a desirable supplement. |
| **Disadvantages** | |
| Low mechanical properties | In general, implants need to have the capacity to withstand a particular load while also resisting deformation. At the moment, the majority of magnesium alloys struggle to satisfy clinical requirements in terms of both their strength and their plasticity |
| High degradation rate | It is simple to induce early loss of mechanical integrity and support of implants, which restricts its utilization in clinical treatment, particularly in orthopedic load-bearing parts. This is especially true when it comes to load-bearing components |
| Hydrogen | The surrounding soft tissue becomes saturated with the hydrogen gas that is produced as magnesium degrades |

*Sources:* Refs. [6, 7].

The surface qualities of Mg alloys have been found to be improved by natural polymeric coatings combined with surface modification, creating a barrier that prevents corrosion from degrading. These breakthroughs have the potential to significantly improve the corrosion resistance, cell adhesion, proliferation, and biodegradability of Mg-based implants. The following types of coating method are discussed in detail.

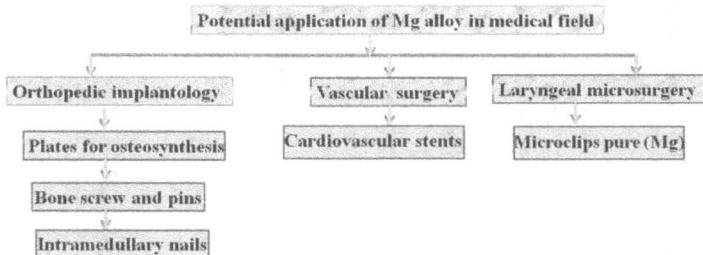

**FIGURE 5.3**   Applications of magnesium and alloys of magnesium in the field of implantology.

## 5.4  CLASSIFICATION OF COATINGS

Coatings can be manufactured on Mg alloys utilizing mechanical, physical, chemical, and biological methods.

1. Shot peening, friction, and attrition are methods that can be used to create mechanical coatings [7, 8].
2. The fabrication of physical coatings can be accomplished by processes such as magnetron sputtering, laser cladding, electron beam, and ion implant [9–12].
3. It is feasible to produce chemical coatings by the techniques of chemical conversion, electrodeposition, sol–gel, electroless plating, micro-arc oxidation (MAO) or plasma electrolyte oxidation (PEO), layer-by-layer assembly, and ionic liquid [13–18].
4. The use of biological approaches involves biomineralization and the identification of molecules.

In addition, surface coatings may be divided into two broad groups based on the mechanics of coating formation: chemical conversion coatings and deposited coatings. Surface coatings for Mg alloys may be divided into three categories: metallic, ceramic, and polymeric. These categories are determined by the chemical composition and atomic structure of the coatings, respectively. In addition, there are several types of coatings that may be applied to biomedical Mg alloys, and these coatings are classified according to the functions shown in Figure 5.4. Biofunctionalized coatings are one such example (i.e., drug-loading and antibacterial coatings). A self-cleaning coating, self-healing coating, or self-repairing coating is a type of highly hydrophobic coating, coatings that are selfless. Self-cleaning and self-healing coatings are classified as smart coatings [19–21].

### 5.4.1  PHYSICAL AND CHEMICAL VAPOR DEPOSITION COATING

A secondary layer on the substrate can also be created using deposition coating methods. The composition of such a layer may be easily modified to provide degradation

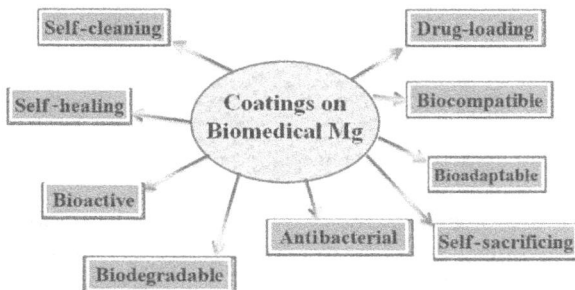

**FIGURE 5.4**  Coating on Mg alloys materials based on their functions.

resistance and improved tissue implant contact. Dip coating, spin coating, sol–gel coating, electrospinning, physical vapor deposition (PVD), chemical vapor deposition (CVD), and thermal spray coatings are among the deposition coatings described on Mg targeting for degradable implant applications. As a result of the well-known fact that the deposition thin-film coating process parameters have a major impact on the overall performance of the deposited films, several research work have made consistent attempts to use various optimization techniques [22, 23].

### 5.4.2 Chemical Conversion Coatings

The electrochemical or chemical reaction of Mg-based materials is what leads to the formation of chemical conversion coatings, which often consist of fluoride, phosphates, carbonate, and chromate. The chemical conversion treatment can result in the formation of an insoluble compound film on the surface of the magnesium, which has a good adhesion. This film can not only protect the Mg alloy from water and other corrosive environments, but it can also improve the adhesion of subsequent coatings.

### 5.4.3 Biomimetic Deposition

Biomimetic deposition is a method that was developed in recent years to simulate the process of physiological apatite mineralization that occurs in nature and to spontaneously deposit bioceramic membranes on the surface of substrates. This was accomplished through the use of a method known as biomimetic deposition. The benefits of the biomimetic approach may be divided into the following categories: first, the crystallinity, phase, and composition of the coating are all quite simple to alter; second, the approach may also be used to generate biomimetic apatite coatings on porous or complex-shaped implants; coprecipitation, as opposed to simple surface adsorption, is the preferred approach for integrating physiologically active chemicals or pharmaceuticals into apatite coatings since it is both easy and effective. As a result, biomimetic techniques have seen widespread use in the modification of metallic biomaterials.

### 5.4.4 MAO Coating

MAO is a high-voltage plasma-assisted anodic oxidation method that evolved from conventional anodizing to create ceramic-like coatings [24].

### 5.4.5 Sol–Gel Coating

The chemical solution deposition technique, more often known as the sol–gel method, has found a lot of usage in the disciplines of materials science and ceramic engineering. It is also known as the chemical solution deposition technique. The method is applied most commonly for the synthesis of materials, and it begins with a chemical solution that acts as the precursor for an integrated network (or gel) of either discrete particles or network polymers. This is the most common application of the method.

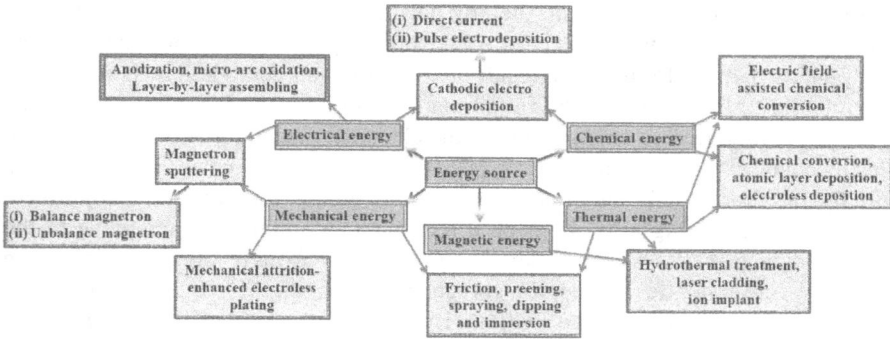

**FIGURE 5.5**   Surface coating techniques for biomedical Mg alloys, including an examination of their classifications and connections.

### 5.4.6   ION IMPLANTATION

Ion implantation is a method of surface modification that begins with the creation of target atoms into an ion beam inside of a vacuum. This step takes place at the beginning of the process. After this, the ions are sputtered onto the material that is being changed, and the process culminates in the development of a layer with a certain chemical composition and structural organization on the surface of the substrate.

Methods for preparing coatings using electricity (including metal-organic oxide, electrolytic deposition [ED], and layer-by-layer assembly [LBL]), chemistry (including chemical conversion and sol–gel), and heat, magnetism, and mechanical force (TMM) are all distinct categories (i.e., physical vapor deposition, friction, and peening). Figure 5.5 depicts the many classifications as well as the interconnections of surface coating processes used on biomedical Mg alloys [25].

## 5.5   EFFECT OF SURFACE COATING MODIFICATION ON BIOCOMPATIBILITY OF Mg ALLOY

The phrase "surface modification technology" refers to the process of creating protective coatings with a variety of functions on the surface of substrate materials using a variety of technological methods in order to accomplish the goal that is desired. This is a very important surface modification method that is used in surface engineering technology [26]. In order to slow down the process of Mg alloy deterioration and create a barrier, a coating treatment can be applied to the surface of the metal [27]. The biocompatibility of Mg alloy primarily indicates that Mg alloy, when used as a bone implant, will not bring any adverse effects to the body on the basis of successfully establishing connection and fixation, as well as preserving normal healing in the body. The Mg alloy used in the healing process must first demonstrate that it can support the fracture site and ensure the normal mending of bones before the fracture can be considered healed [28]. It is also important that Mg alloy corrode and degrade slowly enough in the human body. Excessive quickly will prevent the bone from healing in a reasonable amount of time, which will result in the therapy not being effective. If it is too sluggish, the patient's therapy will take an excessively lengthy amount of time, and the compounds that are formed as a result of corrosion and degradation should not be detrimental to the human body. Inflammation can be caused, for instance, when hydrogen is produced as a by-product of the chemical reaction that occurs when Mg electrochemical potential and electrolytes mix in an aqueous environment [29, 30]. Finally, in order to make sure that the most fundamental functions are maintained, the surface of the Mg alloy is given a treatment that makes it conducive to the development of cells, which makes the material even more biocompatible. The chemical conversion technique, the sol–gel approach, the MAO method, the electrodeposition method, and the hydrothermal treatment method are examples of common surface coating treatment procedures for metals.

## 5.6   EFFECT OF CHEMICAL TRANSFORMATION ON BIOCOMPATIBILITY

The chemical conversion method is a way of turning the surface of the material itself into a coating, which is part of the in situ development of the material and has strong coating adherence. This approach is also known as the chemical conversion technique [31]. During the conversion coating process, the substrate that needs to be protected is submerged in a solution that reacts with the surface. This causes the concentration of metal ions and the pH value of the interface of the metal solution to shift, resulting in the conversion of the substrate material itself into a different material and the formation of a coating that has strong adhesion [32]. The chemical conversion technique is a method that has convenient manufacturing, rapid reaction, a cheap initial investment, and the ability to adjust the production conditions. The surface of the material itself is converted into a coating, which gives the ceramic film a strong bonding force. Additionally, the ceramic film is capable of transforming one nanomaterial into another new nanostructure that is difficult to prepare directly, complex, and possesses properties that are not found elsewhere. As a result, there is a wide range of potential applications for this technology. The phrase "chemical conversion coating" can refer to a variety of different types of coatings, including "chromate coating," "phosphate coating," "fluorine-containing coating," and so on. In light of the fact that chromate will leach out of the coating and cause cancer, chemical conversion coatings concentrate mostly on phosphate coating and fluorine-containing coating.

## 5.7   EFFECT OF MAO ON BIOCOMPATIBILITY

A high-pressure plasma-assisted anodizing technique is referred to as MAO, plasma electrolytic oxidation (PEO), or micro-plasma oxidation (MPO) [33].The following are some of the benefits that come from using MAO: (1) enhanced micro-hardness, ranging from 1000 to 2000 HV and extending as high as 3000 HV, which is equivalent to the micro-hardness of cemented carbide; (2) excellent resistance to wear, which essentially makes up for the deficiencies of soft metal materials such as Mg alloy and Al alloy when used in applications.

## 5.8   EFFECT OF SOL–GEL METHOD ON BIOCOMPATIBILITY

The sol–gel technique is a process in which liquid compounds which include components that have a high level of chemical activity undergo a sequence of chemical reactions to produce gels, which are subsequently oxidized to form solids [34]. The sol–gel technique is a versatile technology with several advantages.

a. The dispersion of the raw materials in the solvent allows for a more thorough and uniform molecular mixing of the reactants. Gel may be formed in such a way that it uniformly coats whatever surface it is applied to, making it ideal for surfaces that are not perfectly smooth.

b. It is simple to incorporate some trace elements in a uniform and quantitative approach due to the process of solution reaction, which makes it possible to accomplish uniform doping at the molecular level.

c. The chemical reaction that occurs in solution is easy to carry out and requires a lower temperature throughout the synthesis process compared to the reaction that takes place in solid phase. It is widely accepted knowledge that the diffusion of components in a sol–gel system occurs in the nanoscale range, but in a solid-phase reaction, it occurs in the micrometer range; hence, the purity of the newly created coating is regarded to be higher. Altering the ratio of precursor to solvent, hydrolysis agent, curing temperature, hydrolysis rate, and deposition time can be used to produce effective coatings with better characteristics [35].

## 5.9   EFFECT OF THERMAL SPRAYING METHOD

The process of thermal spraying involves the use of high temperatures and high speeds in order to melt powder or metal wires, which are used as raw materials, and then deposit one substance on the surface of another material [36]. Thermal spraying can be subdivided into a variety of subcategories, such as flame thermal spraying, arc thermal spraying, plasma spraying, and so on, depending on the type of heat source that is being used. In the field of Mg alloy surface modification, plasma spraying, also known as PSP, is the technique that is used most frequently. Electric control power supplies, plc-based operator control stations, gas mass flow systems, closed-loop water cooling systems, powder feeders, and plasma torches all are part of a complete plasma spraying system. The following are special characteristics of the plasma spraying method:

- It is useful for melting a wide range of metals, ceramics, and composites [37, 38].
- The rate of deposition is quite high [39].
- The resultant coating is consistent and homogeneous [40].
- Depending on how different parameters are configured, the coating may be adjusted to provide the desired effect [41].

The particle velocity of plasma spraying is higher than that of flame spraying and arc spraying, which results in a coating that is denser and has a surface morphology that is finer. This is the most essential benefit of plasma spraying [42].

The most typical method for the manufacture of medicinal Mg alloy coating is spraying HA particles. By plasma spraying hydroxyapatite coating on the Mg alloy, Gao et al. were able to enhance the corrosion resistance and bioactivity of the material. During the past few years, as a result of the expansion of research, everyone has started to develop HA coating [43, 44]. Plasma spraying was used by Singh et al. [45] to effectively apply a coating of Ta/Ti on AZ31B magnesium alloy. This coating has a high level of hardness and a lower rate of wear. This behavior is attributed to the high passivation property of cold-sprayed Ta/Ti coatings and the rough surface (island shape) of these coatings, which can provide proper nucleation sites for the formation and growth of calcium phosphate compounds in Hanks solution, and the dense structure of Ta layer hinders the penetration of corrosive solution [44]. Mohajernia et al. developed a hydroxyapatite covering that included multi-walled carbon nanotubes in their formulation (MWCNTs). The high melting point of MWCNTs allowed them to remain intact during the plasma spraying process. This allowed them to function as a bridge between melted and semi-melted fragments, which improved the fracture toughness of the HAP coating [46].

## 5.10   CONCLUDING REMARK

Due to their biodegradability, good biocompatibility, and biomechanical compatibility, Mg alloys are considered to be a promising biodegradable implant material. The alloying components, chemical composition, and microstructure of Mg materials all have an impact in the alloy's ability to degrade. In most cases, the secondary or intermetallic phases possess a higher degree of purity than the Mg matrix. This might result in the formation of micro-galvanic cells between them. The existence of secondary or intermetallic phases can, depending on their distribution, size, and quantity, accelerate the overall corrosion of the material. As a result, chemical conversion coatings, MAO coatings, and other types of coatings have been applied in an effort to increase the corrosion resistance of Mg alloys. There are still a lot of obstacles to overcome in the process of developing innovative coatings for biomedical Mg alloys. It is possible that corrosion-resistant, self-degradable, biocompatible, and drug-loading properties would make the optimal coatings for biodegradable Mg alloys to be used in clinical applications. So far, it is extremely difficult to create coatings that possess all of the qualities that have been discussed up until this point. Particularly challenging for biodegradable magnesium alloys used as implant materials is the task of developing an effective regulated corrosion rate. Mg alloys are used in a variety of medical applications.

## DECLARATION OF COMPETING INTEREST

The authors have declared that they do not have any competing interests with regard to this study.

## REFERENCES

1. Braszczyńska-Malik, Katarzyna N. "Microstructure and mechanical properties of hybrid AZ91 magnesium matrix composite with Ti and SiC particles." *Materials* 15, no. 18 (2022): 6301.

2. Cesarz-Andraczke, Katarzyna, Aneta Kania, Katarzyna Młynarek, and Rafał Babilas. "Amorphous and crystalline magnesium alloys for biomedical applications." In *Magnesium alloys structure and properties*, pp. 1–21. IntechOpen, 2020.

3. Cuartas-Marulanda, Diego, Laura Forero Cardozo, Adriana Restrepo-Osorio, and Patricia Fernández-Morales. "Natural coatings and surface modifications on magnesium alloys for biomedical applications." *Polymers* 14, no. 23 (2022): 5297.

4. Reginster, Jean-Yves, L. Strause, Rita Deroisy, Marie Paule Lecart, Paul Saltman, and Purnelle Franchimont. "Preliminary report of decreased serum magnesium in post-menopausal osteoporosis." *Magnesium* 8, no. 2 (1989): 106–109.

5. Agarwal, Sankalp, James Curtin, Brendan Duffy, and Swarna Jaiswal. "Biodegradable magnesium alloys for orthopaedic applications: a review on corrosion, biocompatibility and surface modifications." *Materials Science and Engineering: C* 68 (2016): 948–963.

6. Zhang, Ting, Wen Wang, Jia Liu, Liqiang Wang, Yujin Tang, and Kuaishe Wang. "A review on magnesium alloys for biomedical applications." *Frontiers in Bioengineering and Biotechnology* 10 (2022): 953344.

7. Guerrera, Mary P., Stella Lucia Volpe, and Jun James Mao. "Therapeutic uses of magnesium." *American Family Physician* 80, no. 2 (2009): 157–162.

8. Mhaede, Mansour, Filip Pastorek, and Branislav Hadzima. "Influence of shot peening on corrosion properties of biocompatible magnesium alloy AZ31 coated by dicalcium phosphate dihydrate (DCPD)." *Materials Science and Engineering: C* 39 (2014): 330–335.

9. Xiong, Xiaoming, Yan Yang, Jinguang Li, Minmin Li, Jian Peng, Chen Wen, and Xiaodong Peng. "Research on the microstructure and properties of a multi-pass friction stir processed 6061Al coating for AZ31 Mg alloy." *Journal of Magnesium and Alloys* 7, no. 4 (2019): 696–706.

10. Zeng, Rong-Chang, Ke Jiang, Shuo-Qi Li, Fen Zhang, Hong-Zhi Cui, and En-Hou Han. "Mechanical and corrosion properties of Al/Ti film on magnesium alloy AZ31B." *Frontiers of Materials Science* 9 (2015): 66–76.

11. Guo, Yu, Yingqiao Zhang, Zhiyong Li, Shouzheng Wei, Tao Zhang, Liuqing Yang, and Shengyao Liu. "Microstructure and properties of in-situ synthesized ZrC-Al3Zr reinforced composite coating on AZ91D magnesium alloy by laser cladding." *Surface and Coatings Technology* 334 (2018): 471–478.

12. Gao, Yali, Cunshan Wang, Hongjie Pang, Hongbin Liu, and Man Yao. "Broad-beam laser cladding of Al-Cu alloy coating on AZ91HP magnesium alloy." *Applied Surface Science* 253, no. 11 (2007): 4917–4922.

13. Liu, Jiao, Yang Zheng, Yanze Bi, Yan Li, and Yufeng Zheng. "Improved cytocompatibility of Mg-1Ca alloy modified by Zn ion implantation and deposition." *Materials Letters* 205 (2017): 87–89.

14. Wang, Huanxin, Shaokang Guan, Yisheng Wang, Hongjian Liu, Haitao Wang, Liguo Wang, Chenxing Ren, Shijie Zhu, and Kuisheng Chen. "In vivo degradation behavior of Ca-deficient hydroxyapatite coated Mg-Zn-Ca alloy for bone implant application." *Colloids and Surfaces B: Biointerfaces* 88, no. 1 (2011): 254–259.

15. Zhang, Zhao-Qi, Rong-Chang Zeng, Wei Yan, Cun-Guo Lin, Li Wang, Zhen-Lin Wang, and Dong-Chu Chen. "Corrosion resistance of one-step superhydrophobic polypropylene coating on magnesium hydroxide-pretreated magnesium alloy AZ31." *Journal of Alloys and Compounds* 821 (2020): 153515.

16. Gao, Jia Hong, Xing Y. Shi, Bin Yang, Suh S. Hou, Eric C. Meng, Fang Xi Guan, and Su Kin Guan. "Fabrication and characterization of bioactive composite coatings on Mg-Zn-Ca alloy by MAO/sol–gel." *Journal of Materials Science: Materials in Medicine* 22, no. 7 (2011): 1681–1687.

17. Zuleta, Alejandro A., Esteban Correa, Juan Guillermo Castaño, Felix Echeverría, Wanda A. Baron-Wiecheć, Peter Skeldon, and George E. Thompson. "Study of the formation of alkaline electroless Ni-P coating on magnesium and AZ31B magnesium alloy." *Surface and Coatings Technology* 321 (2017): 309–320.

18. White, Leon, Youngmi Koo, Sudheer Neralla, Jagannathan Sankar, and Yeoheung Yun. "Enhanced mechanical properties and increased corrosion resistance of a biodegradable magnesium alloy by plasma electrolytic oxidation (PEO)." *Materials Science and Engineering: B* 208 (2016): 39–46.

19. Kim, Seo-Young, Yu-Kyoung Kim, Kyung-Seon Kim, Kwang-Bok Lee, and Min-Ho Lee. "Enhancement of bone formation on LBL-coated Mg alloy depending on the different concentration of BMP-2." *Colloids and Surfaces B: Biointerfaces* 173 (2019): 437–446.

20. Ji, Xiao-Jing, Qiang Cheng, Jing Wang, Yan-Bin Zhao, Zhuang-Zhuang Han, Fen Zhang, Shuo-Qi Li, Rong-Chang Zeng, and Zhen-Lin Wang. "Corrosion resistance and antibacterial effects of hydroxyapatite coating induced by polyacrylic acid and gentamicin sulfate on magnesium alloy." *Frontiers of Materials Science* 13 (2019): 87–98.

21. Shanaghi, Ali, Ali Reza Souri, Babak Mehrjou, and Paul K. Chu. "Corrosion resistance, nano-mechanical properties, and biocompatibility of Mg-plasma-implanted and plasma-etched Ta/TaN hierarchical multilayered coatings on the nitrided AZ91 Mg alloy." *Biomedical Materials* 16, no. 4 (2021): 045028.

22. Vikram, Kamlendra, Kanak Kalita, and Ranjan Kumar Ghadai. "Multi-attribute optimization of diamond-like carbon thin films." *AIP Conference Proceedings* 2273, no. 1 (AIP Publishing, 2020):040010.

23. Vikram, Kamlendra, Uvaraja Ragavendran, Kanak Kalita, Ranjan Kumar Ghadai, and Xiao-Zhi Gao. "Hybrid metamodel-NSGA-III-EDAS based optimal design of thin film coatings." *Computers, Materials\& Continua* 66, no. 2 (2021): 1771–1784.

24. Chen, Quanzhi, Weizhou Li, Kui Ling, and Ruixia Yang. "Effect of $Na_2WO_4$ addition on formation mechanism and microstructure of micro-arc oxidation coating on Al-Ti double-layer composite plate." *Materials & Design* 190 (2020): 108558.

25. Yin, Zheng-Zheng, Wei-Chen Qi, Rong-Chang Zeng, Xiao-Bo Chen, Chang-Dong Gu, Shao-Kang Guan, and Yu-Feng Zheng. "Advances in coatings on biodegradable magnesium alloys." *Journal of Magnesium and Alloys* 8, no. 1 (2020): 42–65.

26. Zhao, Yanbin, Xueyang Chen, Shuoqi Li, Rongchang Zeng, Fen Zhang, Zhenlin Wang, and Shaokang Guan. "Corrosion resistance and drug release profile of gentamicin-loaded polyelectrolyte multilayers on magnesium alloys: effects of heat treatment." *Journal of Colloid and Interface Science* 547 (2019): 309–317.

27. Surmeneva, Maria A., Anna A. Ivanova, Qiaomu Tian, Rebekah Pittman, Wensen Jiang, Jiajia Lin, Huinan H. Liu, and Roman A. Surmenev. "Bone marrow derived mesenchymal stem cell response to the RF magnetron sputter deposited hydroxyapatite coating on AZ91 magnesium alloy." *Materials Chemistry and Physics* 221 (2019): 89–98.

28. Surmeneva, Maria A., Timur M. Mukhametkaliyev, Hadis Khakbaz, Roman A. Surmenev, and M. Bobby Kannan. "Ultrathin film coating of hydroxyapatite (HA) on a magnesium–calcium alloy using RF magnetron sputtering for bioimplant applications." *Materials Letters* 152 (2015): 280–282.

29. Tian, Li, Ning Tang, To Ngai, Chi Wu, Yechun Ruan, Le Huang, and Ling Qin. "Hybrid fracture fixation systems developed for orthopaedic applications: a general review." *Journal of Orthopaedic Translation* 16 (2019): 1–13.

30. Chandra, Girish, and Ajay Pandey. "Biodegradable bone implants in orthopedic applications: a review." *Biocybernetics and Biomedical Engineering* 40, no. 2 (2020): 596–610.

31. Wan, Peng, Lili Tan, and Ke Yang. "Surface modification on biodegradable magnesium alloys as orthopedic implant materials to improve the bio-adaptability: a review." *Journal of Materials Science & Technology* 32, no. 9 (2016): 827–834.

32. Hornberger, Helga, Sannakaisa Virtanen, and Aldo R. Boccaccini. "Biomedical coatings on magnesium alloys: a review." *Acta Biomaterialia* 8, no. 7 (2012): 2442–2455.

33. Chen, Xiao Bo, Nick Birbilis, and Trevor B. Abbott. "Review of corrosion-resistant conversion coatings for magnesium and its alloys." *Corrosion* 67, no. 3 (2011): 035005-1.
34. Zhu, Yuanyuan, Weidong Gao, Huade Huang, Wenhui Chang, Shufang Zhang, Rongfa Zhang, Rongfang Zhao, and Yijia Zhang. "Investigation of corrosion resistance and formation mechanism of calcium-containing coatings on AZ31B magnesium alloy." *Applied Surface Science* 487 (2019): 581–592.
35. Talha, Mohd, Yucong Ma, Mingjie Xu, Qi Wang, Yuanhua Lin, and Xiangwei Kong. "Recent advancements in corrosion protection of magnesium alloys by silane-based sol–gel coatings." *Industrial & Engineering Chemistry Research* 59, no. 45 (2020): 19840–19857.
36. Qiu, Zhaozhong, Bo Yin, Jianyong Wang, Jia Sun, Yunxiang Tong, Li, and Rui Wang. "Theoretical and experimental studies of sol–gel electrodeposition on magnesium alloy." *Surface and Interface Analysis* 53, no. 4 (2021): 432–439.
37. Berndt, C. C., Fahad Hasan, U. Tietz, and K-P Schmitz. "A review of hydroxyapatite coatings manufactured by thermal spray." In Advances in *calcium phosphate biomaterials*, pp. 267–329. Springer, 2014.
38. Bansal, Puneet, Gurpreet Singh, and Hazoor Singh Sidhu. "Investigation of surface properties and corrosion behavior of plasma sprayed HA/ZnO coatings prepared on AZ31 Mg alloy." *Surface and Coatings Technology* 401 (2020): 126241.
39. Mardali, Marzieh, Hamidreza SalimiJazi, Fathallah Karimzadeh, Berengere Luthringer, Carsten Blawert, and Sheyda Labbaf. "Comparative study on microstructure and corrosion behavior of nanostructured hydroxyapatite coatings deposited by high velocity oxygen fuel and flame spraying on AZ61 magnesium-based substrates." *Applied Surface Science* 465 (2019): 614–624.
40. Yao, Hai-Long, Xiao-Zhen Hu, Hong-Tao Wang, Qing-Yu Chen, Xiao-Bo Bai, Meng-Xian Zhang, and Gang-Chang Ji. "Microstructure and corrosion behavior of thermal-sprayed hydroxyapatite/magnesium composite coating on the surface of AZ91D magnesium alloy." *Journal of Thermal Spray Technology* 28 (2019): 495–503.
41. Daroonparvar, Mohammadreza, MU Farooq Khan, Y. Saadeh, Charles, M. Kay, R. K. Gupta, Ashish Kumar Kasar, Pankaj Kumar, Manoranjan Misra, Pradeep L. Menezes, Hamid Reza, and Bakhsheshi-Rad. "Enhanced corrosion resistance and surface bioactivity of AZ31B Mg alloy by high pressure cold sprayed monolayer Ti and bilayer Ta/Ti coatings in simulated body fluid." *Materials Chemistry and Physics* 256 (2020): 123627.
42. Wang, Qiang, Qi Sun, Ming-Xing Zhang, Wen-Juan Niu, Chang-Bin Tang, Kuai-She Wang, Xing Rui, Le Zhai, and Lu Wang. "The influence of cold and detonation thermal spraying processes on the microstructure and properties of Al-based composite coatings on Mg Alloy." *Surface and Coatings Technology* 352 (2018): 627–633.
43. García-Rodríguez, Sonia, Antonio Julio López, Victoria Bonache, Belén Torres, and Joaquín Rams. "Fabrication, wear, and corrosion resistance of HVOF sprayed WC-12Co on ZE41 magnesium alloy." *Coatings* 10, no. 5 (2020): 502.
44. Gao, Ya Li, Yu Liu, and Xue Ying Song. "Plasma-sprayed hydroxyapatite coating for improved corrosion resistance and bioactivity of magnesium alloy." *Journal of Thermal Spray Technology* 27 (2018): 1381–1387.
45. Singh, Balraj, Gurpreet Singh, and Buta Singh Sidhu. "Analysis of corrosion behaviour and surface properties of plasma-sprayed composite coating of hydroxyapatite–tantalum on biodegradable Mg alloy ZK60." *Journal of Composite Materials* 53, no. 19 (2019): 2661–2673.
46. Mohajernia, Shiva, Sadegh Pour-Ali, Seyedsina Hejazi, Mohsen Saremi, and Ali-Reza Kiani-Rashid. "Hydroxyapatite coating containing multi-walled carbon nanotubes on AZ31 magnesium: mechanical-electrochemical degradation in a physiological environment." *Ceramics International* 44, no. 7 (2018): 8297–8305.

# 6 Surface Modification of Mg Alloys
## An Insight into Friction Stir–Based Techniques

Sufian Raja
University of Malaya, Kuala Lumpur, Malaysia

Farazila Yusof
University of Malaya, Kuala Lumpur, Malaysia
and
Centre of Advanced Manufacturing and Material Processing
(AMMP Centre), University of Malaya, Kuala Lumpur, Malaysia
and
Centre for Foundation Studies in Science,
University of Malaya, Kuala Lumpur, Malaysia

Ridha bin Muhamad
Centre of Advanced Manufacturing and Material Processing
(AMMP Centre), University of Malaya, Kuala Lumpur, Malaysia

Mohd Fadzil Jamaludin
Centre of Advanced Manufacturing and Material
Processing (AMMP Centre), University of Malaya,
Kuala Lumpur, Malaysia

Md. F. Khan
College of Engineering, King Faisal University,
Al-Ahsa, Saudi Arabia

Mohd Bilal Naim Shaikh and Sajjad Arif
ZHCET, Aligarh Muslim University, Uttar Pradesh, India

Mohammad Azad Alam
Universiti Teknologi PETRONAS, Seri Iskandar, Malaysia

DOI: 10.1201/9781003400462-6

## 6.1  INTRODUCTION

When humans have biological structures that have been damaged or lost, biomedical components made of materials that are synthetic or natural are routinely implanted as replacements to enhance the overall quality of life of the patient. These biomedical components may be manufactured from a variety of materials. People who are older have a higher risk of developing conditions such as joint discomfort and arthritis, which has led to an increase in the need for medical devices fabricated from biomaterials that can substitute malfunctioning tissues (Navarro et al. 2008). Because of this, a lot of attention has been paid to materials that have biological functioning during the last several years. Depending on the particular use, biomaterials may be placed in many sections of the human body (Barba, Alabort, and Reed 2019; Martinez-Marquez et al. 2020; Dobrzański, Dobrzańska-Danikiewicz, and Dobrzański 2021). Reports indicate that orthopaedic procedures have contributed significantly to the fast growth of the prosthetics industry (H. Singh, Singh, and Prakash 2019). As a result, biomedical implants that are used need to possess a variety of trustworthy features, including appropriate mechanical, corrosion, tribological, and osseointegration characteristics (H. Singh, Singh, and Prakash 2019).

Researchers have created a wide range of metal-based and polymer-based biomaterials for application in orthopaedics purposes, including scaffolding, hard tissue implantation, and stents (Wang et al. 2016; Sezer et al. 2018; Yuan, Zhu, and Chung 2018; Warburton et al. 2020). To date, the metal-based biomaterial implant that has seen the most widespread use is magnesium and its alloys, titanium and its alloys, and stainless steel chromium-based alloys (Hu et al. 2014; Chen and Thouas 2015). Additive manufacturing techniques, friction stir–based procedures, arc melting, and powder metallurgy are only some of the manufacturing methods that have been used in the fabrication of biomedical materials (M. Zhu et al. 2017; Ho et al. 2020; Prakash, Singh, and Ramakrishna 2020; Prakash et al. 2020).

Processing biomedical materials is a challenging endeavour as it requires not solely the maintaining of the material's mechanical characteristics but additionally the retention of the material's unique biological features. Therefore, friction-based approaches are potential strategies for the development of biomaterials with increased characteristics (T et al. 2018; Mani Prabu et al. 2019; Perumal, Grewal, and Arora 2020). The regulation of biomedical materials manufacturing involves the utilisation of heat and pressure in conjunction with friction stir–based methodologies, which are classified as solid-state methods (Raja et al. 2020; Muhamad et al. 2021; Raja et al. 2022; bin Ariffin et al. 2022). Friction stir–based approaches operate through severe plastic deformation, resulting in the refinement of the grain shape of the prepared materials. The components with fine grains typically demonstrate enhanced mechanical properties, elevated tribocorrosion characteristics, and superior biocompatibility in comparison to components with coarse grains. Materials with fine grains, especially those combined with nanograins, exhibit a reduced number of atomic particles per grain, leading to an increased number of atoms and, consequently, elevated surface energy. Consequently, the cells of bone exhibit a greater tendency to attach to the outermost layer of said materials, thereby leading to a heightened level of osseointegration. Moreover, prior studies have demonstrated that these surfaces impede the attachment of bacteria, resulting in a decrease in the formation of biofilms. The significant impact of the refinement of grains has led to an increasing interest in friction stir–based techniques. Friction stir processing (FSP) is a technique utilised for the purpose of refining the size of the grains of materials. This technique involves rotating tools containing a shoulder and pin. With regard to this discovery, scholars have ascertained that the utilisation of FSP could potentially facilitate the enhancement of the refinement of grains as well as the microstructural characteristics of the material (Misra et al. 2009; Bagherifard et al. 2014; Thangaraj et al. 2015; Yamani et al. 2022).

Magnesium is a type of biomedical material that has been found to have advantages over currently utilised biomaterial. Specifically, Mg has been shown to prevent the need for secondary surgical procedures after wounds have healed completely and to alleviate patient discomfort. The biological significance of Mg, including its ability to enhance bone formation, facilitate vascular development, and promote the healing of wounds, has been scientifically demonstrated (Zhang et al. 2018). Mg has the ability to biodegrade in vivo, thereby imparting structural integrity. The corroded outermost layer of magnesium-based implants has been found to be toxic-free, making it suitable for temporary tissue functions. Moreover, in light of prior affirmative findings, biomaterials containing Mg have the potential to stimulate the regeneration of fresh bone tissue, thereby facilitating the mending of bone fractures. The experimental results indicate that AZ91 alloy exhibits remarkable resistance to corrosion and biocompatibility in vivo. The adoption of microstructure modification via FSP presents a viable means of enhancing the ability to resist corrosion of AZ91, as it does not involve the introduction or disintegration of new phase materials into the alloy's matrix (R. V. Vignesh, Padmanaban, and Govindaraju 2019). AZ31B alloy, which was manufactured by FSAM utilising hydroxyapatite, is an appropriate alternative for real bone owing to its improved strength and greater biocorrosion resistance, both of which are due to the result of grain size reduction (Ho et al. 2020).

The utilisation of friction stir–based methodologies has witnessed a surge in popularity owing to their eco-friendly attributes and superior efficacy in producing robust products. The lack of comprehensive research on the application of friction stir–based approaches to enhance various characteristics, particularly those composed of magnesium and utilised in biomedical applications, presents a significant challenge. Hence, it is imperative to acquire a comprehensive understanding of the utilisation of friction stir–based techniques in biomedical domains concerning magnesium and its alloys. This chapter has been assembled based on an extensive analysis of various published articles. This chapter aims to delineate diverse aspects of friction-based biological purposes and compare them within the field.

## 6.2   FSP: A PROMISING FRICTION STIR–BASED TECHNIQUE FOR SURFACE MODIFICATION OF Mg IMPLANTS

Following the breakthroughs of the FSW, researchers modified this method in order to change the surface of the primary materials by introducing severe plastic deformation mechanisms at the outermost surface, as seen in Figure 6.1(a) (Mishra et al. 1999; Vaira Vignesh et al. 2019). When compared to more traditional methods of

SPD, such as HPT and ECAP, it was shown that this method might produce super-plasticity at higher strain rates while maintaining the temperature at which it occurs (Harwani et al. 2021; Mirzadeh 2021). The characteristics of superplastic development in other processes, including the ability to produce a near-net structure without intermediary phases, are limited, which results in a greater amount of time needed for the operation. In addition to this, FSP may be used especially to change the outermost layer of the base material, thereby improving the surface qualities that are needed for a wide variety of applications, including those involving biological implants and equipment (Zhu et al. 2016). It has been discovered that following FSP, the size of the grains becomes significantly smaller as well as more homogenised than it was in the base material. For instance, the size of the grains of base AZ31 was found to be anywhere between 0.2 μm and 53.5 μm, having an average dimension of 10 μm. On the other hand, the grain that was the size of the same AZ31 material

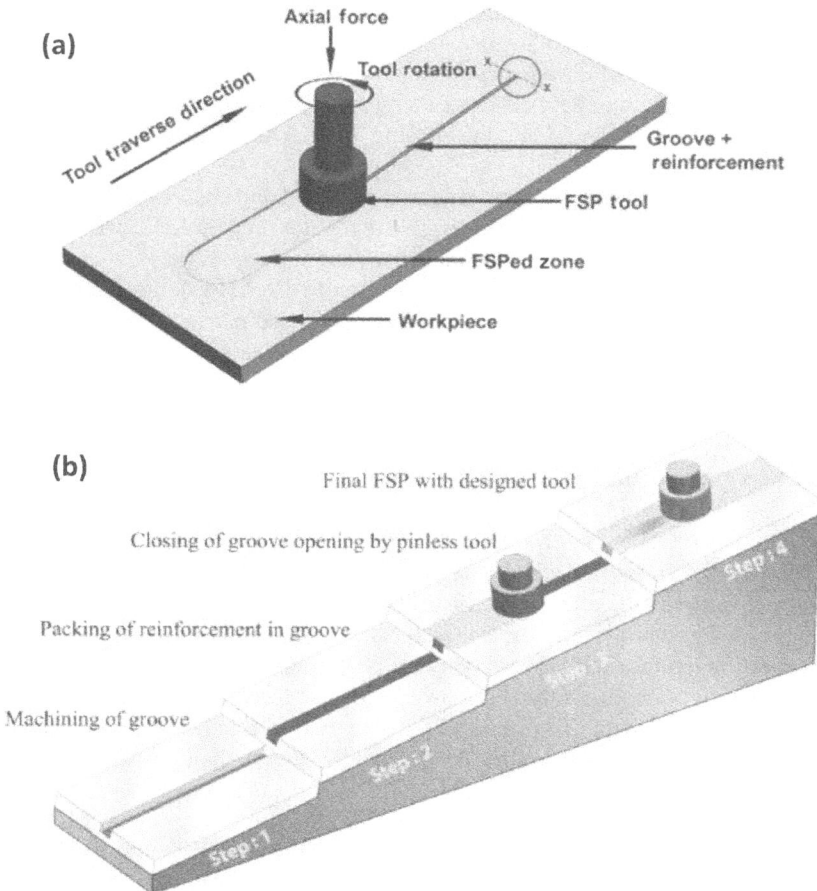

FIGURE 6.1    (a) Illustration of FSP (Vaira Vignesh et al. 2019). (b) Introduction of the additives by using grooves during FSP (Rathee et al. 2018).

following FSP was anywhere between 0.1 μm and 15 μm, having an average dimension of 4.0 μm (Qiao et al. 2021).

Introducing reinforcement materials onto the outermost layer of the base material may result in an additional specific improvement to the surface characteristics of the material. In general, there are three ways that reinforcement particles may be incorporated into the base material. These techniques are (i) coating with epoxy that contains reinforcing particles; (ii) making grooves at the base materials; and (iii) drilling numerous holes on the outermost layer and then filling the grooves and holes with reinforcing particles, as depicted in Figure 6.1(b) (Zhu et al. 2016; Rathee et al. 2018; Rana and Badheka 2019; Almasi et al. 2020).

In FSP, a rotating tool is introduced into the material being processed. This causes materials in the area of the processing zone to be stirred and generates intense heat as a result of the frictional force. As a direct consequence of this, an SPD takes place, and the base material grains are modified into finer sizes (Rana and Badheka 2019; Mirzadeh 2021). Four unique areas – SZ, TMAZ, HAZ, and base material – can be seen owing to the thermal and strain energies in the zone, which resemble grain morphologies found in the FSWed specimen. The mechanical characteristics exhibited by composites, including hardness and strength, are improved due to the diminutive sized grains present in the SZ and the ensuing restriction on atomic motion provided by its reinforcement.

To attain optimal reinforcement materials dispersal and ensure favourable performance of processed material, it is imperative to regulate and optimise various parameters throughout the process. Although an increase in the number of passes may lead to longer processing times, multiple welding tool runs have demonstrated greater efficacy in generating more widely dispersed reinforced particles and finer-grained structures, ultimately resulting in improved material characteristics (Navazani and Dehghani 2016; Orozco-Caballero et al. 2017).

Extensive research has been conducted on using FSP in biomedical fields, with a particular emphasis on improving its biofunctional and mechanical characteristics. While maximising strength is typically a desirable goal for numerous purposes, the biomedical field requires properties that closely correspond to those of the body's organ in concern. The modulus of elasticity intended for application in the implanting bone should closely match that of natural bone cellular tissue. Failure to do so may result in stress shielding, which is the non-uniform transfer of stress generated by the implantation device to the bones. This can ultimately result in implant loosening, bone fractures, and bone atrophy (Niinomi and Nakai 2011; Ho et al. 2020). Several materials are currently being investigated as substrates for biomedical uses. These materials are depicted in Figure 6.2. The research indicates that magnesium alloys receive significant attention from scholars due to their distinctive material characteristics, including biodegradability. Conversely, titanium alloys have become recognised for their exceptional mechanical strength and low weight. In addition, polymers have garnered attention in recent times because of their versatility during manufacturing, which facilitates the improvements of particular characteristics, including mechanical integrity and biodegradability (Amirtharaj Mosas et al. 2022; Moghadasi et al. 2022; Wang et al. 2022). The implementation of FSP enables additional improvement of surface properties on said materials, including but not limited to enhanced bioactivity and resistance to wear.

## MATERIALS

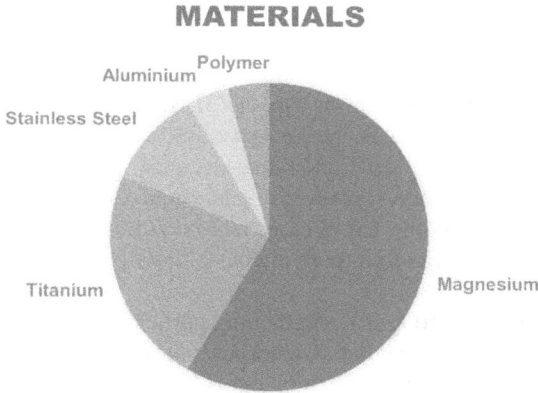

**FIGURE 6.2** Application of FSP in various materials for biomedical implant.

### 6.2.1 Effect of FSP on Mechanical and Tribological Properties

Magnesium is widely recognised for its exceptional biodegradability, rendering it a viable option for targeted applications within the human body where implant degradation is desirable, obviating the need for subsequent surgical intervention for removal (Ho et al. 2020). The resistance to corrosion exhibited by magnesium and its associated alloys in biological settings is notably inadequate. Consequently, the majority of research endeavours have centred on the incorporation of materials for reinforcement as a means of enhancing characteristics.

Several research investigations have explored the utilisation of toughness and high-strength ceramics such as $ZrO_2$. The study investigated the impact of the number of passes on the microstructural characteristics during the processing of AZ31 alloy using $ZrO_2$ particles with a range of sizes of 30–40 nm. Distinct SZ, TMAZ, HAZ, and BM regions were discernible based on grain morphology (Mazaheri et al. 2020). When compared to the BM, which had an average size of grains of 10.7 m, the result of increasing the number of FSP passes is also apparent in the size of the grain, which was reported to be 4.1 m with a single pass and further decreased to 2.1 m with four passes.

The aforementioned ceramic materials $ZrO_2$ were evaluated using three distinct volume fractions as follows: 2.14%, 4.29%, and 6.43%. It was found that the strength improves with a more significant $ZrO_2$ content in the base AZ31, and reported as 234 MPa, 258 MPa, and 262 MPa, respectively. The researcher discovered that additional FSP passes might be conducted in order to attain greater strength using the same set-up for experimentation (Zang et al. 2020). Navazani and Dehghani (2016) experimented with blended reinforcing particles comprising $Y_2O_3$ and $ZrO_2$, having a mean particle size of 40 nm, and producing a similar effect. It was discovered that the four-pass FSP has the ability to attain superior surface micro-hardness. This is in comparison to single-pass FSP, which can attain 310 MPa in terms of strength, while four-pass FSP can reach 340 MPa. This may be understood by referring to the microstructure specifically how a more refined size of grains increases the imped-ance of the dislocation movement. In addition to this, increasing the number of times the FSP is run leads to an improved particle distribution and prevents agglomeration.

Research on tribological characteristics has been carried out to explore the correlation between the sliding distance and the decrease in mass under stability force and sliding speed. The findings indicate that the base AZ31 incurred the most significant loss of mass subsequent to the FSP of base AZ31, single-pass FSPed specimen. The lowest mass loss was observed in the four-pass FSPed specimen. The rate of wear, defined as the total mass lost per unit sliding distance, was found to be the least in the four-pass FSPed workpiece, recording a value approximately 50% lower than that of the base AZ31. This finding has demonstrated that improved wear behaviour can be achieved using finer grains and more effective alloying elements in base materials (Mazaheri et al. 2020).

In addition to utilising $ZrO_2$ as strengthening particles for Mg materials, researchers have also explored the potential of incorporating more prevalent elements found within the human body, including calcium and HA. Upon application of calcium onto the ZE41 alloy surface, Ca particle consolidation was observed within the processes zone. This study has revealed an upsurge in the mechanical characteristics, specifically hardness, up to 73.70 HV from 60.98 HV, as well as an improvement in the corrosion behaviour of ZE41 following processing, in comparison to its unprocessed ZE41 Mg alloy (Vasu et al. 2019). Numerous investigations have been conducted on the incorporation of HA onto Mg alloys substrate, owing to the material's bioactivity and biocompatibility, which are properties that are inherent to teeth and bone tissues. According to investigations, the composite's hardness has been found to rise as a result of the refinement of grains and intensified movement of dislocations due to the inclusion of secondary phase particles. Additionally, exhibiting greater strength compared to the base substrate, HA's surface agglomeration was marginally diminished in the FSPed Mg alloys. Furthermore, the resistance to corrosion and biocompatibility exhibited substantial improvements due to the inclusion of HA (Sodhi and Singh 2018; Cao et al. 2019).

The dominant factors influencing the wearing mechanisms of Mg alloys subjected to FSP are its working conditions. Bhadouria et al. (2017) conducted FSP on

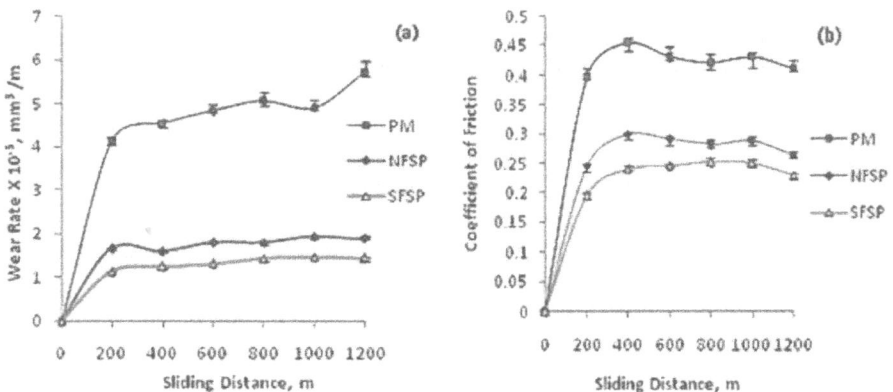

FIGURE 6.3    (a) Wear rate comparison of parent metal (PM) and conventional FSPed (denoted by NFSPed abbreviation) and SFSPed workpieces. (b) Friction coefficient (Bhadouria et al. 2017).

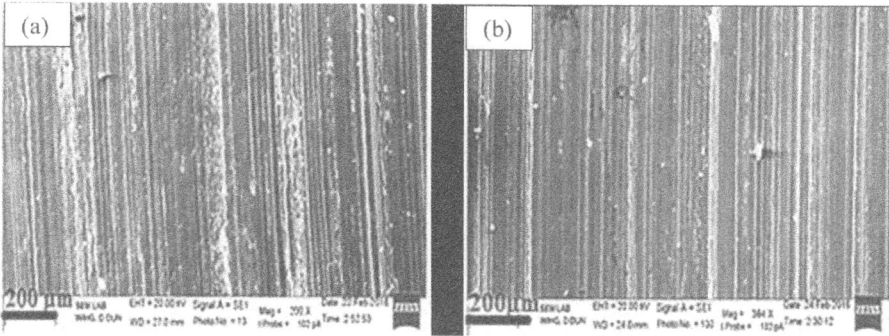

**FIGURE 6.4**  SEM image of the worn surfaces of the (a) base AZ91 and (b) SFSPed workpiece (Bhadouria et al. 2017).

AZ91 in two distinct settings: conventional FSP and SFSP. The graphical representation in Figure 6.3 illustrates the relationship between the rate at which wear occurs and the friction coefficient concerning the sliding distance. The results indicate that the rate of wear and friction coefficient are notably reduced for the FSP conducted under NFSP. The study found that as the sliding distance increased, the rate of wear in the base AZ91 exhibited corresponding increases as well. However, in the case of conventional FSP and SFSP specimens, there was no notable enhancement observed in the rate of wear.

The scanning electron microscopy (SEM) of the worn facet of the base AZ91 and submerged friction stir processed workpiece is depicted in Figure 6.4. The base AZ91 exhibits tracks that are comparatively broader and more pronounced when contrasted with those of the SFSPed sample.

The findings depicted in Figure 6.5 demonstrate that an oxide layer has developed on the base material in the SFSP workpiece. This is supported by the results of the EDS examination, which indicate the existence of both iron and oxide. The formation

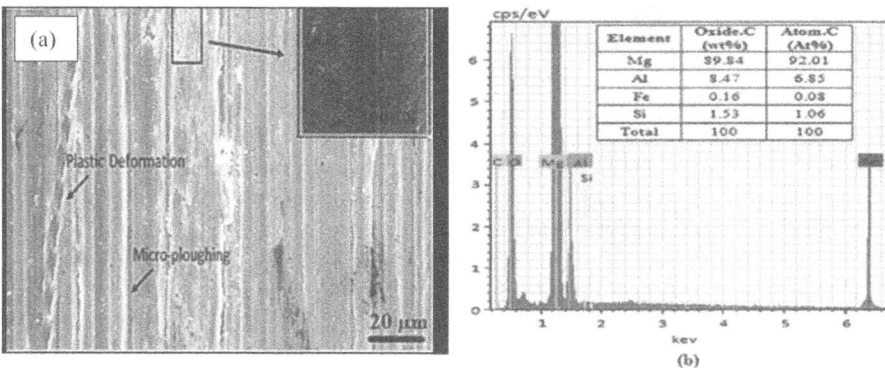

**FIGURE 6.5**  (a) SEM images of the worn surfaces at higher magnification. (b) SFSPed workpiece EDS (Bhadouria et al. 2017).

of a stable oxide layer throughout the process of SFSP results in an enhancement of resistance to wear, leading to a reduction in the rate of wear. The results indicate that the influence of the ambient liquid while performing FSP is noteworthy.

Asadi et al. (2012) conducted a study on applying underwater FSP. The results indicated that this method led to a surge in the oxide particles within the FSPed region. Additionally, the cooling action of the water resulted in a reduction in the resulting size of the grains, which in turn enhanced the material's hardness and decreased its frictional coefficient. The average grain size was decreased from 150 μm to 4 μm by altering the direction of tool rotation following each successive pass.

Likewise, Iwaszko and Kudła (2021) used jet-cooled nozzles to execute FSP on the AZ91 in order to cool down the FSPed region. The base AZ91, the conventionally cooled FSPed workpiece, as well as the jet of air-cooled FSPed workpieces underwent tribological testing. The findings showed that the FSPed workpiece's resistance to wear rose while its coefficient of friction dropped. These may be ascribed to a rise in AZ91 hardness in the stirring region as an outcome of the thorough grain refining, which reduces the surface area that comes into contact with the counterpart sample. It is important to note that the resulting frictional coefficient for the jet of air-cooled friction stir processed workpiece was 0.72, the frictional coefficient for the conventionally cooled FSPed workpiece was 0.76, and the frictional coefficient for the base AZ91 was 0.78. According to Figure 6.6, the FSPed workpiece cooled with a jet of air has a little lesser frictional coefficient than the conventionally cooled FSPed workpiece, which is explained by its higher refinement of the grains.

Arora et al. (2012) conducted FSP to produce a surface composite consisting of AZ31 as substrate and TiC as reinforcement. The results of the EDS investigation of the FSPed workpiece revealed the existence of particles of TiC of small size all over the surface. Additionally, the reduced size of the grains was achieved through the FSP, which resulted in an improved hardness of the AZ31 in the stirred zone. Consequently, the ability to withstand the wear of the FSPed workpiece was enhanced in comparison to the base AZ31.

The shape and size of the FSP tool is an additional feature that has a role in determining the tribological characteristics of the FSPed workpiece. FSP was done on the AZ31B using an SST and a CST at three different tool rotational speeds and three different tool traverse speeds. The workpiece that was processed by the SST seems to have far less wear loss, as is evident from close inspection. When the tool traverse speed is set to 14 mm/min, with 1000 rpm tool rotational speed, the wear loss is at its lowest. According to the findings, using an SST with a slow traverse speed and a fast rotating speed results in more refined grains, which in turn enhances the workpiece's resistance to wear and raises its level of hardness. The SST has an exceptionally small size of grains when the tool rotational speed is set to 1000 rpm, and the traverse speed is set to 14 mm/min (Balamurugan and Mahadevan 2013).

Magnesium alloys have been the subject of several investigations in the present day for FSP, emphasising microstructural characteristics, parameters, mechanical characteristics, etc., and their potential uses are expanding rapidly. FSP is generally believed to be among the most efficient methods for modifying a material's surface characteristics, so Mg and its alloys may be employed in biomedical uses. It is anticipated that a greater variety of combinations of materials will be accessible

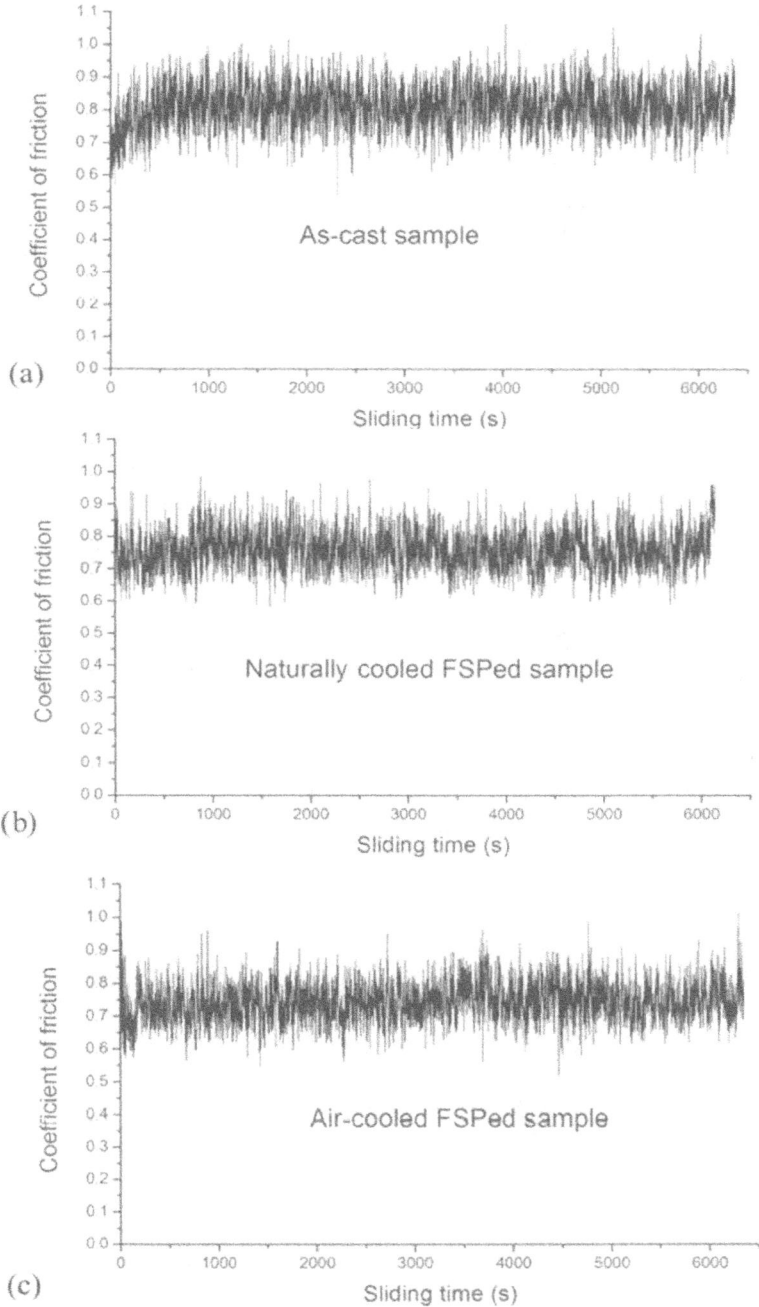

(a)

(b)

(c)

**FIGURE 6.6**  Plot of frictional coefficient of (a) base AZ91 Mg alloy, (b) conventionally cooled friction stir processed workpiece, (c) air jet–cooled friction stir processed workpiece (Iwaszko and Kudła 2021).

as a choice that precisely matches the characteristics of the human being's organ as research advancements in this field continues. It is feasible to create unconventional material combinations utilising FSP employing a more inventive approach.

### 6.2.2 Effect of FSP on Corrosion Properties

The degradation and corrosion of an implant is one of the major considerations in designing a well-established biomaterial. Depending on the applications, the process of degradation inside the biological environment can either be desirable or undesirable. Desirable degradation, which is intended for biodegradable implants, works in the sense that they are expected to fulfil desired functions for only a temporary period while supporting the regenerative process of wounded tissues and gradually degrade thereafter (Hermawan, Dubé, and Mantovani 2010). Surface corrosion as well as implant material wear and tear constitutes unwanted deterioration. Degradation may weaken the implant, unleash ions of metal, and lead to debris from wear that can harm nearby tissues.

The fundamental idea behind implants that biodegrade is to break down the components of metal in an environment of biological activity so that they may be eliminated from the body via physiological routes while simultaneously maintaining a level of toxicity that is below the threshold at which they would corrode (Witte 2010). It is one of the primary problems connected with biodegradable implants to ensure that injured tissues are completely restored before the implant is completely dissolved in vivo. This may be accomplished by ensuring that the implant demonstrates an adequate rate of deterioration. Typically, significant breakdown rates are linked with biodegradable magnesium alloys, especially in the early period after implantation (Xin, Hu, and Chu 2010). It is required to change the outermost layer of the Mg implant so that correct tissue repair and development is able to take place. This is essential for preventing Mg from degrading too quickly. During the last few years, many FSP surface modification strategies have been successfully used in order to realise the mitigation of the Mg degradation at the very beginning (Qin et al. 2018). In their study, Qin et al. employed FSP to fabricate a nano-hydroxyapatite surface composite upon ZK60 Mg alloy. The objective of this approach was to develop a biodegradable implantation that exhibits a suitable degradation rate. The research findings indicated that the inclusion of nano-hydroxyapatite particulates had a dual effect upon the material's properties. Firstly, it enhanced the biological compatibility of the product by facilitating the formation of sites of nucleation for apatite advancement. Secondly, it promoted the formation of biomineralised films on the outermost layer of the material, thereby slowing down the degradation process (Qin et al. 2018).

Several researchers have utilised the method of potentiodynamic polarisation in their investigations on the corrosion behaviour of FSPed of magnesium alloys. Owing to the uniform dispersal of reinforcing particles onto the surface of the base Mg alloys, it was discovered that the resistance to corrosion is 4.469-fold greater than the base (Vaira Vignesh et al. 2019; Qiao et al. 2021). Qiao et al. have reported a comparable outcome, wherein the surface composite material exhibits superior resistance to corrosion in comparison to the base Mg material. In comparison to the FSP of the base Mg material absent of $ZrO_2$, the resistance to corrosion of the

(a)

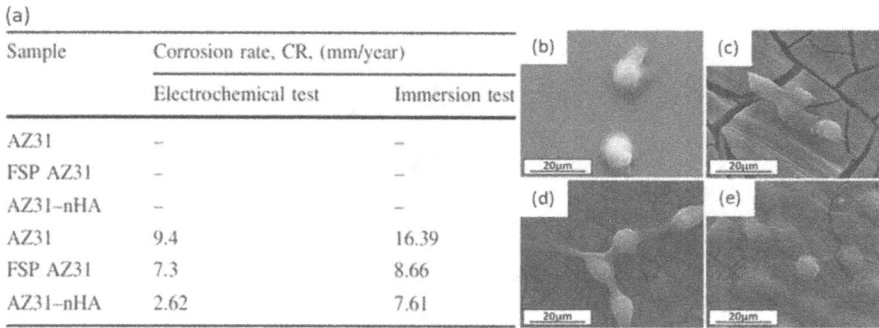

| Sample | Corrosion rate, CR, (mm/year) | |
|--------|---------------------|----------------|
| | Electrochemical test | Immersion test |
| AZ31 | – | – |
| FSP AZ31 | – | – |
| AZ31–nHA | – | – |
| AZ31 | 9.4 | 16.39 |
| FSP AZ31 | 7.3 | 8.66 |
| AZ31–nHA | 2.62 | 7.61 |

**FIGURE 6.7**   (a) FSPed AZ31 Mg alloy corrosion characteristics. (b) TCPS. (c) Adhesion of cell upon the base material. (d) FSPed AZ31 Mg alloy. (e) FSPed AZ31Mg alloy using HA additive after incubation (Ratna Sunil et al. 2014).

surface composite specimen exhibits a decrease in value. The microstructural analysis revealed a notable elevation in the density of dislocations surrounding $ZrO_2$ particles, resulting in galvanic corrosion due to the significant increase in the nucleation sites (Qiao et al. 2021).

In addition, the cell adhesion analysis was conducted utilising a typical TCPS. The findings suggest that the cells exhibited poor adhesion when placed together. In contrast, the cells within FSPed AZ31 and FSPed AZ31-HA surface composite demonstrated strong interconnectivity, elongation, and adhesion on the facet. The proliferation of the cells in FSPed AZ31 Mg alloy with HA surface composite remains significantly higher in the wake of the higher wetting characteristics of HA that facilitate protein adsorption, enhance osteointegration, and reduce the rate of degradation, as illustrated in Figure 6.7 (Ratna Sunil et al. 2014).

The investigation of the corrosion morphological structures, subsequent to the elimination of corrosion products, revealed that FSPed WE43 Mg Alloy using HA exhibited a notably finer texture. This observation implies that the surface composite possesses greater resistance to corrosion characteristics (Cao et al. 2019).

## 6.3   ADDITIONAL FRICTION STIR–BASED APPROACH FOR MANUFACTURING Mg-BASED IMPLANTS

### 6.3.1   Friction Stir Welding (FSW) and Its Effect on Various Properties

In 1991, The Welding Institute (UK) developed the FSW technique and demonstrated favourable results in the welding of various combinations of materials. The technique of extreme plastic deformation of the adjacent surface of the materials to be joined is initiated by the heat produced due to the frictional force between a non-consumable tool and the workpiece. This leads to an interaction of the workpiece and offers several advantages over conventional joining techniques (Raja, Hasan, and Ansari 2016; Ivanov, Panchenko, and Mikhailov 2018; K. Singh, Singh, and Singh 2018; Naumov et al. 2019; Casanova et al. 2020; Ariffin et al. 2022; Raja et al.

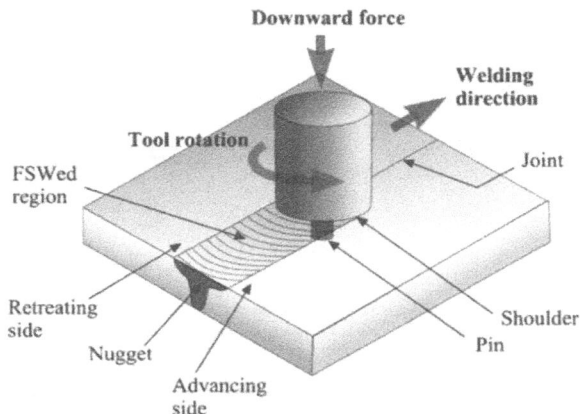

**FIGURE 6.8**  Schematic illustration of the FSW process (Ogunsemi et al. 2021).

2022). Figures 6.8 and 6.9 (Ogunsemi et al. 2021) illustrate the basic diagram and microstructural features of the FSW procedure, respectively.

FSW is utilised in various biomedical implant joints owing to its exceptional joint characteristics. The utilisation of FSW has demonstrated efficacy in welding biomaterials, including Mg-based alloys (Sunil et al. 2015; K. Singh, Singh, and Singh 2018).

For purposes of manufacturing sustainable bioimplants, alloys of Mg are being studied since they have desirable mechanical properties and are biologically compatible. UaFSW was done on AZ91 alloy by Baradarani et al. (Baradarani, Mostafapour, and Shalvandi 2019). They reported that the method of ultrasonic assisting during FSW did not discover any defects in the welded specimen. Additionally, it was noted that traditional FSW decreased the size of the grains to 4 µm from 80 µm in comparison to the base AZ91. Furthermore, UaFSW reduced the grains' size to 1.8 µm from 4 µm. As well, reducing the grain's size improves the interaction that occurs between implantation and the tissue of the bone.

The refinement of grains in AZ31 and AZ91 was observed, along with additional enhancements achieved through employing the post-weld heat treatment approach. Following the post-weld treatment, strength and efficiency of joints were found to have significantly increased (K. Singh, Singh, and Singh 2019). The dissimilar FSW

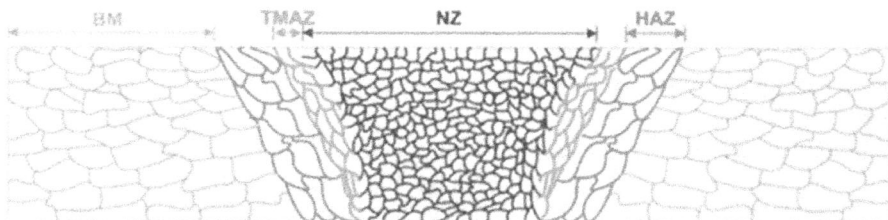

**FIGURE 6.9**  Schematic illustration of the different zones of the cross section of the FSWed specimen (Ogunsemi et al. 2021).

of AZ31 and AZ91 promoted minute quantities of $Mg_{17}Al_{12}$ IMC and finer grains. The development of IMC might have been responsible for the noticeable increase in hardness (Sunil et al. 2015).

Dissolution and coarsening of precipitate and recrystallisation are the three types of microstructural modifications that may occur when different alloys are welded together using FSW. The characteristics of dissimilar welding prone to corrosion are profoundly affected by the generation of precipitates. It may be possible to increase the resistance to corrosion of such joints by adjusting the dispersion of the precipitates. The corrosion properties of FSWed joints were investigated by Xie et al. (2021). It has been shown that increasing the speed of the welding process while reducing the amount of heat input results in a joint that is more resistant to corrosion. They came to the conclusion that when it comes to immersion corrosion, larger precipitates tend to induce pitting corrosion more than smaller ones. On the contrary, pitting corrosion may be delayed by using the solid solution, which can be achieved by heat caused by FSW. In order to attain electrochemical uniformity, they developed a technique that would reduce the amount of heat during the FSW process. This would make joints more resistant to corrosion.

### 6.3.2 FRICTION STIR ADDITIVE MANUFACTURING (FSAM) AND ITS EFFECT ON VARIOUS PROPERTIES

One of the processes that may be used while manufacturing a variety of products into a three-dimensional form is known as AM. The approach has found widespread use in the realm of medical care, particularly in the production of metallic implants used for a variety of applications, including fracture healing, replacement of joints, etc. It is acknowledged that the fabrication of an implant by using the traditional approach may have an effect on the functionality, physical characteristics, and chemical characteristics of the materials, which in turn can limit the lifespan of the implants in the first place. There are just a few parameters that require to be taken into consideration in order to make implants compatible with the tissue of humans they will surround. Among these requirements is the utilisation of acceptable materials that are high in bio-functioning, have adequate mechanical characteristics, and have a compatible morphology (Griffiths et al. 2019). The AM method, namely FSAM, is most likely to be successful in meeting the requirements that have been outlined (A. K. Srivastava, Kumar, and Dixit 2021). The FSAM technique involves the material's layer-by-layer joining by utilising thermo-mechanical stirring caused by the rotating tool. This leads to substantial material deformation due to the intense heat developed (M. Vignesh et al. 2021).

Figure 6.10 depicts the sequential schematic presentation of the FSAM process, which comprises several layers of materials, beginning with a couple of layers and progressing to a total of four layers. First, the evenness of each material plate and the accuracy of its measurements are checked and adjusted as necessary. The subsequent action is to clean up these plates. At the beginning of the process, two plates are stacked on top of one another in the manner that would ultimately be used for the manufacturing. After the layers have been arranged in a suitable fashion, the FSAM is carried out employing suitable process parameters. Following the initial pass, the

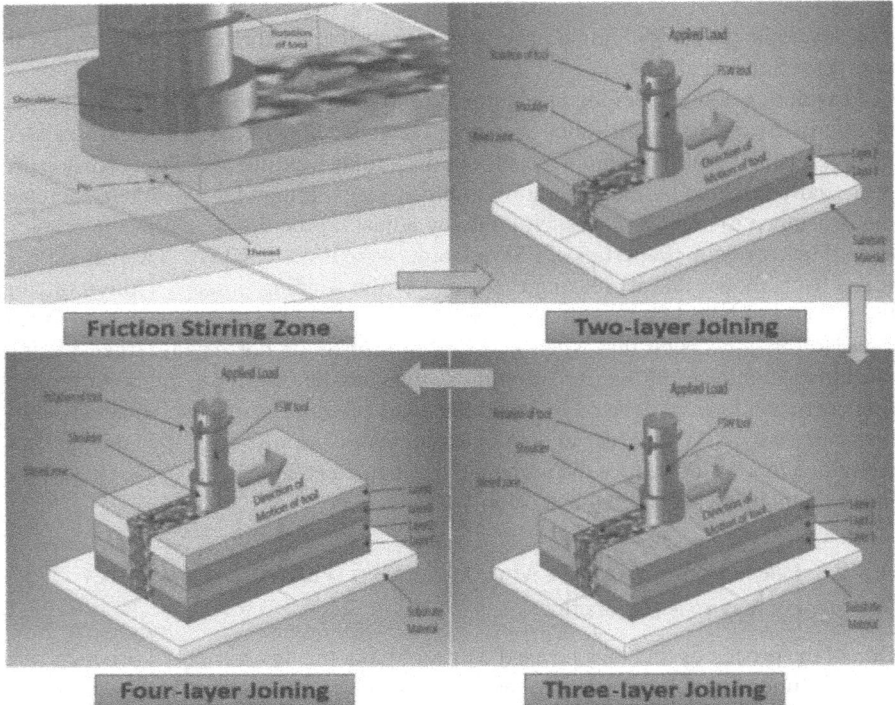

**FIGURE 6.10**   Schematic illustration of the FSAM method (A. K. Srivastava et al. 2021).

procedure of incorporating extra layers is halted until the desired finished structure elevation has been reached. Nevertheless, if the requisite construct height fails to be attained, the upper layer of the part that is being processed must be completed first. Necessary steps must be taken in order to eliminate any flash that forms throughout the FSAM operation. After that, a fresh panel is installed on top of the previous panel. These stages are repeated as often as necessary until the structure reaches the appropriate build-up elevation (M. Srivastava et al. 2019; A. K. Srivastava, Kumar, and Dixit 2021).

There have only been a few studies that have concentrated on the microstructural characteristics of Mg alloy. The structure of the grains and the behaviour of the AZ31B were investigated by Ho et al., who used the FSAM technique to include HA. A profound equiaxed grain arrangement can be seen in Figure 6.11, with a reported size of 7.7 μm. With the addition of 10% HA during FSAM of AZ31B alloy, the grain size reached up to 2.2 μm from without the addition of HA, which was found to be 7.7 μm (Ho et al. 2020).

In addition to this, Palanivel et al. (2015) investigated the properties of WE43 alloy using two distinct sets of FSAM conditions and workpieces. The formation of Mg2Y IMC has been detected. Due to the fact that the topmost layer has generated a significant amount of strain, the size of the grains and dimensions of the topmost layers have become finer than those of the layer underneath.

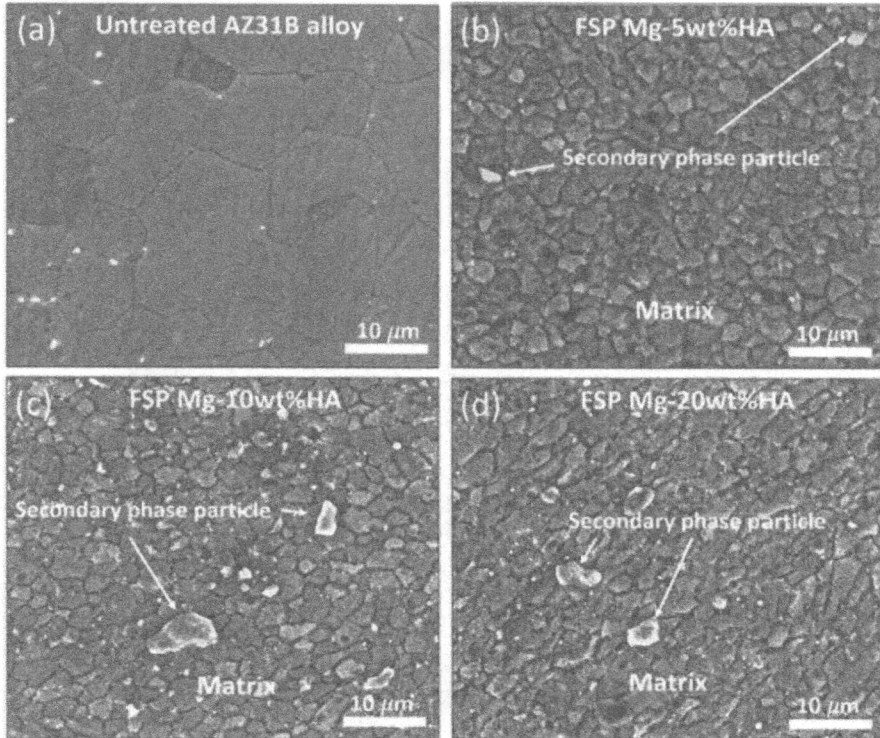

**FIGURE 6.11** Microstructural illustration. (a) Base AZ31B. (b–d) FSAM of AZ31B alloy with different HA percentages (Ho et al. 2020).

The FSAM process has the ability to produce components with superior structural qualities that are suitable for usage in the biomedical sector. It has been shown that, in addition to creating superior and outstanding performance materials, it is also possible to produce a more refined and homogeneous morphology by making use of the necessary parameters during the setting up process. This, in turn, leads to an improvement in the mechanical characteristics of the components. As a consequence of this, more clinical applications and tests may be conducted in the interest of developing a wide range of high-quality biomaterials in the not-too-distant future.

### 6.3.3 FRICTION SURFACING (FS) AND ITS EFFECT ON VARIOUS PROPERTIES

An axial force is applied to the material during the FS process, which causes the consumable rotating rod to rub against the surface of the substrate. As a result of the raised temperature generated by the frictional interaction, a metallic connection is created between the processed consumable rod and the substrate. Because of the high temperature generated by the frictional contact, a coating of viscoplastic material develops at the blunt end of the consumable rod. Because of the elevated temperature and pressure involved, a process known as inter-diffusion takes place, which ultimately results

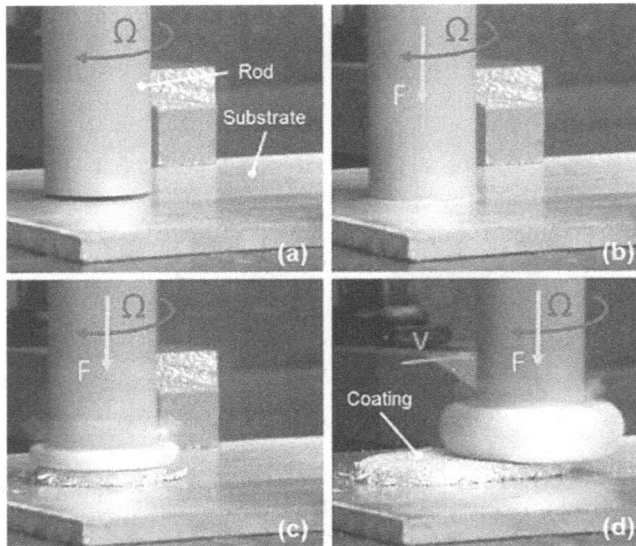

**FIGURE 6.12** Various phases of friction surfacing. (a) Rotation of rod. (b) Starting of contact. (c) Beginning of deformation. (d) Material build-up phase (Gandra et al. 2014).

in the formation of a metallurgical relationship between the substrate and the plasticised material. Figure 6.12 illustrates a graphical representation of frictional surfacing (Gandra et al. 2014; Gopan, Leo Dev Wins, and Surendran 2021).

A larger depositing height and speed, morphology with more refined grains, chemically stable surfaces, and the capacity to process a broad range of substrate types are some of the benefits of FS. Other benefits include the ability to process a wide range of materials. The substrate material's corrosion resistance was significantly increased by the application of friction FS. However, because of limitations imposed by the technology at the time, this strategy could only be used in a select few contexts (Bararpour, Jamshidi Aval, and Jamaati 2019; Stegmüller, Grant, and Schindele 2019).

## 6.4 CONCLUSIONS

The metallurgical and compositional features of Mg-based biomaterials have been scrutinised in order to fulfil the criteria for applications in biomedical science, specifically, implant that used friction-stir based processes. The efficiency with which friction stir–based approaches may increase mechanical and microstructural characteristics, along with corrosion and tribological properties, has been discussed. Reduced size of grains and an enhanced basal texture are two potential outcomes of FSP, which has the potential to increase the anti-corrosion properties of an Mg alloy. The inherent mechanism of corrosion in pure metal is altered when the metal microstructural characteristics are modified using FSP. Because of the change in the microstructural characteristics, fresh layers of corrosion-related substances will form, which will serve as an inhibitor to prevent further damage. The research indicates that the FSP of Mg alloy with HA has improved the biomineralisation and anti-corrosion properties when compared with the FSP of Mg alloy without HA.

Because of its exceptional joint qualities, FSW is applied in Mg-based biomedical implantation joints. Mg alloys underwent the recrystallisation procedure when they were subjected to extreme conditions and considerable deformation that was present throughout the FSW procedure. Grain refining results in a significant increase in the joint's tensile strength compared to the base Mg.

FSAM is the approach that should be used since it is optimal for ensuring the functionality of Mg implants that are surrounded by human tissue. Once layers are joined sequentially in the FSAM procedure, unique microstructural features among the subsequent layers arise as a result of the creation of temperature and deformation that occurs throughout this procedure. The size of the grains was reportedly reduced by a technique termed dynamic recrystallisation as a result of the deformation. This, in turn, had an effect on the FSAM workpieces' mechanical qualities.

When processing biomedical implants made of lightweight alloys such as magnesium alloy, the FS approach combined with different biomaterials such as titanium alloy and stainless steel as the consumables rod may be used to strengthen the interaction between the implants and the surrounding tissue.

## ACKNOWLEDGEMENTS

The authors would like to acknowledge the University of Malaya, Malaysia, for providing the necessary facilities and resources for this research. This research is supported by the Konsortium Kecemerlangan Penyelidikan Grant Scheme from the Ministry of Higher Education (MOHE) in Malaysia (No. KKP001A-2021) and EU-project H2020-MSCA-RISE-2018 Number 823786, i-Weld.

## REFERENCES

Almasi, Davood, Woei Jye Lau, Sajad Rasaee, Roohollah Sharifi, and Hamid Reza Mozaffari. 2020. "Fabrication of a Novel Hydroxyapatite/Polyether Ether Ketone Surface Nanocomposite via Friction Stir Processing for Orthopedic and Dental Applications." *Progress in Biomaterials* 9 (1): 35–44. https://doi.org/10.1007/s40204-020-00130-7

Amirtharaj Mosas, Kamalan Kirubaharan, Ashok Raja Chandrasekar, Arish Dasan, Amirhossein Pakseresht, and Dušan Galusek. 2022. "Recent Advancements in Materials and Coatings for Biomedical Implants." *Gels* 8 (5): 323. https://doi.org/10.3390/gels8050323

Ariffin, Mohammad Ashraf bin, Mohd Ridha bin Muhamad, Sufian Raja, Mohd Fadzil Jamaludin, Farazila Yusof, Tetsuo Suga, Huihong Liu, Yoshiaki Morisada, and Hidetoshi Fujii. 2022. "Friction Stir Alloying of AZ61 and Mild Steel with Cu-CNT Additive." *Journal of Materials Research and Technology* 21: 2400–415. https://doi. org/10.1016/j.jmrt.2022.10.082

Arora, H. S., Harpreet Singh, Brij Kumar Dhindaw, and Harpreet S. Grewal. 2012. "Improving the Tribological Properties of Mg Based AZ31 Alloy Using Friction Stir Processing." *Advanced Materials Research* 585: 579–83.

Asadi, P., M. K. Besharati Givi, N. Parvin, A. Araei, M. Taherishargh, and S. Tutunchilar. 2012. "On the Role of Cooling and Tool Rotational Direction on Microstructure and Mechanical Properties of Friction Stir Processed AZ91." *The International Journal of Advanced Manufacturing Technology* 63: 987–97.

Bagherifard, Sara, Ramin Ghelichi, Ali Khademhosseini, and Mario Guagliano. 2014. "Cell Response to Nanocrystallized Metallic Substrates Obtained through Severe Plastic Deformation." *ACS Applied Materials & Interfaces* 6 (11): 7963–85. https://doi.org/10.1021/am501119k

Balamurugan, K. Ganesa, and K. Mahadevan. 2013. "Investigation on the Changes Effected by Tool Profile on Mechanical and Tribological Properties of Friction Stir Processed AZ31B Magnesium Alloy." *Journal of Manufacturing Processes* 15 (4): 659–65.

Baradarani, Faraz, Amir Mostafapour, and Maghsoud Shalvandi. 2019. "Effect of Ultrasonic Assisted Friction Stir Welding on Microstructure and Mechanical Properties of AZ91-C Magnesium Alloy." *Transactions of Nonferrous Metals Society of China* 29 (12): 2514–22. https://doi.org/10.1016/S1003-6326(19)65159-9

Bararpour, Seyedeh Marjan, Hamed Jamshidi Aval, and Roohollah Jamaati. 2019. "Mechanical Alloying by Friction Surfacing Process." *Materials Letters* 254: 394–97. https://doi.org/10.1016/j.matlet.2019.07.113

Barba, D., E. Alabort, and R. C. Reed. 2019. "Synthetic Bone: Design by Additive Manufacturing." *Acta Biomaterialia* 97: 637–56. https://doi.org/10.1016/j.actbio.2019.07.049

Bhadouria, N., L. Thakur, P. Kumar, and Navneet Arora. 2017. "An Investigation of Normal and Submerged Condition on Microstructural and Tribological Properties of Friction Stir Processed AZ91-D Magnesium Alloy." *Canadian Metallurgical Quarterly* 56 (1): 94–103.

Cao, Genghua, Lu Zhang, Datong Zhang, Yixiong Liu, Jixiang Gao, Weihua Li, and Zhenxing Zheng. 2019. "Microstructure and Properties of Nano-hydroxyapatite Reinforced WE43 Alloy Fabricated by Friction Stir Processing." *Materials* 12 (18): 2994.

Casanova, Jaime, Gonçalo Sorger, Pedro Vilaça, and Sérgio Duarte Brandi. 2020. "Microstructure and Mechanical Properties of 9% Nickel Steel Welded by FSW." *The International Journal of Advanced Manufacturing Technology* 111 (11): 3225–40. https://doi.org/10.1007/s00170-020-06313-7

Chen, Qizhi, and George A. Thouas. 2015. "Metallic Implant Biomaterials." *Materials Science and Engineering: R: Reports* 87: 1–57. https://doi.org/10.1016/j.mser.2014.10.001

Dobrzański, Leszek A., Dobrzańska-Danikiewicz, Anna D. and Dobrzański, Lech B. 2021. "Effect of Biomedical Materials in the Implementation of a Long and Healthy Life Policy." *Processes* 9 (5): 865. https://doi.org/10.3390/pr9050865

Gandra, J., H. Krohn, R. M. Miranda, P. Vilaça, L. Quintino, and J. F. dos Santos. 2014. "Friction Surfacing: A Review." *Journal of Materials Processing Technology* 214 (5): 1062–93. https://doi.org/10.1016/j.jmatprotec.2013.12.008

Gopan, Vipin, K. Leo Dev Wins, and Arun Surendran. 2021. "Innovative Potential of Additive Friction Stir Deposition among Current Laser Based Metal Additive Manufacturing Processes: A Review." *CIRP Journal of Manufacturing Science and Technology* 32: 228–48. https://doi.org/10.1016/j.cirpj.2020.12.004

Griffiths, R. Joey, Dylan T. Petersen, David Garcia, and Hang Z. Yu. 2019. "Additive Friction Stir-enabled Solid-state Additive Manufacturing for the Repair of 7075 Aluminum Alloy." *Applied Sciences* 9 (17): 3486.

Harwani, Deepika, Vishvesh Badheka, Vivek Patel, Wenya Li, and Joel Andersson. 2021. "Developing Superplasticity in Magnesium Alloys with the Help of Friction Stir Processing and Its Variants: A Review." *Journal of Materials Research and Technology* 12: 2055–75.

Hermawan, H., D. Dubé, and D. Mantovani. 2010. "Developments in Metallic Biodegradable Stents." *Acta Biomaterialia* 6 (5): 1693–97.

Ho, Yee-Hsien, Sameehan S Joshi, Tso-Chang Wu, Chu-Mao Hung, New-Jing Ho, and Narendra B Dahotre. 2020. "In-Vitro Bio-Corrosion Behavior of Friction Stir Additively Manufactured AZ31B Magnesium Alloy–Hydroxyapatite Composites." *Materials Science and Engineering: C* 109: 110632. https://doi.org/10.1016/j.msec.2020.110632

Hu, Xuefeng, Koon Gee Neoh, Jieyu Zhang, and En-Tang Kang. 2014. "Bacterial and Osteoblast Behavior on Titanium, Cobalt–Chromium Alloy and Stainless Steel Treated with Alkali and Heat: A Comparative Study for Potential Orthopedic Applications." *Journal of Colloid and Interface Science* 417: 410–19. https://doi.org/10.1016/j.jcis.2013.11.062

Ivanov, S. Yu., O. V. Panchenko, and V. G. Mikhailov. 2018. "Comparative Analysis of Non-uniformity of Mechanical Properties of Welded Joints of Al-Mg-Si Alloys during Friction Stir Welding and Laser Welding." *Metal Science and Heat Treatment* 60 (5): 393–98. https://doi.org/10.1007/s11041-018-0289-z

Iwaszko, Józef, and Krzysztof Kudła. 2021. "Microstructure, Hardness, and Wear Resistance of AZ91 Magnesium Alloy Produced by Friction Stir Processing with Air-Cooling." *The International Journal of Advanced Manufacturing Technology* 116: 1309–23.

Mani Prabu, S. S., Chandra S Perugu, H. C. Madhu, Ashutosh Jangde, Sohel Khan, S. Jayachandran, M. Manikandan, P. Ajay Kumar, Satish V. Kailas, and I. A. Palani. 2019. "Exploring the Functional and Corrosion Behavior of Friction Stir Welded NiTi Shape Memory Alloy." *Journal of Manufacturing Processes* 47: 119–28. https://doi.org/10.1016/j.jmapro.2019.09.017

Martinez-Marquez, Daniel., Delmar, Ylva, Sun, Shoujin and Stewart, Rodney A. 2020. "Exploring Macroporosity of Additively Manufactured Titanium Metamaterials for Bone Regeneration with Quality by Design: A Systematic Literature Review." *Materials* 13 (21): 1–44. https://doi.org/10.3390/ma13214794

Mazaheri, Yousef, Mohammad Mahdi Jalilvand, Akbar Heidarpour, and Amir Reza Jahani. 2020. "Tribological Behavior of AZ31/$ZrO_2$ Surface Nanocomposites Developed by Friction Stir Processing." *Tribology International* 143: 106062.

Mirzadeh, Hamed. 2021. "High Strain Rate Superplasticity via Friction Stir Processing (FSP): A Review." *Materials Science and Engineering: A* 819: 141499.

Mishra, Rajiv S., M W Mahoney, S X McFadden, N A Mara, and A K Mukherjee. 1999. "High Strain Rate Superplasticity in a Friction Stir Processed 7075 Al Alloy." *Scripta Materialia* 42 (2): 163–68.

Misra, R. D. K., W. W. Thein-Han, T. C. Pesacreta, K. H. Hasenstein, M. C. Somani, and L. P. Karjalainen. 2009. "Cellular Response of Preosteoblasts to Nanograined/Ultrafine-Grained Structures." *Acta Biomaterialia* 5 (5): 1455–67. https://doi.org/10.1016/j.actbio.2008.12.017

Moghadasi, Kaveh, Mohammad Syahid Mohd Isa, Mohammad Ashraf Ariffin, Muhammad Zulhiqmi Mohd Jamil, Sufian Raja, Bo Wu, and Mehrdad Yamani et al. 2022. "A Review on Biomedical Implant Materials and the Effect of Friction Stir Based Techniques on Their Mechanical and Tribological Properties." *Journal of Materials Research and Technology* 17: 1054–121. https://doi.org/10.1016/j.jmrt.2022.01.050

Muhamad, Mohd Ridha, Sufian Raja, Mohd Fadzil Jamaludin, Farazila Yusof, Yoshiaki Morisada, Tetsuo Suga, and Hidetoshi Fujii. 2021. "Enhancements on Dissimilar Friction Stir Welding between AZ31 and SPHC Mild Steel with Al-Mg as Powder Additives." *Journal of Manufacturing Science and Engineering* 143 (July): 1–22. https://doi.org/10.1115/1.4049745

Naumov, Anton, Iuliia Morozova, Evgenii Rylkov, Aleksei Obrosov, Fedor Isupov, Vesselin Michailov, and Andrey Rudskoy. 2019. "Metallurgical and Mechanical Characterization of High-Speed Friction Stir Welded AA 6082-T6 Aluminum Alloy." *Materials* 12 (24). https://doi.org/10.3390/ma12244211

Navarro, M., A. Michiardi, O. Castaño, and J. A. Planell. 2008. "Biomaterials in Orthopaedics." *Journal of the Royal Society Interface* 5 (27): 1137–58. https://doi.org/10.1098/rsif.2008.0151

Navazani, Mohammad, and Kamran Dehghani. 2016. "Fabrication of Mg-$ZrO_2$ Surface Layer Composites by Friction Stir Processing." *Journal of Materials Processing Technology* 229: 439–49.

Niinomi, Mitsuo, and Masaaki Nakai. 2011. "Titanium-based Biomaterials for Preventing Stress Shielding between Implant Devices and Bone." *International Journal of Biomaterials* 2011: 836587.

Ogunsemi, B. T., T. E. Abioye, T. I. Ogedengbe, and H. Zuhailawati. 2021. "A Review of Various Improvement Strategies for Joint Quality of AA 6061-T6 Friction Stir Weldments." *Journal of Materials Research and Technology* 11: 1061–89. https://doi.org/10.1016/j.jmrt.2021.01.070

Orozco-Caballero, Alberto, Marta Álvarez-Leal, David Verdera, Pilar Rey, Oscar A. Ruano, and Fernando Carreño. 2017. "Evaluation of the Mechanical Anisotropy and the Deformation Mechanism in a Multi-pass Friction Stir Processed Al-Zn-Mg-Cu Alloy." *Materials & Design* 125: 116–25.

Palanivel, S., P. Nelaturu, B. Glass, and R. S. Mishra. 2015. "Friction Stir Additive Manufacturing for High Structural Performance through Microstructural Control in an Mg Based WE43 Alloy." *Materials & Design (1980–2015)* 65: 934–52.

Perumal, G., H. S. Grewal, and H. S. Arora. 2020. "Enhanced Durability, Bio-Activity and Corrosion Resistance of Stainless Steel through Severe Surface Deformation." *Colloids and Surfaces B: Biointerfaces* 194: 111197. https://doi.org/10.1016/j.colsurfb.2020.111197

Prakash, Chander, Sunpreet Singh, and Seeram Ramakrishna. 2020. "Characterization of Indigenously Coated Biodegradable Magnesium Alloy Primed through Novel Additive Manufacturing Assisted Investment Casting." *Materials Letters* 275: 128137. https://doi.org/10.1016/j.matlet.2020.128137

Prakash, Chander, Sunpreet Singh, Seeram Ramakrishna, Grzegorz Królczyk, and Chi H. Le. 2020. "Microwave Sintering of Porous Ti-Nb-HA Composite with High Strength and Enhanced Bioactivity for Implant Applications." *Journal of Alloys and Compounds* 824: 153774. https://doi.org/10.1016/j.jallcom.2020.153774

Qiao, Ke, Ting Zhang, Kuaishe Wang, Shengnan Yuan, Shengyi Zhang, Liqiang Wang, Zhi Wang, Pai Peng, Jun Cai, and Chaozong Liu. 2021. "Mg/ZrO$_2$ Metal Matrix Nanocomposites Fabricated by Friction Stir Processing: Microstructure, Mechanical Properties, and Corrosion Behavior." *Frontiers in Bioengineering and Biotechnology* 9: 605171.

Qin, Dingqiang, Haorui Shen, Zhikang Shen, Haiyan Chen, and Li Fu. 2018. "Manufacture of Biodegradable Magnesium Alloy by High Speed Friction Stir Processing." *Journal of Manufacturing Processes* 36: 22–32.

Raja, Sufian, Faisal Hasan, and Akhter Husain Ansari. 2016. "Effect of Friction Stir Welding on the Hardness of Al-6061 T6 Aluminium Alloy." *International Conference on Advanced Production and Industrial Engineering, 9–10 December, 2016*, no. August 2017: 9–13.

Raja, Sufian, Mohd Ridha Muhamad, Mohd Fadzil Jamaludin, and Farazila Yusof. 2020. "A Review on Nanomaterials Reinforcement in Friction Stir Welding." *Journal of Materials Research and Technology* 9 (6): 16459–87.

Raja, Sufian, Mohd Ridha Muhamad, Farazila Yusof, Mohd Fadzil Jamaludin, Tetsuo Suga, Huihong Liu, Yoshiaki Morisada, and Hidetoshi Fujii. 2022. "Friction Stir Alloying of AZ61 and Mild Steel with Al-CNT Additive." *Science and Technology of Welding and Joining* 27 (7): 533–40. https://doi.org/10.1080/13621718.2022.2080449

Rana, Harikrishna, and Vishvesh Badheka. 2019. "Elucidation of the Role of Rotation Speed and Stirring Direction on AA 7075-B4C Surface Composites Formulated by Friction Stir Processing." *Proceedings of the Institution of Mechanical Engineers, Part L: Journal of Materials: Design and Applications* 233 (5): 977–94.

Rathee, Sandeep, Sachin Maheshwari, Arshad Noor Siddiquee, and Manu Srivastava. 2018. "A Review of Recent Progress in Solid State Fabrication of Composites and Functionally Graded Systems via Friction Stir Processing." *Critical Reviews in Solid State and Materials Sciences* 43 (4): 334–66.

Ratna Sunil, B., T. S. Sampath Kumar, Uday Chakkingal, V. Nandakumar, and Mukesh Doble. 2014. "Nano-hydroxyapatite Reinforced AZ31 Magnesium Alloy by Friction Stir Processing: A Solid State Processing for Biodegradable Metal Matrix Composites." *Journal of Materials Science: Materials in Medicine* 25 (4): 975–88. https://doi. org/10.1007/s10856-013-5127-7

Sezer, Nurettin., Evis, Zafer, Kayhan, Said Murat, Tahmasebifar, Aydin and Koç, Muammer. 2018. "Review of Magnesium-based Biomaterials and Their Applications." *Journal of Magnesium and Alloys* 6 (1): 23–43. https://doi.org/10.1016/j.jma.2018.02.003

Singh, Harjit, Sunpreet Singh, and Chander Prakash. 2019. "Current Trends in Biomaterials and Bio-Manufacturing." In *Biomanufacturing*, edited by Chander Prakash, Sunpreet Singh, Rupinder Singh, Seeram Ramakrishna, B S Pabla, Sanjeev Puri, and M S Uddin, 1–34. Cham: Springer International Publishing. https://doi.org/ 10.1007/978-3-030-13951-3_1

Singh, Kulwant, Gurbhinder Singh, and Harmeet Singh. 2018. "Review on Friction Stir Welding of Magnesium Alloys." *Journal of Magnesium and Alloys* 6 (4): 399–416. https://doi.org/10.1016/j.jma.2018.06.001

———. 2019. "Microstructure and Mechanical Behaviour of Friction-Stir-Welded Magnesium Alloys: As-Welded and Post Weld Heat Treated." *Materials Today Communications* 20: 100600. https://doi.org/10.1016/j.mtcomm.2019.100600

Sodhi, Gurvinder Pal Singh, and Harpreet Singh. 2018. "Development of Corrosion Resistant Surfaces via Friction Stir Processing for Bio Implant Applications." *IOP Conference Series: Materials Science and Engineering*, 284:012026.

Srivastava, Ashish Kumar, Nilesh Kumar, and Amit Rai Dixit. 2021. "Friction Stir Additive Manufacturing: An Innovative Tool to Enhance Mechanical and Microstructural Properties." *Materials Science and Engineering: B* 263: 114832.

Srivastava, Manu, Sandeep Rathee, Sachin Maheshwari, Arshad Noor Siddiquee, and T. K. Kundra. 2019. "A Review on Recent Progress in Solid State Friction Based Metal Additive Manufacturing: Friction Stir Additive Techniques." *Critical Reviews in Solid State and Materials Sciences* 44 (5): 345–77.

Stegmüller, Michael J. R., Richard J. Grant, and Paul Schindele. 2019. "Quantification of the Interfacial Roughness When Coating Stainless Steel onto Aluminium by Friction Surfacing." *Surface and Coatings Technology* 375: 22–33.

Sunil, B. Ratna, G. Pradeep Kumar Reddy, A. S. N. Mounika, P. Navya Sree, P. Rama Pinneswari, I. Ambica, R. Ajay Babu, and P. Amarnadh. 2015. "Joining of AZ31 and AZ91 Mg Alloys by Friction Stir Welding." *Journal of Magnesium and Alloys* 3 (4): 330–34.

Thangaraj, Balusamy, Sankara Narayanan T. S. Nellaiappan, Ravichandran Kulandaivelu, Min Ho Lee, and Toshiyasu Nishimura. 2015. "A Facile Method to Modify the Characteristics and Corrosion Behavior of 304 Stainless Steel by Surface Nanostructuring toward Biomedical Applications." *ACS Applied Materials & Interfaces* 7 (32): 17731–47. https://doi.org/10.1021/acsami.5b03877

Tharayil, Hanas, T. S. Sampath Kumar, Govindaraj Perumal, Mukesh Doble, and Seeram Ramakrishna. 2018. "Electrospun PCL/HA Coated Friction Stir Processed AZ31/HA Composites for Degradable Implant Applications." *Journal of Materials Processing Technology* 252: 398–406. https://doi.org/10.1016/j.jmatprotec.2017.10.009

Vaira Vignesh, R., R. Padmanaban, M. Govindaraju, and G. Suganya Priyadharshini. 2019. "Investigations on the Corrosion Behaviour and Biocompatibility of Magnesium Alloy Surface Composites AZ91D-ZrO₂ Fabricated by Friction Stir Processing." *Transactions of the IMF* 97 (5): 261–70.

Vasu, Ch, K. J. A. Naga Durga, I. Srinivas, Shaik Dariyavali, B. Venkateswarlu, and B. Ratna Sunil. 2019. "Developing Composite of ZE41 Magnesium Alloy–Calcium by Friction Stir Processing for Biodegradable Implant Applications." *Materials Today: Proceedings* 18: 270–77.

Vignesh, M, G. Ranjith Kumar, M. Sathishkumar, M. Manikandan, G. Rajyalakshmi, R. Ramanujam, and N. Arivazhagan. 2021. "Development of Biomedical Implants through Additive Manufacturing: A Review." *Journal of Materials Engineering and Performance* 30 (7): 4735–44. https://doi.org/10.1007/s11665-021-05578-7

Vignesh, R. Vaira, R. Padmanaban, and M. Govindaraju. 2019. "Investigations on the Surface Topography, Corrosion Behavior, and Biocompatibility of Friction Stir Processed Magnesium Alloy AZ91D." *Surface Topography: Metrology and Properties* 7 (2): 25020.

Wang, Jing, Jinhe Dou, Zhongchao Wang, Cheng Hu, Huijun Yu, and Chuanzhong Chen. 2022. "Research Progress of Biodegradable Magnesium-based Biomedical Materials: A Review." *Journal of Alloys and Compounds* 923: 166377. https://doi.org/10.1016/j.jallcom.2022.166377

Wang, Xiaojian, Shanqing Xu, Shiwei Zhou, Wei Xu, Martin Leary, Peter Choong, M. Qian, Milan Brandt, and Yi Min Xie. 2016. "Topological Design and Additive Manufacturing of Porous Metals for Bone Scaffolds and Orthopaedic Implants: A Review." *Biomaterials* 83: 127–41. https://doi.org/10.1016/j.biomaterials.2016.01.012

Warburton, Andrew., Girdler, Steven J, Mikhail, Christopher M, Ahn, Amy and Cho, Samuel K. 2020. "Biomaterials in Spinal Implants: A Review." *Neurospine* 17 (1): 101–10. https://doi.org/10.14245/ns.1938296.148

Witte, Frank. 2010. "The History of Biodegradable Magnesium Implants: A Review." *Acta Biomaterialia* 6 (5): 1680–92.

Xie, Yuming, Xiangchen Meng, Feifan Wang, Yimeng Jiang, Xiaotian Ma, Long Wan, and Yongxian Huang. 2021. "Insight on Corrosion Behavior of Friction Stir Welded AA2219/AA2195 Joints in Astronautical Engineering." *Corrosion Science* 192: 109800. https://doi.org/10.1016/j.corsci.2021.109800.

Xin, Yunchang, Tao Hu, and Paul K. Chu. 2010. "Influence of Test Solutions on In Vitro Studies of Biomedical Magnesium Alloys." *Journal of the Electrochemical Society* 157 (7): C238.

Yamani, Seyed Mehrdad, Sufian Raja, Mohammad Ashraf bin Ariffin, Mohammad Syahid Mohd Isa, Mohd Ridha Muhamad, Mohd Fadzil Jamaludin, Farazila Yusof, and Muhammad Khairi Faiz bin Ahmad Hairuddin. 2022. "Effects of Preheating on Microstructural and Mechanical Properties of Friction Stir Welded Thin Low Carbon Steel Joints." *Journal of Engineering Materials and Technology* 145 (2): 021001. https://doi.org/10.1115/1.4055909

Yuan, Bin., Zhu, Min and Chung, Chi Yuen. 2018. "Biomedical Porous Shape Memory Alloys for Hard-Tissue Replacement Materials." *Materials* 11 (9): 1716. https://doi.org/10.3390/ma11091716

Zang, Qianhao, Xiaowen Li, Hongmei Chen, Jing Zhang, Ling Wang, Shujin Chen, Yunxue Jin, and Sheng Lu. 2020. "Microstructure and Mechanical Properties of AZ31/ZrO$_2$ Composites Prepared by Friction Stir Processing with High Rotation Speed." *Frontiers in Materials* 7: 278.

Zhang, Ruixia, Xianfeng Zhou, Hongyu Gao, Steven Mankoci, Yang Liu, Xiahan Sang, Haifeng Qin, Xiaoning Hou, Zhencheng Ren, and Gary L. Doll. 2018. "The Effects of Laser Shock Peening on the Mechanical Properties and Biomedical Behavior of AZ31B Magnesium Alloy." *Surface and Coatings Technology* 339: 48–56.

Zhu, Chenyuan, Yuting Lv, Chao Qian, Haixin Qian, Ting Jiao, Liqiang Wang, and Fuqiang Zhang. 2016. "Proliferation and Osteogenic Differentiation of Rat BMSCs on a Novel Ti/SiC Metal Matrix Nanocomposite Modified by Friction Stir Processing." *Scientific Reports* 6 (1): 38875.

Zhu, Min., Huang, Ting, Du, Xiaoyu and Zhu, Yufang. 2017. "Progress of the 3D Printing Technology for Biomaterials." *Journal of University of Shanghai for Science and Technology* 39 (5): 473–83 and 489. https://doi.org/10.13255/j.cnki.jusst.2017.05.011

# 7 Biological and Chemical Stability of Coatings

*Fatima Jalid and Aravi Muzaffar*
National Institute of Technology, Srinagar, India

## 7.1 INTRODUCTION

Magnesium (Mg) alloys have received considerable attention in the biomedical field for clinical applications owing to their excellent mechanical properties, biocompatibility, and biodegradability (Yang, Cui, and Lee 2011; Tian and Liu 2015). Mg alloys exhibit high strength and their elastic modulus and density are close to that of natural bone, thus, making them a viable option for implant materials (Tian and Liu 2015). The density of Mg is 1.74 g/cm$^3$, which is equivalent to that of natural bone ranging from 1.8 g/cm$^3$ to 2.1 g/cm$^3$, whereas the elastic modulus of Mg and human bone is 45 GPa and 40–57 GPa, respectively (Tian and Liu 2015). However, the major limitation posed by the usage of Mg alloys in a physiological environment is that of corrosion, as they show high degradation rates, especially in the early stages of the healing process (Zhang et al. 2020). This results in subsequent loss of mechanical stability of Mg alloys which eventually leads to premature rupture of the implant. On corrosion, the formation of loose magnesium hydroxide (Mg(OH)$_2$) as degradation product takes places, which is easily destroyed by the presence of corrosive chloride anions found in body fluid in its interlayer space (Tian and Liu 2015; Tong et al. 2022; Singh et al. 2023). Additionally, the corrosion of Mg alloys produces hydrogen which increases the pH of the local tissues. This rise in alkalinity ultimately harms the surrounding tissues, in turn, hampering the healing process (Wu, Ibrahim, and Chu 2013). The overall corrosion reaction of Mg in aqueous medium is given as follows:

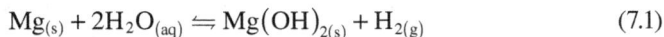

$$Mg_{(s)} + 2H_2O_{(aq)} \leftrightharpoons Mg(OH)_{2(s)} + H_{2(g)} \tag{7.1}$$

This may be further divided into the following reactions:

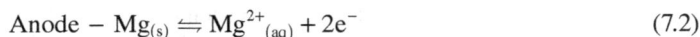

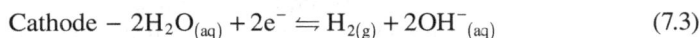

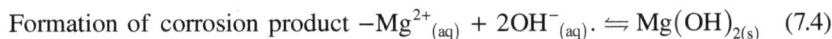

$$Anode - Mg_{(s)} \leftrightharpoons Mg^{2+}_{(aq)} + 2e^- \tag{7.2}$$

$$Cathode - 2H_2O_{(aq)} + 2e^- \leftrightharpoons H_{2(g)} + 2OH^-_{(aq)} \tag{7.3}$$

$$Formation\ of\ corrosion\ product - Mg^{2+}_{(aq)} + 2OH^-_{(aq)}. \leftrightharpoons Mg(OH)_{2(s)} \tag{7.4}$$

DOI: 10.1201/9781003400462-7

In order to combat the degradation of Mg alloys, surface modifications are considered to be an attractive approach to tackle their early degradation as the deposition of coating over Mg alloys allows for modulation of corrosion rates such that the implant does not show any failure (Tong et al. 2022). In principle, the coating layer prevents the corrosive ions from diffusing to the magnesium alloy substrate, thus diminishing the corrosion rate. As these materials are to be used in implants and stents, the surface modifications should exhibit the requisite biological and chemical properties which essentially is the corrosion resistance and biocompatibility in the biological environment. For surface biomodifications, the alloy should meet certain perquisites, i.e., self-cleaning, self-healing, bioadaptable, biocompatible, biodegradable, bioactive, antibacterial, etc. (Tan, Balan, and Birbilis 2021). The alloy should be nontoxic and ions released from the coatings must not harm the surrounding cells, tissues, blood circulation, and immune system and also not cause any metal allergy. Furthermore, it should be degradable and absorbable inside the human body. It must also exhibit biocompatibility with the coating material having the required bioactivity so that the cells can easily adhere to and spread over the surface, which will speed up the healing process. Most importantly, the degradation rate of the alloy must be tailored such that it meets the requisite healing rate.

Surface modifications of Mg alloys are classified into metallic coatings, inorganic coatings, polymer coatings, and composite coatings (Tong et al. 2022). The methods involved in deposition of these coatings include mechanical methods, magnetron sputtering, chemical conversion, ion implantation technology, micro-arc oxidation, sol–gel, layer-by-layer assembly, etc. (Tong et al. 2022). The primary focus of the process of applying metallic coatings is on deposition of metal oxide and metal hydroxide layer onto Mg alloy which act as an inert phase, thereby enhancing the resistance to degradation. Besides, layered double hydroxide (LDH) coatings are also employed for combating corrosion, as they trap the chloride ions (Guo et al. 2018; Tan, Balan, and Birbilis 2021). Inorganic surface modifications include the nonmetallic coatings of magnesium fluoride ($MgF_2$), phosphate, and graphene oxide (GO) coating. The protectiveness by $MgF_2$ layers does not hold for long time which is attributable to the presence of cracks and holes in the coatings. Polymer coatings are further classified into natural polymer and synthetic polymer coatings. These show enhanced biocompatibility due to their semblance with soft biological tissues (Tong et al. 2022). Lastly, composite coatings are explored, which are a combination of a number of coatings and usually consist of an inner layer that is firmly attached to the substrate, while the second layer consists of coatings displaying better biological properties (Lin et al. 2013; Li et al. 2018; Yu et al. 2018; Liu et al. 2021).

On the whole, surface modifications are seen as the way through for applications of Mg alloys in biomedical field owing to the enhanced biological compatibility and resistance toward corrosion. However, their chemical and biological characteristics and in vivo behavior are what dictates their applicability in implants and stents. Their chemical and biological stability may also be tuned by altering the chemical constitution of coating, thickness of the layer, or combining two or more layers in order to achieve the desired properties.

## 7.2 METALLIC COATINGS

Surface modifications involving metallic coatings primarily consist of deposition of metal oxide and metal hydroxide layer which act as an inert phase imparting protection to Mg alloys by enhancing the resistance toward corrosion.

### 7.2.1 METAL OXIDE COATINGS

Metal oxide coatings over the Mg alloys mainly comprise magnesium oxide, titanium dioxide, and zirconium oxide. For coatings of MgO, the preparation methods include micro-arc oxidation (MAO), anionic oxidation (AO), and steam oxidation (SO). The formation of MgO coatings by means of anodic electrodeposition has been found to boost the corrosion resistance as compared to bare metallic Mg as well as Mg alloy (Lei et al. 2010b, 2010a). Xu et al. conducted a comparative study in the enhancement of corrosion resistance and biocompatibility of surface-modified Mg alloys by means of SO and MAO methods of deposition of MgO coating (Xu et al. 2020). The coatings formed by both the procedures were observed to combat the initial degradation of Mg implants; however, the MAO coating exhibited better biocompatibility and osteoinductivity (Xu et al. 2020). Furthermore, a number of studies are indicative of the fact that using concentrated electrolytes for MAO coatings results in improved resistance to corrosion owing to the increased compactness and volume fraction of coatings as well as decrease in porosity (Barchiche et al. 2007; Ko, Namgung, and Shin 2010). Another study based on MAO coating of MgO over AZ31 Mg alloy showed good cytocompatibility and anticorrosive properties when tested in simulated body fluid (Jian et al. 2019). Overall, SO and MAO coatings show better corrosion resistance than AO coatings; however, the biocompatibility of MAO coatings has been observed to be the highest among the three.

Besides MgO coatings, $TiO_2$ coatings prepared by magnetron sputtering and atomic layer deposition (ALD) have also been experimentally found to show reduced corrosion rates and good biocompatibility. $TiO_2$ coating prepared over MgZn alloy by magnetron sputtering has shown a two order of magnitude decrease in the corrosion current density as well as improved biocompatibility in terms of reduced hemolysis and platelet adhesion, and increased endothelial cell viability and adhesion (Hou et al. 2020). Another study based on $TiO_2$ nanotube coating over AZ91D Mg alloys by magnetron sputtering $TiO_2$ has shown to effectively decrease the degradation rate of magnesium alloy (Li et al. 2017). Kania et al. showed that $TiO_2$ coating over $MgCa_2Zn_1Gd_3$ by ALD effectively protects this alloy from corrosion, with greater thickness of the film showing greater resistance, as depicted in Figure 7.1 (Kania, Szindler, and Szindler 2021). A comparative analysis between $TiO_2$ coatings over AZ31 Mg alloy produced by magnetron sputtering and ALD by means of potentiodynamic polarization and hydrogen evolution tests showed higher corrosion protection by ALD owing to superior integrity of the coating so formed, with smoother surfaces showing better degradation resistance than rough ones (Peron et al. 2020). To enhance the biocompatibility of $TiO_2$-based coatings, these are clubbed with organic coating material or polymeric coatings (Tang et al. 2020; Karthega et al. 2021).

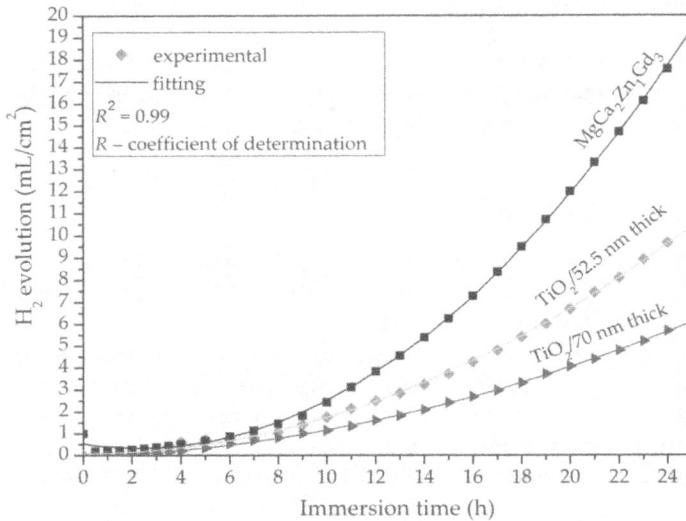

**FIGURE 7.1** Hydrogen evolution volume as a function of immersion time in Ringer's solution for $TiO_2$ thin films deposited onto the $MgCa_2Zn_1Gd_3$ alloy and bare alloy (Kania, Szindler, and Szindler 2021).

$ZrO_2$ has been widely explored as a biomedical implant material due to its excellent mechanical properties – ability to osseointegrate, high strength, high compression resistance, and resistance to crack propagation as well as good biocompatibility and antibacterial properties (Sennerby et al. 2005; Langhoff et al. 2008; Al-Radha et al. 2012; Tong et al. 2022). $ZrO_2$ coating over AZ31B Mg alloy has been found to inhibit the rate of corrosion as tested in simulated body fluids (SBF), with the porous structure of $ZrO_2$ further enabling the bond between the bone and implant (Gao et al. 2018). $ZrO_2$ nanofilm deposited over Mg-Sr alloy by means of ALD has shown effective reduction in corrosion whereby the presence of $ZrO_2$ led to an enhancement in the activity and adhesion of osteoblasts to the alloy surface as shown by cell culture experiments (Yang et al. 2017). Further, similar to $TiO_2$ coatings, with increased thickness of $ZrO_2$ which was controlled by the number of ALD cycles, the resistance to degradation is also observed to increase (Yang et al. 2017). $ZrO_2$ coating deposited over AZ91D Mg alloys via electrophoretic deposition technique has been found to significantly combat the bio-corrosion as per the in vitro tests conducted in SBF solution (Amiri, Mohammadi, and Afshar 2017). A study comparing the MgO and $ZrO_2$ coating over AZ31 Mg alloy by MAO showed improved anticorrosion properties attributable to its higher density and homogeneity (Wang et al. 2018). Further, the in vitro cytotoxicity tests showed that the presence of $ZrO_2$ did not induce any cytotoxic reaction in L-929 cells, thus promoting cell growth (Wang et al. 2018). Another study comparing the two coatings over AM50 Mg alloy revealed that the resistance of MgO coatings was higher than $ZrO_2$ for 0.5 h, after which it faced much higher deterioration (Liang et al. 2009). As opposed to that, the $ZrO_2$ coating exhibited higher stability in the 50-h immersion tests due to higher microstructural integrity

(Liang et al. 2009). Apart from pure zirconia coatings, the addition of other coatings, for instance, poly(L-lactic acid) (PLLA), $Y_2O_3$, CaO, etc., has shown considerable enhancement in the resistance toward degradation and improved cell viability (Liu et al. 2018; Istrate et al. 2020).

## 7.2.2 METAL HYDROXIDE COATINGS

The metal hydroxide coatings are focused on the deposition of dense $Mg(OH)_2$ layer over Mg alloys in order to accentuate its corrosion resistance. Loose $Mg(OH)_2$ layer is also formed as a product of corrosion of Mg alloy (Equation 7.5); however, it is easily destroyed by chloride ions, thereby enhancing the corrosion rate. Thus, making the layer denser can potentially provide resistance to corrosion.

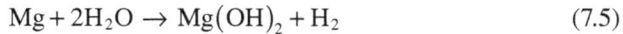

$$Mg + 2H_2O \rightarrow Mg(OH)_2 + H_2 \tag{7.5}$$

The traditional method for the preparation of $Mg(OH)_2$ coating over Mg alloys is the hydrothermal treatment (Zhu et al. 2011; Feng et al. 2013; Xu et al. 2017). Protective $Mg(OH)_2$ layer synthesized by one step hydrothermal treatment over ZK60 Mg alloy exhibited improved resistance to degradation (Xu et al. 2017). Similar observations were made when AZ31 Mg alloy was coated with $Mg(OH)_2$ (Zhu et al. 2011). Feng et al. also evaluated the performance of $Mg(OH)_2$ film over AZ91 alloy whereby they observed the formation of compact and uniform films resulting in superior corrosion resistance (Feng et al. 2013). To further accentuate the performance of $Mg(OH)_2$, it has been combined with other coatings showing better biocompatibility. The introduction of $Mg(OH)_2$ particles into PLLA has shown a decline in corrosion rate while limiting the formation of gas pockets under the polymer layer over hydrofluoric acid pretreated Mg-Nd-Zn-Zr alloy, thus resulting in improved adhesion of coating (Shi et al. 2017). The coating so formed exhibited excellent cytocompatibility in terms of proliferation of endothelial cells (Shi et al. 2017). A composite coating of $Mg(OH)_2$/graphene oxide/hydroxyapatite developed over ZQ71 Mg alloy has shown enhanced bonding strength, hydrophilicity, and significantly reduced rate of degradation of the alloy (Yuan et al. 2022). Furthermore, the coated alloy has increased cell viability, bone regeneration, and antibacterial activity leading to a more biocompatible implant material (Yuan et al. 2022). Surface modifications comprising Mg–phenolic networks have shown improved in vitro osteocompatibility which was observed to rise with increasing concentration of Mg. The corrosion resistance was noted to be three times as that of uncoated samples achieved by mitigating the formation of gas pockets around the implantation area (Asgari et al. 2019). Zhu et al. also observed a significant enhancement in the resistance to corrosion upon the addition of a thin film of silicate over $Mg(OH)_2$-coated AZ31 Mg alloy (Zhu et al. 2019). Besides this increase, the silicate film also led to an improvement in the hydrophilicity of the alloy (Zhu et al. 2019).

Another category of metal hydroxide coatings is the layered double hydroxide (LDH) coating which consists mainly of the hydrotalcite or hydrotalcite like compounds, with divalent or trivalent metal cations positioned in the octahedral holes of alternate pairs of hydroxides planes (Guo et al. 2018). The generalized formula of LDHs is $[M^{2+}_{(1-x)}M^{3+}_x(OH)_2]^{x+}(A^{m-})_{x/m}/.nH_2O$, where $M^{2+}$, $M^{3+}$, $A^{m-}$, and $m$ represent a divalent metal cation, a trivalent metal cation, a layer of intercalated anions between two cation layers, and the charge of the inter-layer anion, respectively (Guo et al. 2018; Tan et al. 2021). The alternating double-layered structure of LDH is what traps the corrosive anion by replacing the intercalated anions, thus limiting the rate of corrosion. Additionally, the ions replaced from the anion layer form stable precipitates over the coating upon binding with the metal ions. The rate of decline in the corrosion is dictated by the ion-exchange rate of the intercalated ions. It therefore is more suitable to have LDH coatings over anions possessing greater corrosion resistance, self-cleaning, self-healing, antibacterial properties, and biocompatibility for applications as surface modifications in the biomedical field (Singh et al. 2023). Zn-Al LDH coatings over AZ31 Mg alloy with different intercalated anions showed corrosion resistance in the following order: $ZnAl-VO_4^{3-}-LDH > ZnAl-MoO_4^{2-}-LDH > ZnAl-PO_4^{3-}-LDH > ZnAl-Cl^{-}-LDH > ZnAl-NO_3^{-}-LDH$ (Tang et al. 2019). The excellent performance of $ZnAl-VO_4^{3-}-LDH$ is attributable to the large basal spacing distance which facilitates the increased ability to release anions (Tang et al. 2019). The most common synthesis methods for the in situ growth of LDH films over Mg alloys are hydrothermal treatment and dip coating. Chen et al. conducted an in situ growth of Mg-Fe LDH coating with $CO_3^{2-}$ anions over MgCa alloy exploring the effect of temperature, time, and pH. Whereas all the coatings did bring down the corrosion current, the coating prepared at 55°C, at pH 11 for 24 h was found to be best (Chen et al. 2021). An Ag-MgAl-LDH coating produced over Mg-3Zn-0.5Zr-0.5Sr alloy was found to exhibit increased resistance to corrosion with enhanced cytocompatibility of MC3TC cells and antibacterial response (Zhao et al. 2020). Zhang et al. fabricated a Mg-Fe LDH film over Mg-Nd-Zn-Zr alloy which showed a reduction in the corrosion current density while simultaneously enhancing the biocompatibility reflected in terms of higher degree of spreading of MC3T3-E1 cells with improved adhesiveness (Zhang et al. 2019). Modifications in the LDH coatings have shown further enhancement in the biological front with improved cytocompatibility and biodegradability (Peng et al. 2017, 2018; Sun et al. 2020; Wu et al. 2020). Sun et al. fabricated a composite coating of Mg-Al LDH and PLLA which showed a reduction of corrosion current density by three orders of magnitude as compared to bare AZ31 alloy (Sun et al. 2020). The addition of PLLA to Mg-Al LDH was shown to prolong the service life of the coating (Sun et al. 2020). Besides, the biocompatibility toward mouse embryonic fibroblasts (NIH3T3) was also observed to increase (Sun et al. 2020). A similar study by the same group revealed analogous results for Mg-Al LDH sealed by poly-L-glutamic acid whereby the cytocompatibility of NIH3T3 cell line was significantly improved (Wu et al. 2020). Peng et al. explored the sealing of pores of plasma electrolytic oxidation (PEO) coating over AZ31 Mg alloy by means of Mg-Al LDH coating (Peng et al. 2017). The LDH coating not only enhanced the corrosion resistance but also improved the cell adhesion and proliferation of rat bone marrow stem cells, reducing the hemolysis rate along with favorable drug delivery ability (Peng et al. 2017). The authors further incorporated Zn into the composite coating which led to a further decline in the corrosion current density (Peng et al. 2018). Moreover, the addition of Zn resulted in stronger antimicrobial ability, no cytotoxicity, and significantly improved osteogenic activity (Peng et al. 2018).

## 7.3 NONMETALLIC COATINGS

Surface modifications involving inorganic nonmetallic coatings primarily consist of $MgF_2$, phosphate, and graphene oxide coating.

### 7.3.1 MgF$_2$ Coatings

$MgF_2$ coatings are deposited chiefly by traditional method of fluorination treatment wherein hydrofluoric acid is used to form a protective layer of $MgF_2$ over the surface of the alloy, given by Equation 7.6. This reaction shows a negative Gibbs free energy change, indicating the predominance of formation of product as noted by Wagman et al. (1989).

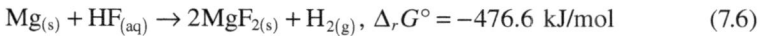

$$Mg_{(s)} + HF_{(aq)} \rightarrow 2MgF_{2(s)} + H_{2(g)}, \Delta_r G^\circ = -476.6 \text{ kJ/mol} \tag{7.6}$$

These coatings are widely employed in biomedical field owing to its compact structure and compatibility with the base alloy. Li et al. deposited an $MgF_2$ layer over Mg-Ca alloy by means of vacuum evaporation deposition, and the protective layer so formed showed lower rates of corrosion as tested by immersion and electrochemical tests (Li et al. 2013). Human osteosarcoma cells and mouse osteoblast-like cells showed enhanced adherence and spreading over the coated alloys as opposed to uncoated ones (Li et al. 2013). Similar results were reported by Drynda et al. for smooth muscle cells over Mg-Ca alloys, showing improved degradation resistance as well as in vitro biocompatibility (Drynda et al. 2010). Another study by Drynda et al. over Mg-Ca alloys of varying compositions having $MgF_2$ coatings showed a decrease in the rate of corrosion (Drynda et al. 2013). The alloys when tested using in vivo subcutaneous mouse model did not exhibit any inflammatory reactions or extensive proliferating effects, thus establishing the biocompatibility (Drynda et al. 2013). Coatings of $MgF_2$ over Mg-Nd-Zn-Zr alloy have also shown improvement in the resistance to corrosion as well as good antiplatelet adhesion and decrease in homolysis ratio (Mao et al. 2013). Fluoride-coated AZ31B Mg alloys have revealed considerable improvement in the degradation of alloy while exhibiting good osteogenic activity in a rabbit model with reduced inflammatory reaction, as depicted in Figure 7.2 (Sun et al. 2016). The performance of Mg-3Zn-0.8Zr rods coated with $MgF_2$ implanted in the femur of white rabbits have been reported by Sun et al. and compared with the uncoated samples and samples coated with calcium phosphates. The results show that after three months of implantation, the sample coated with $MgF_2$ has the least corrosion attack and volume loss (Figure 7.3), with enhanced cell adherence and formation of new bone mass (Sun et al. 2013). These studies elucidate the effective role of $MgF_2$ coating over Mg alloys implants toward corrosion resistance in biological environments. However, fluoride coatings display inadequate stability with prolonged immersion in physiological media (Fintová et al. 2019).

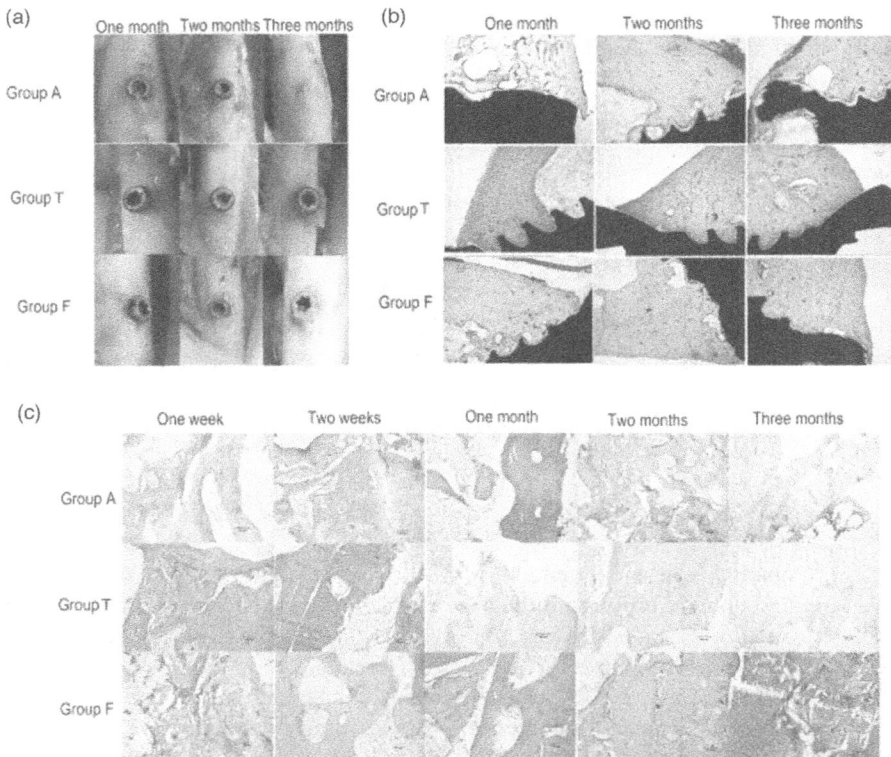

**FIGURE 7.2** Effects of implantation in Group A, untreated AZ31 magnesium alloy screw; group T, titanium alloy screw; group F, AZ31 magnesium alloy screw coated with fluorine at different intervals of implantation. (a) Specimens of bone tissue reaction around implantations. (b) Hard tissue section of the interface of implantation and bone. (c) Hematoxylin-eosin (HE)-stained sections surrounding implantation (Sun et al. 2016).

### 7.3.2 PHOSPHATE COATINGS

Phosphate coatings have shown great potential as surface modifications in Mg alloys for biomedical applications as their chemical structure is similar to that of natural bone (Liu et al. 2018), with good stability at higher temperatures and insolubility in water. Particularly, it is the salts of calcium-phosphate, which include brushite, octacalcium phosphate, tricalcium phosphate, and hydroxyapatite (HAP), that have been widely explored as bone implant materials as these involve formation of a layer which is similar to the mineral phase of natural bone, thus inducing the growth of bone tissue (Yin et al. 2017). A study by Wang et al. showed that HAP coating over ZK60 Mg alloys promoted resistance to corrosion in neutral environment as determined by immersion and electrochemical tests (Wang et al. 2021). Additionally, the cell culture experiments performed over the Ca-P coated alloys exhibited improved biocompatibility (Wang et al. 2021). Gao et al. also observed the improvement of biocompatibility and corrosion resistance of Ca-P (dicalcium

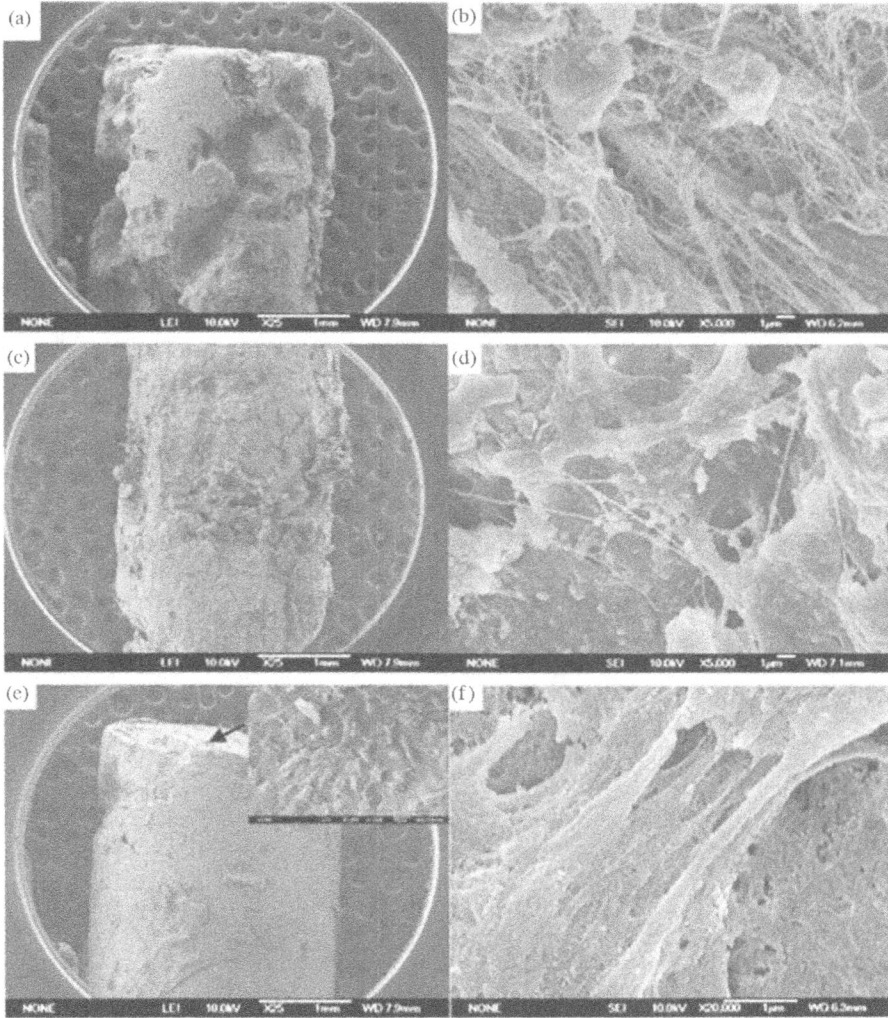

**FIGURE 7.3** Images of untreated (a and b), phosphate coated (c and d), and MgF$_2$ coated (e and f) implants of the alloy Mg-3Zn-0.8Zr after three months of implantation in white rabbits (Sun et al. 2013).

phosphate dihydrate)-coated AZ60 magnesium alloy, showing an in vivo degradation rate required to match the bone-healing process (Figure 7.4) (Gao, Su, and Qin 2021). Further, the coating enhanced the cell adhesion, proliferation, and differentiation of osteoblasts promoting new bone formation without inducing any adverse effect (Gao, Su, and Qin 2021). Another research based on Ca-P coatings over Mg alloys demonstrated better surface cytocompatibility and a great enhancement in the osteoconductivity and osteogenesis in the first four weeks post-implantation (Xu et al. 2009). A study reporting the micro-computed tomography images of an in vivo study of Ca-P-coated AZ60 Mg alloy showed threefold reduction in corrosion rate as compared to bare alloys (Xiao et al. 2013). The osteointegration response of Ca-P coatings is largely dependent upon the surface morphology whereby it has been observed that nanoplate- and nanosphere-like structures greatly enhance the cell attachment compared to whisker or flake-like structures (Lin, Wu, and Chang 2014). Despite the controlled morphology, the fabrication of these coatings free from the fragile surface and spatial defects is still a challenge. Toward this, doping the Ca-P-coated Mg alloys with other elements and formation of composite coatings have been observed to further enhance the corrosion resistance as well as the biocompatibility of the implant (Bakhsheshi-Rad et al. 2014; Zhou et al. 2020).

### 7.3.3   GRAPHENE OXIDE COATINGS

The GO coatings are observed to be chemically inert and resistant toward permeation of corrosive ions, resulting in a boost in corrosion resistance (Plachá and Jampilek 2019). The two-dimensional single layer structure leads to high surface area which makes it widely applicable in fields of drug delivery, tissue engineering, and cancer therapy (Xia et al. 2019). The functional groups present in GO coatings – epoxy, carboxyl and hydroxyl – can capture, anchor, and immobilize polymers and various biologically active substances, thus exhibiting the requisite biocompatibility in terms of inhibiting the antiviral, antibacterial, or anticancer activities (Tiwari et al.

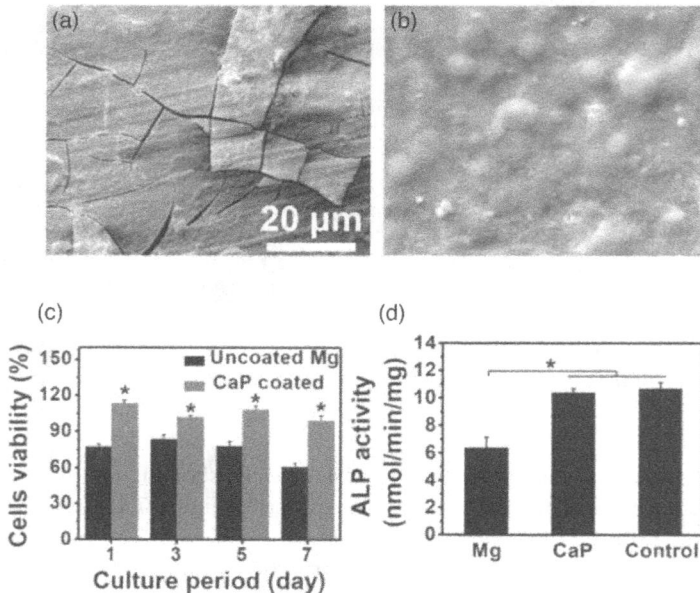

**FIGURE 7.4**   Osteoblast cell morphologies after three days of culture on (a) uncoated and (b) CaP-coated samples, (c) cell viability, and (d) alkaline phosphate activity when cells were cultured with sample extracts. *$p < 0.05$, compared to uncoated group (Gao et al. 2021).

2019). These also result in improved hydrophilicity and dispersibility (Lawal 2019). Furthermore, it has shown great potential in biomedical field, particularly in the facets of bone repair and augmentation, and cell proliferation (Akhavan 2016; Zhang et al. 2018). GO has reported appreciable compatibility with the red blood cells and organs in the body and no pathological changes have been noted in blood circulation for a long time (Zhang et al. 2011). Maqsood et al. noted an enhancement in the resistance to degradation in GO-coated AZ31B Mg alloy as compared to bare Mg alloys, thus showing the potential of GO coatings in modulating the corrosion rate for applications in biomedical field (Maqsood et al. 2020). Another study explored the formation of reduced GO coating over Mg sheets by means of electrochemical and chemical methods, wherein both methods exhibited a significant decline in the corrosion rates with chemically modified alloys showing a reduction of 80% (Fernández et al. 2019). The major drawback faced with GO coatings over Mg alloys is the weak interfacial bonding strength, which may result in premature detachment of the protective GO layer (Liu et al. 2015; Zhao et al. 2020). To overcome this predicament, GO may be combined with other coatings to enhance the bonding strength. In this direction, Shuai et al. used $TiO_2$ nanoparticles deposited on the surface of GO coating over AZ61 Mg alloy which led to a significant improvement in slowing down the corrosion rate by a factor of 25.6% as compared to AZ61-GO biocomposite (Shuai et al. 2020). Thus, composite coatings are the way forward in the application of GO coatings over Mg alloys.

## 7.4 POLYMER COATINGS

Coatings showing good biodegradability and biocompatibility comprise polymer coatings; however, these pose limitation of weak binding force to the substrate and restricted mechanical properties. They are classified into natural polymer and synthetic polymer coatings.

### 7.4.1 NATURAL POLYMER COATINGS

Natural polymers inherently possess biological activity, which serves as templates for cell attachment and growth, and can stimulate cellular response in the meanwhile. Owing to their excellent biocompatibility and bioactivity, natural polymers have been utilized in biomedical fields for a long period. Natural polymer coatings employed for surface modifications of Mg-based alloys for applications in the biomedical field mainly consist of hyaluronic acid (HA), collagen, and chitosan.

#### 7.4.1.1 Hyaluronic Acid

HA is a biologically derived natural polymer consisting of repeating poly-disaccharide structure which exhibits good antibacterial properties (Kim et al. 2019). Being one of the constituents of extracellular matrix where it is involved in cell adhesion, wound repair, proliferation, and differentiation, it therefore is nonallergenic, showing minimal side effects upon introduction inside the human body (Tong et al. 2022). Experimentally, covalent grafting of HA-lysozyme (HA-LZ) coating onto the silane-coated AZ31 Mg has been observed to boost the osteoinductive and antibacterial effects as compared to LZ coated and uncoated AZ31 alloys, thus improving the biocompatibility of the implant (Agarwal et al. 2017). The coating of polydopamine (PDA)/ HA over the Mg-Zn-Y-Nd alloy has shown effective protection of the substrate under in vivo conditions (Li et al. 2020). Furthermore, the authors observed that the PDA/HA coating with HA molecular weight of $1 \times 10^5$ Da showed better corrosion resistance, enhanced blood compatibility, anti-hyperplasia, and anti-inflammation functions than the bare substrate (Li et al. 2020). Kim et al. evaluated the performance of cerium and HA multilayer coating which showed that $Ce(OH)_3/CeO_2$ penetrating HA had a self-healing ability and enhanced resistance to local damage and initial corrosion, thus imparting better biodegradation to the magnesium implant (Kim et al. 2020).

### 7.4.1.2 Collagen
Collagen formulates one of the main constituents of extracellular matrix of bones, tendons, and ligaments that enables for cell attachment and migration, and provides mechanical support (Nudelman et al. 2010). The protein finds applications as coating material for implants due to its ability to enhance tissue integration between the surface of the implant and the surrounding tissues (Tong et al. 2022). The interaction of collagen monomer with Mg and AZ31 alloy was studied by Zhao et al. wherein they observed that base materials with higher surface roughness resulted in stronger absorption of collagen and higher similarity to natural bone collagen, although with compromised bone cell attachment (Zhao and Zhu 2014). They noted that collagen fibrils form on the surface once the collagen concentration reaches a minimum threshold level, which is further affected by the pH and the assembly time (N. Zhao and Zhu 2014). A study on the coatings of HAP/collagen over AZ31 Mg alloys showed significant drop in corrosion of coated alloys which was measured by the amount of $H_2$ produced (Bao et al. 2017). Additionally, the hydrogen evolution for HAP/collagen coating was lesser than that of pure HAP coating, hinting at the role of collagen toward better biocompatibility (Bao et al. 2017). A similar study reported enhancement in corrosion resistance upon coating AZ31 Mg alloy with poly(L-lactic acid)/hydroxyapatite/collagen (PLLA/HCA) layer which was determined from electrochemical measurements (Wang et al. 2013). The polarization analysis further indicated toward a drop in corrosion with increasing mass ratio of PLLA/HAC as compared to pure PLLA, suggesting better mechanical properties upon introduction of HAC to PLLA (Wang et al. 2013).

### 7.4.1.3 Chitosan
Chitosan is obtained upon the removal of acetyl group from chitin and consists of glucoside linkages between glucosamine and *N*-acetylglucosamine units (Roman, Ostafe, and Isvoran 2020). Chitosan has many physiological functions, such as bacteriostasis, biocompatibility, biodegradability, anticancer, and nontoxicity. Further, its decomposition does not affect the pH in physiological environment (Singh et al. 2023). Moreover, it shows a good antibacterial property due to the large amount of positive charges on its surface (Xu et al. 2018). These properties make it biocompatible for applications in biomedical field, in addition to enhancing

the corrosion resistance. In vitro tests have shown that chitosan-coated magnesium alloys exhibited lower immersion corrosion rate, pH values of the SBF, and the released metal ion concentration as compared to uncoated alloys (Liangjian et al. 2015). Another study exploring the role of chitosan coating on Mg-6%Zn-10%Ca$_3$(PO$_4$)$_2$ implant by means of in vivo tests revealed lower metal ion concentration in the venous blood of New Zealand rabbits as opposed to uncoated alloy (J. Zhao et al. 2015). Chitosan has also been found to attribute self-healing ability to shield Mg alloys from biocorrosion (Jia et al. 2016). The active corrosion inhibition in Mg alloys with coatings of nanosized cerium oxides containing chitosan multilayers was observed to be lower than bare alloys as indicated by immersion degradation tests with respect to Mg$^{2+}$ release, pH alteration, crack development, and scanning Kelvin potential (Jia et al. 2016).

## 7.4.2 SYNTHETIC POLYMER COATINGS

Synthetic polymer coatings mainly comprise polylactic acid (PLA), poly(lactic-*co*-glycolic) acid (PLGA), polycaprolactone (PCL), and PDA. As compared to the natural polymer coatings, their biocompatibility is not as good due to formation of highly acidic products upon degradation (Tong et al. 2022).

### 7.4.2.1 Polylactic Acid

PLA is a lactic acid polymer that has been researched extensively for applications in medical field – surgical devices, tissue engineering, bone fixation, and drug delivery applications – owing to biocompatibility which is attributable to formation of non-toxic products upon degradation in physiological environment (Nair and Laurencin 2007). Alabbasi et al. explored the effect of coating AZ91 Mg alloy with a coating of PLA by means of electrochemical impedance spectroscopy in SBF whereby they observed significant enhancement in the resistance to degradation, although the resistance decreased with increasing exposure time (Alabbasi, Liyanaarachchi, and Kannan 2012). They also noted that the resistance increased with increasing PLA thickness, but led to weaker adhesion, thus directing toward the use of a thin film of PLA (~2–3 μm) showing a balance between the opposing forces (Figure 7.5) (Alabbasi, Liyanaarachchi, and Kannan 2012). To overcome the drawbacks of poor strength and adhesion posed by PLA coatings, multifunctional composite layers consisting of PLA have also been explored (Zhang et al. 2017). A study in this direction used a bilayer coating of PLA/brushite over a Mg-Nd-Zn-Zr alloy which showed high interfacial bonding strength, enhanced cytocompatibility, and in vitro tests indicated a considerable reduction in the resistance to corrosion (Zhang et al. 2017). Reinforced composites consisting of PLA with high-strength Mg alloy wires have shown excellent strength, toughness, and impact strength due to the unidirectional reinforcing in addition to prevention of corrosion, thus being a promising material in load-bearing applications (Li et al. 2015). A coating of nano-amorphous magnesium phosphate and PLA over AZ31 Mg alloy has shown significant reduction in corrosion in the SBF as well as enhanced bioactivity, suggested by the formation of massive bone-like apatite precipitates over the coated implant (Ren, Babaie, and Bhaduri 2018).

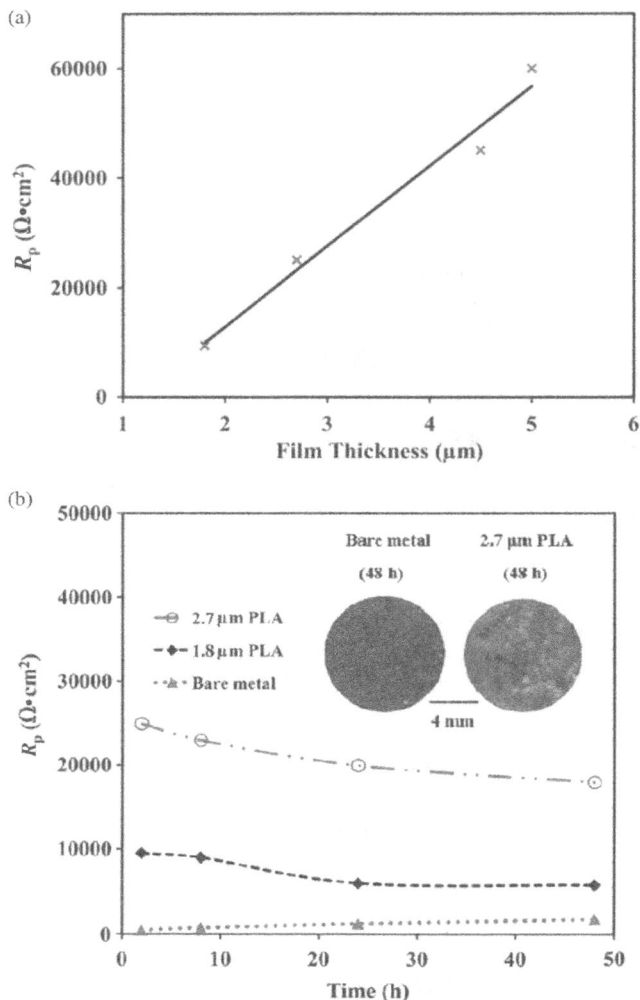

**FIGURE 7.5** (a) Polarization resistance of PLA-coated (different thickness) alloy samples after a 2-h immersion in SBF. (b) Polarization resistance of AZ91 magnesium alloy and PLA-coated magnesium alloy samples, after different immersion intervals in SBF (Alabbasi et al. 2012).

## 7.4.2.2 Poly(lactic-*co*-glycolic) Acid

PLGA is formed by the random polymerization of lactic acid and glycolic acid and is the most commonly used copolymer of PLA. It shows good biocompatibility, drug release effects, and controllable degradability (Zhang et al. 2014). The possibility of alteration of lactic acid/glycolic acid ratio in PLGA opens opportunity to tailor its physical, chemical, as well as mechanical properties, which further allows for tuning its resistance to degradation, thus making it a preferred choice in biomedical applications (Zhu, Liu, and Ngai 2022). The application of PLGA coating over Mg-6Zn alloy showed a significant decrease in the corrosion rate as measured by immersion tests and electrochemical tests, in addition to enhanced cell adhesion, spreading, and migration when compared with the bare alloy (Li et al. 2010). Micro-arc oxidation sealed with PLGA also exhibited improved inhibition to corrosion, coupled with enhanced mechanical stability (Chen et al. 2019). PLGA coatings over two Mg alloys – AZ31 and Mg4Y – showed reduced corrosion for three days, beyond which there was no reduction in corrosion rate due to the onset of aqueous corrosion attack (Ostrowski et al. 2013). The coatings also showed gas pocket formations which led to eventual detachment of the coating from the alloy surface (Ostrowski et al. 2013). Despite efficient corrosion inhibition of PLGA coatings, these show high susceptibility toward hydrolysis forming lactic acid and glycolic acid, entrapment of $H_2$ during in vitro immersion, and poor adhesion toward Mg substrate, which can potentially be improved by introduction of other components. A PLGA and gallic acid coating with gallic acid sandwiched between two PLGA layers over ZK60 Mg alloy has been observed to show uniform film structure with enhanced degradation resistance when used as coronary artery stent (Lin, Lee, and Yeh 2020). As compared to PLGA, the sandwich coating led to promotion of endothelial cell proliferation, significant suppression of smooth muscle cells over-proliferation, anti-hemolysis ability, and antioxidation effects compared to PLGA (Lin, Lee, and Yeh 2020). PLGA also finds applications in prevention of implant-related infections after an orthopedic surgery by incorporating a sustained release of antibiotics as has been observed in coating enoxacin with PLGA on a porous pure Mg scaffold which led to effective inhibition of bacterial adhesion and biofilm formation (Li et al. 2016).

### 7.4.2.3 Polycaprolactone

PCL is a highly explored surface modification for Mg alloys exhibiting good biocompatibility and biodegradability. Huang et al. studied the electrografting of PCL over Mg-Zn-Y-Nd alloy and observed reduction in the degradation of Mg alloy in SBF, and better cytocompatibility in terms of improved cell adhesion and enhancement in the ability to maintain cell viability (Huang et al. 2021). The corrosion resistance for the electrografted PCL coating was noted to be higher as compared to that prepared from traditional methods (Huang et al. 2021). Further, electrospun PCL over AZ31B Mg alloy has exhibited lower rates of corrosion as well as enhanced cytocompatibility, which was measured in terms of cell viability of osteoblastic MC3T3-E1 cells (Cusanno et al. 2020). Electrochemical tests of copper-based metal–organic frameworks incorporated with PCL have also shown a reduction in the corrosion current density by three orders of magnitude (Zheng et al. 2019). However, PCL coatings show weak adhesion with Mg substrates due to a limited number of oxygen sites in PCL structure; recent studies have therefore suggested addition of inorganic components in order to enhance the adhesion. In this direction, a research based on formation of composite coatings of PCL/HAP has shown a tenfold reduction in the rate of corrosion as opposed to HAP-coated AZ31 alloy (Chunyan et al. 2022). Moreover, the addition of PCL to HAP coating has displayed improved cytocompatibility measured in terms of better bone marrow–derived mesenchymal stem cells compatibility (Chunyan et al. 2022).

However, there is scope for improvement in the antibacterial properties for applications in the biomedical field (Chunyan et al. 2022).

### 7.4.2.4 Polydopamine

PDA is formed upon oxidation of dopamine and is widely employed for the surface modification of Mg alloys owing to the presence of diverse functional groups – catechol, amine, and imine – which facilitates adherence to all kinds of substates, by means of covalently immobilizing biomolecules and anchoring metal ions, without altering the bulk properties of the bare alloy (Jia et al. 2019). A number of studies have shown that coating a PDA layer can effectively enhance the attachment, proliferation, and migration of endothelial cells (Yang et al. 2012; Zhang et al. 2021). The deposition of PDA coating over Mg alloys has shown strong improvement in the corrosion properties when compared to bare Mg as observed from Tafel analysis conducted by Singer et al. (2015). A study based on the formulation of composite coating of PDA with PCL over Mg alloys has also shown significant enhancement in the initial corrosion resistance and has led to improvement in the adhesion of PCL layer, thus resulting in a more stable coating (Choi et al. 2019). A $MgF_2$/PDA/HA coating over ZE21B alloy has not only enhanced the corrosion performance but also exhibited great cytocompatibility in terms of anticoagulant functions and antihemolytic properties (Yu et al. 2021).

## 7.5 COMPOSITE COATINGS

Composite coatings are the way forward in the development of Mg-based alloys for applications in the biomedical field as these alloys combine the properties of different coatings, thus enabling much better performance of the alloy in a physiological environment. This serves as a promising alternative to fulfill the diverse functionalities required in the implant such as improved resistance to degradation, cell viability, osteogenesis, antibacterial and anti-inflammatory response along with the added advantage of target drug delivery at the implantation site. Generally, the inner layer of the composite is made up of coatings which adhere strongly to the substrate, whereas the outer layer exhibits better biological functionalities as shown by organic coatings (Lin et al. 2013; Li et al. 2018; Yu et al. 2018; Liu et al. 2021). Based on the constitution of the composite coatings, these may be further categorized, as depicted in Figure 7.6 (Singh et al. 2023).

**Class (a)** represents the composite coatings with inner layer–outer layer on Mg substrate as inorganic–organic (Figure 7.6(a)). Abdal-hay et al. fabricated a composite coating of this category for biomedical applications with Ti-O and PLA as inorganic and organic layers, respectively (Abdal-hay et al. 2014). This coating exhibited remarkable reduction in the corrosion rate, especially in the initial stages with improved biocompatibility measured in terms of attachment of seeded MC3T3 osteoblasts (Abdal-hay et al. 2014). To tailor the properties of AZ31 alloy for temporary implant applications, Hanas et al. coated the bare alloy with $Mg(OH)_2$ followed by PCL which led to enhancement in cell viability, adhesion, as well as proliferation in addition to reduction in the corrosion rate, the mechanism of which is illustrated in Figure 7.7 (Hanas et al. 2016). Li and group also manufactured a coating of this

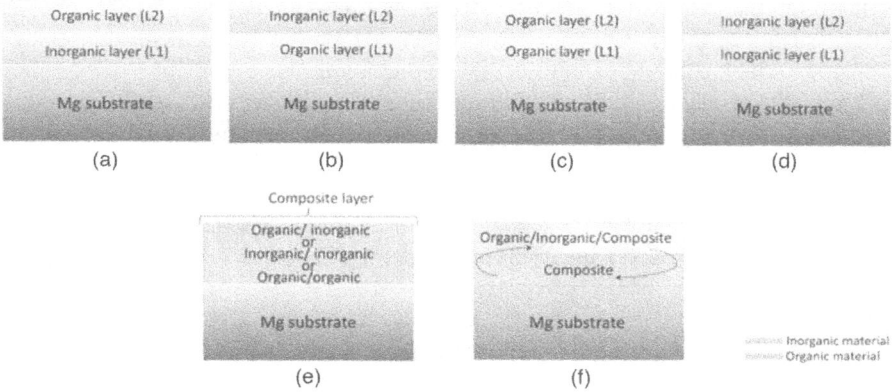

FIGURE 7.6 Composite coatings based on (a) organic–inorganic layers, (b) inorganic–organic layers, (c) organic–organic layers, (d) inorganic–inorganic layers, (e) organic/inorganic or inorganic/inorganic or organic/organic composite layers, (f) organic/inorganic/composite–composite–organic/inorganic/composite layer assemblies on Mg-based alloys (Singh et al. 2023).

category with MAO-sealed PLGA coating that revealed significantly improved resistance toward corrosion and stress corrosion cracking of bare alloy (Chen et al. 2019). **Class (b)** denotes the coatings with organic–inorganic layer deposited over the Mg alloy. The composite coating prepared with PDA and HA being the inner and outer layers over AZ31 Mg alloy showed a decrease in the corrosion rate while promoting

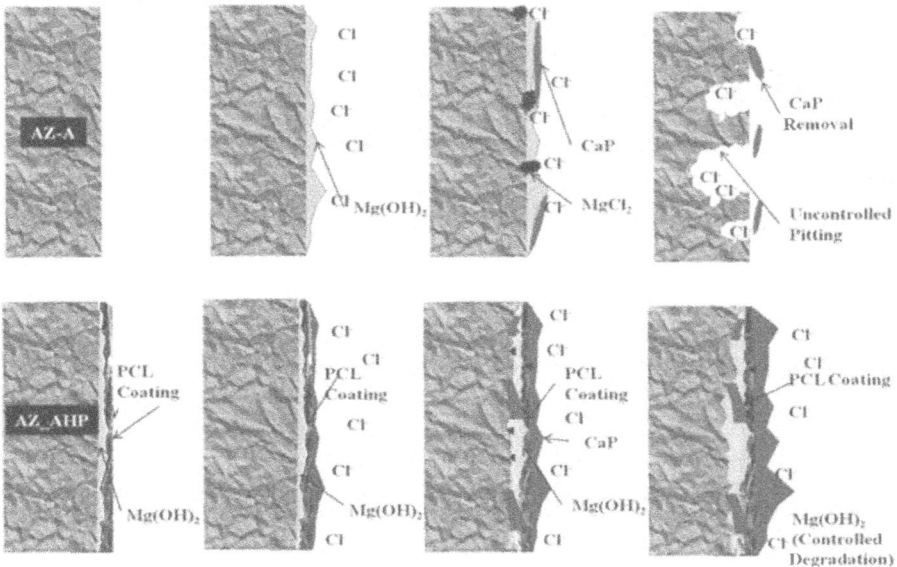

FIGURE 7.7 Schematic representation of degradation control in AZ-A (uncoated) samples compared with AZ-AHP (coated) samples (Hanas et al. 2016).

cell growth for L-929 cells without showing any toxic effects on the same (Lin et al. 2015). Zhang et al. prepared a coating of PLA followed by dicalcium phosphate dihydrate which exhibited a considerable reduction in the degradation of Mg alloy as measured by electrochemical and immersion tests (Zhang et al. 2017). The composite coating revealed an enhanced osteoinductive potential as it did not show any toxicity to MC3TC-E1 osteoblastic cells but promoted cell attachment, proliferation, and osteogenic differentiation (Zhang et al. 2017). Enhanced biofunctionality has also been observed when Mg is coated with $TiO_2$ incorporated over phytic acid which resulted in improved hydrophilicity, anticoagulation ability, and cell adhesion (Tang et al. 2020).

**Class (c)** represents the composite coatings made up of two organic layers. Biopoylmeric coating of PLGA and PCL prepared over AZ31 Mg alloy displayed the ability for controlled delivery of antibiotics, improved corrosion control, and biocompatibility (Zomorodian et al. 2017). Zeng et al. fabricated a layer-by-layer assembly of gentamicin sulfate and poly(sodium 4-styrene sulfonate) that exhibited excellent antibacterial property as well as improved resistance to degradation (Zeng et al. 2015). The assembled multilayers were observed to be more effective in inhibiting the in vitro growth of *Staphylococcus aureus* when the number of layers is increased (Zeng et al. 2015). Esophageal stent implantation has also been explored using Class (c) coatings made up of PCL and poly(trimethylene carbonate) which revealed that long-term mechanical stability as well decreased the degradation rates with no complications such as esophageal perforation, bleeding, and stent translocation even after 48 compression cycles (Yuan et al. 2016).

**Class (d)** represents the combination of two inorganic layers. Coatings of $ZrO_2$ over PEO-coated Mg-Ca alloy has exhibited a reduction in the corrosion current density by two orders of magnitude as compared to bare alloy (Daroonparvar et al. 2018). The addition of $ZrO_2$ accentuates the decrease of corrosion in PEO-coated alloy (Daroonparvar et al. 2018). Furthermore, the multilayer coating shows enhanced antibacterial activity against *Escherichia coli* as compared to bare and PEO-coated alloys as the $ZrO_2$ top coat which completely seals the PEO bond, thus preventing and delaying transportation of aggressive ions (Daroonparvar et al. 2018). A layer-by-layer assembly of $SiO_2$ and $CeO_2$ fabricated over AZ31 alloy has shown a tenfold reduction in the current density as compared to bare alloy, exhibiting good long-term corrosion resistance (Zhao et al. 2019). The study proposed that $SiO_2$ was forming the physical barrier against corrosion solution, while $CeO_2$ was considered as a corrosion inhibitor to heal the physical damage, enabling it to self-heal even after immersing for 72 h (Zhao et al. 2019). Combination of MgO followed by $Mg(OH)_2$ over AZ31 alloy led to a reduction of corrosion current by three and one order of magnitude as compared to bare alloy and MgO-coated alloy, respectively (Li et al. 2019).

**Class (e)** of composite coatings consists of amalgamated organic and inorganic layers over Mg alloy substrate which may comprise individual coatings, as depicted in Figure 7.6(e). Abdal-hay et al. formulated a hybrid matrix of HA and PCL over AM50 Mg alloy by means of dip coating technique, which showed a 34% enhancement in the mechanical integrity of the alloy (Abdal-hay, Amna, and Lim 2013). The corrosion tests revealed better and uniform performance of the composite coating for extended incubation time as opposed to bare alloy and PCL-coated alloy (Abdal-hay,

Amna, and Lim 2013). The coating exhibited better cell attachment, proliferation, migration, and growth inside the bone tissue as well as improved absorption of extracellular matrix proteins as measured for MC3T3 cells (Abdal-hay et al. 2013). Another study on HA/PCL coating over AM50 showed an enhancement in the mechanical properties – improved Young's modulus of elasticity and ultimate tensile strength of PCL upon the addition of 20 wt% HA. Bioactive glass nanoparticles containing copper (Cu-BGN) when incorporated into PCL have shown enhancement of anticorrosion properties, bioactivity, as well as antibacterial properties, under physiological conditions (Yang et al. 2018). The release of $Cu^{2+}$ ions led to the inhibition of the growth of *Staphylococcus carnosus* and *E. coli* (Yang et al. 2018). The cytocompatibility measured in terms of viability and proliferation of MG-63 cells was observed to enhance as compared to bare alloy, although an additional increase of Cu-BGN concentration led to a slight decrease of cell proliferation and cell activity (Yang et al. 2018).

**Class (f)** of composite coatings comprise complex multifunctional coatings having layers of composite coating and organic or inorganic or another composite coating which offers the alloy enhanced biocompatibility, better self-healing, and targeted drug delivery for biomedical applications (Singh et al. 2023). Wei et al. fabricated a PDA-assisted heparinized PEO/PLLA composite coating over AZ31 alloy which resulted in a three orders of magnitude increase in the corrosion resistance as compared to AZ31 coated with PEO/PLLA (Wei et al. 2014). However, the PDA addition and heparinization of the coated alloy improved hemocompatibility evaluated in terms of hemolysis ratio and platelet adhesion tests (Wei et al. 2014). The composite so formed showed no cytotoxicity and improved proliferation of human umbilical vein endothelial cells while simultaneously inhibiting the human umbilical artery smooth muscle cells proliferation (Wei et al. 2014). A composite coating consisting of a fluoride precoating, followed by silk-phytic acid coating in the middle, and silk fibroin coating at the top was observed to endow the Mg-1Ca alloy with active, biocorrosion-responsive self-healing capacity with pH responsiveness, thus enhancing the resistance to corrosion (Xiong et al. 2019). The authors noted an increase in cytocompatibility toward MC3TC-E1 cells quantified by favorable responses in multiple cellular behaviors, i.e., adherence, spreading, proliferation, and differentiation of cells (Xiong et al. 2019). Jia et al. also manufactured a self-healing, pH-responsive coating made up of MAO-precoated substrate covered by nanosized cerium oxides containing chitosan multilayers over Mg-1Ca (Jia et al. 2016). The in vitro tests revealed an effective reduction in the corrosion as well as excellent cytocompatibility evaluated using MC3T3-E1 preosteoblasts (Jia et al. 2016).

Overall, it has been observed that Class (a) lacks necessary biological functionalities such as self-healing, super-hydrophobicity, drug delivery, etc., whereas Class (b) provides additional hydrophobicity and drug release features compared to Class (a), although with lower corrosion resistance due to the inorganic layer at the top. Class (c) composite coatings have lower resistance to degradation as compared to Class (b) and (b). Nevertheless, these have a distinguished drug release feature where the inner layer offers corrosion resistance, while the outer layer acts as a drug reservoir. Class (d) composite coatings are similar to Class (b) with significant corrosion resistance but lacking in performing biofunctionalities. Class (e) demonstrated improved anticorrosion potential along with mechanical properties of the alloys. Lastly, Class (f) composite coatings have shown remarkable self-healing capability, drug delivery, and biocompatibility.

## 7.6 CONCLUSIONS

Surface modifications are considered to be an attractive approach for the enhancement of corrosion resistance and biocompatibility of the Mg alloy as these alter the surface properties of the material to achieve the desired functionalities while retaining the bulk properties of the base alloy. As these surface modifications are what are directly exposed inside the human body, it is essential that they are stable in the major three facets of their operation: mechanical, chemical, and biological. The coatings have been majorly classified into four classes – metallic coatings, inorganic coatings, polymer coatings, and composite coatings. Metallic coatings offer resistance to corrosion based on the formation of metal oxide or metal hydroxide layer over the alloy surface which acts as a physical barrier between the physiological media and implant/stent material. These coatings require further development in the area of biocompatibility and long-term integrity as well as protection of the alloy substrate. LDH coatings facilitate the entrapment of corrosive anions between the cationic layers allowing for enhanced degradation resistance. Inorganic coatings consist of $MgF_2$, phosphate, and GO coatings. $MgF_2$ coatings exhibit short-term stability, which may be amplified by combining with other stable coating materials, leading to fabrication of composite coatings. Phosphate coatings also have potential applications in biomedical field as their chemical structure is similar to the inorganic components of bone tissue, exhibiting chemical stability even at high temperatures (Liu et al. 2018). Particularly, Ca-P salts have been widely used as implants owing to their ability to induce bone growth and strong bone bonding (Yin et al. 2017). Apart from these nonmetallic coatings, the GO coatings are observed to be chemically inert and resistant toward permeation of corrosive ions, resulting in a boost in corrosion resistance (Plachá and Jampilek 2019). But their poor wettability with metal matrix and weak interfacial bonding strength are causes of concern which may be overcome by combining the GO coating with other coatings (Liu et al. 2015; Zhao et al. 2020). While employing the metallic and inorganic coatings, emphasis has to be on the biosafety aspect, such that the coatings also enable cell biocompatibility which includes cell attachment and proliferation without producing any harmful compounds in addition to providing protection against corrosion.

To tailor the requisite biological properties, amalgamation with organic coatings is seen as the way forward. Of the organic coatings, the polymer coatings are the most broadly explored. These comprise the natural and synthetic polymer coatings which have an innate tendency of being biocompatible. The major drawbacks faced by these coatings are the lack of mechanical integrity and weak adhesion to the substrate material, thus requiring addition of other elements to enhance the mechanical and chemical properties for biomedical applications. All the individual surface modifications are limited in their properties, whether mechanical, chemical, or biological. Thus, it is important to form composite coatings as these facilitate the modification of the properties of the implant material so that it can easily meet the requirements of various biological functions, with different layers attributing different properties to the implant. A number of self-healing composite coatings have also been studied. However, the composite coatings pose with the predicament of weak interfacial adhesion and complex degradation patterns which have to be investigated in detail in order to come up with implant materials having controllable release, self-repairing, biosafety, good bioactivity, biocompatibility, and stability while showing improved attachment to the substrate.

# REFERENCES

Abdal-hay, Abdalla, Touseef Amna, and Jae Kyoo Lim. 2013. "Biocorrosion and Osteoconductivity of PCL/NHAp Composite Porous Film-based Coating of Magnesium Alloy." *Solid State Sciences* 18: 131–40. https://doi.org/10.1016/j.solidstatesciences.2012.11.017

Abdal-hay, Abdalla, Montasser Dewidar, Juhyun Lim, and Jae Kyoo Lim. 2014. "Enhanced Biocorrosion Resistance of Surface Modified Magnesium Alloys Using Inorganic/Organic Composite Layer for Biomedical Applications." *Ceramics International* 40 (1, Part B): 2237–47. https://doi.org/10.1016/j.ceramint.2013.07.142

Agarwal, Sankalp, Mathieu Riffault, David Hoey, Brendan Duffy, James Curtin, and Swarna Jaiswal. 2017. "Biomimetic Hyaluronic Acid–Lysozyme Composite Coating on AZ31 Mg Alloy with Combined Antibacterial and Osteoinductive Activities." *ACS Biomaterials Science & Engineering* 3 (12): 3244–53. https://doi.org/10.1021/acsbiomaterials.7b00527

Akhavan, Omid. 2016. "Graphene Scaffolds in Progressive Nanotechnology/Stem Cell-based Tissue Engineering of the Nervous System." *Journal of Materials Chemistry B* 4 (19): 3169–90. https://doi.org/10.1039/C6TB00152A

Al-Radha, Afya Sahib Diab, David Dymock, Charles Younes, and Dominic O'Sullivan. 2012. "Surface Properties of Titanium and Zirconia Dental Implant Materials and Their Effect on Bacterial Adhesion." *Journal of Dentistry* 40 (2): 146–53. https://doi.org/10.1016/j.jdent.2011.12.006

Alabbasi, Alyaa, S. Liyanaarachchi, and M. Bobby Kannan. 2012. "Polylactic Acid Coating on a Biodegradable Magnesium Alloy: An In Vitro Degradation Study by Electrochemical Impedance Spectroscopy." *Thin Solid Films* 520 (23): 6841–44. https://doi.org/10.1016/j.tsf.2012.07.090

Amiri, Hamed, Iman Mohammadi, and Abdollah Afshar. 2017. "Electrophoretic Deposition of Nano-zirconia Coating on AZ91D Magnesium Alloy for Bio-corrosion Control Purposes." *Surface and Coatings Technology* 311: 182–90. https://doi.org/10.1016/j.surfcoat.2016.12.103

Asgari, Mohammad, Ying Yang, Shuang Yang, Zhentao Yu, Prasad K. D. V. Yarlagadda, Yin Xiao, and Zhiyong Li. 2019. "Mg–Phenolic Network Strategy for Enhancing Corrosion Resistance and Osteocompatibility of Degradable Magnesium Alloys." *ACS Omega* 4 (26): 21931–44. https://doi.org/10.1021/acsomega.9b02976

Bakhsheshi-Rad, H. R., E. Hamzah, M. Daroonparvar, R. Ebrahimi-Kahrizsangi, and M. Medraj. 2014. "In-vitro Corrosion Inhibition Mechanism of Fluorine-doped Hydroxyapatite and Brushite Coated Mg-Ca Alloys for Biomedical Applications." *Ceramics International* 40 (6): 7971–82. https://doi.org/10.1016/j.ceramint.2013.12.147

Bao, Quan He, Li Qing Zhao, He Min Jing, and Qiang Xu. 2017. "Microstructure of Hydroxyapatite/Collagen Coating on AZ31 Magnesium Alloy by a Solution Treatment." *Journal of Biomimetics, Biomaterials and Biomedical Engineering* 30: 38–44. https://doi.org/10.4028/www.scientific.net/JBBBE.30.38

Barchiche, C.-E., E. Rocca, C. Juers, J. Hazan, and J. Steinmetz. 2007. "Corrosion Resistance of Plasma-anodized AZ91D Magnesium Alloy by Electrochemical Methods." *Electrochimica Acta* 53 (2): 417–25. https://doi.org/10.1016/j.electacta.2007.04.030

Chen, Jun, Ju Feng, Lei Yan, Huan Li, Changqi Xiong, and Sude Ma. 2021. "In Situ Growth Process of Mg-Fe Layered Double Hydroxide Conversion Film on MgCa Alloy." *Journal of Magnesium and Alloys* 9 (3): 1019–27. https://doi.org/10.1016/j.jma.2020.05.019

Chen, Lianxi, Yinying Sheng, Hanyu Zhou, Zhibin Li, Xiaojian Wang, and Wei Li. 2019. "Influence of a MAO + PLGA Coating on Biocorrosion and Stress Corrosion Cracking Behavior of a Magnesium Alloy in a Physiological Environment." *Corrosion Science* 148: 134–43. https://doi.org/10.1016/j.corsci.2018.12.005

Choi, Ji Bong, Yong Seok Jang, Seon Mi Byeon, Jong Hwa Jang, Yu Kyoung Kim, Tae Sung Bae, and Min Ho Lee. 2019. "Effect of Composite Coating with Poly-dopamine/PCL on the Corrosion Resistance of Magnesium." *International Journal of Polymeric Materials and Polymeric Biomaterials* 68 (6): 328–37. https://doi.org/10.1080/00914037.2018.1455678

Chunyan, Zhang, Cheng Lan, Lin Jiajia, Sun Dongwei, Zhang Jun, and Liu Huinan. 2022. "In Vitro Evaluation of Degradation, Cytocompatibility and Antibacterial Property of Polycaprolactone/Hydroxyapatite Composite Coating on Bioresorbable Magnesium Alloy." *Journal of Magnesium and Alloys* 10 (8): 2252–65. https://doi.org/10.1016/j.jma.2021.07.014

Cusanno, Angela, Nicola Contessi Negrini, Tomaso Villa, Silvia Farè, Maria Luisa Garcia-Romeu, and Gianfranco Palumbo. 2020. "Post Forming Analysis and In Vitro Biological Characterization of AZ31B Processed by Incremental Forming and Coated with Electrospun Polycaprolactone." *Journal of Manufacturing Science and Engineering* 143 (1). https://doi.org/10.1115/1.4048741

Daroonparvar, Mohammadreza, Muhamad Azizi Mat Yajid, Rajeev Kumar Gupta, Noordin Mohd Yusof, Hamid Reza Bakhsheshi-Rad, Hamidreza Ghandvar, and Ehsan Ghasemi. 2018. "Antibacterial Activities and Corrosion Behavior of Novel PEO/Nanostructured $ZrO_2$ Coating on Mg Alloy." *Transactions of Nonferrous Metals Society of China* 28 (8): 1571–81. https://doi.org/10.1016/S1003-6326(18)64799-5

Drynda, Andreas, Thomas Hassel, René Hoehn, Angela Perz, Friedrich-Wilhelm Bach, and Matthias Peuster. 2010. "Development and Biocompatibility of a Novel Corrodible Fluoride-coated Magnesium–Calcium Alloy with Improved Degradation Kinetics and Adequate Mechanical Properties for Cardiovascular Applications." *Journal of Biomedical Materials Research Part A* 93A (2): 763–75. https://doi.org/10.1002/jbm.a.32582.

Drynda, Andreas, Juliane Seibt, Thomas Hassel, Friedrich Wilhelm Bach, and Matthias Peuster. 2013. "Biocompatibility of Fluoride-coated Magnesium–Calcium Alloys with Optimized Degradation Kinetics in a Subcutaneous Mouse Model." *Journal of Biomedical Materials Research Part A* 101A (1): 33–43. https://doi.org/10.1002/jbm.a.34300

Feng, Jing, Yan Chen, Xiaohan Liu, Tiandi Liu, Linyi Zou, Yuting Wang, Yueming Ren, Zhuangjun Fan, Yanzhuo Lv, and Milin Zhang. 2013. "In-situ Hydrothermal Crystallization $Mg(OH)_2$ Films on Magnesium Alloy AZ91 and Their Corrosion Resistance Properties." *Materials Chemistry and Physics* 143 (1): 322–29. https://doi.org/10.1016/j.matchemphys.2013.09.005

Fernández, Javier, Y. El Ouardi, José Bonastre, José M. Molina-Jordá, and Francisco Cases. 2019. "Modification of the Magnesium Corrosion Rate in Physiological Saline 0.9 Wt % NaCl via Chemical and Electrochemical Coating of Reduced Graphene Oxide." *Corrosion Science* 152: 75–81. https://doi.org/10.1016/j.corsci.2019.01.025.

Fintová, Stanislava, Juliána Drábiková, Filip Pastorek, Jakub Tkacz, Ivo Kuběna, Libor Trško, and Branislav Hadzima et al. 2019. "Improvement of Electrochemical Corrosion Characteristics of AZ61 Magnesium Alloy with Unconventional Fluoride Conversion Coatings." *Surface and Coatings Technology* 357: 638–50. https://doi.org/10.1016/j.surfcoat.2018.10.038

Gao, Julia, Yingchao Su, and Yi-Xian Qin. 2021. "Calcium Phosphate Coatings Enhance Biocompatibility and Degradation Resistance of Magnesium Alloy: Correlating In Vitro and In Vivo Studies." *Bioactive Materials* 6 (5): 1223–29. https://doi.org/10.1016/j. bioactmat.2020.10.024

Gao, Yue'e, Lianfu Zhao, Xiaohong Yao, Ruiqiang Hang, Xiangyu Zhang, and Bin Tang. 2018. "Corrosion Behavior of Porous $ZrO_2$ Ceramic Coating on AZ31B Magnesium Alloy." *Surface and Coatings Technology* 349: 434–41. https://doi.org/10.1016/j.surfcoat. 2018.06.018

Guo, Lian, Wei Wu, Yongfeng Zhou, Fen Zhang, Rongchang Zeng, and Jianmin Zeng. 2018. "Layered Double Hydroxide Coatings on Magnesium Alloys: A Review." *Journal of Materials Science & Technology* 34 (9): 1455–66. https://doi.org/10.1016/j. jmst.2018.03.003

Hanas, T., T. S. Sampath Kumar, Govindaraj Perumal, and Mukesh Doble. 2016. "Tailoring Degradation of AZ31 Alloy by Surface Pre-treatment and Electrospun PCL Fibrous Coating." *Materials Science and Engineering* C 65: 43–50. https://doi.org/10.1016/ j.msec.2016.04.017

Hou, Shusen, Weixin Yu, Zhijun Yang, Yue Li, Lin Yang, and Shaoting Lang. 2020. "Properties of Titanium Oxide Coating on MgZn Alloy by Magnetron Sputtering for Stent Application." *Coatings* 10 (10): 999. https://doi.org/10.3390/coatings10100999

Huang, Wenjiang, Di Mei, Junlong Zhang, Dongfang Chen, Jingan Li, Liguo Wang, Yifan Zhou, Shijie Zhu, and Shaokang Guan. 2021. "Improved Corrosion Resistance and Cytocompatibility of Mg-Zn-Y-Nd Alloy by the Electrografted Polycaprolactone Coating." *Colloids and Surfaces A: Physicochemical and Engineering Aspects* 629: 127471. https://doi.org/10.1016/j.colsurfa.2021.127471

Istrate, Bogdan, Julietta V. Rau, Corneliu Munteanu, Iulian V. Antoniac, and Vicentiu Saceleanu. 2020. "Properties and In Vitro Assessment of $ZrO_2$-based Coatings Obtained by Atmospheric Plasma Jet Spraying on Biodegradable Mg-Ca and Mg-Ca-Zr Alloys." *Ceramics International* 46 (10, Part B): 15897–906. https://doi.org/10.1016/j. ceramint.2020.03.138

Jia, Luanluan, Fengxuan Han, Huan Wang, Caihong Zhu, Qianping Guo, Jiaying Li, Zhongliang Zhao, Qiang Zhang, Xuesong Zhu, and Bin Li. 2019. "Polydopamine-assisted Surface Modification for Orthopaedic Implants." *Journal of Orthopaedic Translation* 17: 82–95. https://doi.org/10.1016/j.jot.2019.04.001

Jia, Zhaojun, Pan Xiong, Yuying Shi, Wenhao Zhou, Yan Cheng, Yufeng Zheng, Tingfei Xi, and Shicheng Wei. 2016. "Inhibitor Encapsulated, Self-healable and Cytocompatible Chitosan Multilayer Coating on Biodegradable Mg Alloy: A PH-responsive Design." *Journal of Materials Chemistry* B 4 (14): 2498–2511. https://doi.org/10.1039/C6TB00117C

Jian, Shun-Yi, Mei-Ling Ho, Bing-Ci Shih, Yue-Jun Wang, Li-Wen Weng, Min-Wen Wang, and Chun-Chieh Tseng. 2019. "Evaluation of the Corrosion Resistance and Cytocompatibility of a Bioactive Micro-Arc Oxidation Coating on AZ31 Mg Alloy." *Coatings* 9 (6): 396. https://doi.org/10.3390/coatings9060396

Kania, Aneta, Magdalena M. Szindler, and Marek Szindler. 2021. "Structure and Corrosion Behavior of $TiO_2$ Thin Films Deposited by ALD on a Biomedical Magnesium Alloy." *Coatings* 701: 137945. https://doi.org/10.3390/coatings11010070

Karthega, Mani, Mogan Pranesh, Chockalingam Poongothai, and Nagarajan Srinivasan. 2021. "Poly Caprolactone/Titanium Dioxide Nanofiber Coating on AM50 Alloy for Biomedical Application." *Journal of Magnesium and Alloys* 9 (2): 532–47. https://doi. org/10.1016/j.jma.2020.07.003

Kim, Yu-Kyoung, Young-Seok Jang, Seo-Young Kim, and Min-Ho Lee. 2019. "Functions Achieved by the Hyaluronic Acid Derivatives Coating and Hydroxide Film on Bio-absorbed Mg." *Applied Surface Science* 473: 31–39. https://doi.org/10.1016/j.apsusc. 2018.12.139

Kim, Yu-Kyoung, Seo-Young Kim, Yong-Seok Jang, Il-Song Park, and Min-Ho Lee. 2020. "Bio-corrosion Behaviors of Hyaluronic Acid and Cerium Multi-layer Films on Degradable Implant." *Applied Surface Science* 515: 146070. https://doi.org/10.1016/j.apsusc.2020.146070

Ko, Young Gun, Seung Namgung, and Dong Hyuk Shin. 2010. "Correlation between KOH Concentration and Surface Properties of AZ91 Magnesium Alloy Coated by Plasma Electrolytic Oxidation." *Surface and Coatings Technology* 205 (7): 2525–31. https://doi.org/10.1016/j.surfcoat.2010.09.055

Langhoff, J. D., K. Voelter, D. Scharnweber, M. Schnabelrauch, F. Schlottig, T. Hefti, K. Kalchofner, K. Nuss, and B. von Rechenberg. 2008. "Comparison of Chemically and Pharmaceutically Modified Titanium and Zirconia Implant Surfaces in Dentistry: A Study in Sheep." *International Journal of Oral and Maxillofacial Surgery* 37 (12): 1125–32. https://doi.org/10.1016/j.ijom.2008.09.008

Lawal, Abdulazeez T. 2019. "Graphene-based Nano Composites and Their Applications: A Review." *Biosensors and Bioelectronics* 141: 111384. https://doi.org/10.1016/j.bios.2019.111384

Lei, Ting, Chun Ouyang, Wei Tang, Lian-Feng Li, and Le-Shan Zhou. 2010a. "Enhanced Corrosion Protection of MgO Coatings on Magnesium Alloy Deposited by an Anodic Electrodeposition Process." *Corrosion Science* 52 (10): 3504–8. https://doi.org/10.1016/j.corsci.2010.06.028

――――. 2010b. "Preparation of MgO Coatings on Magnesium Alloys for Corrosion Protection." *Surface and Coatings Technology* 204 (23): 3798–3803. https://doi.org/10.1016/j.surfcoat.2010.04.060

Li, Chang-Yang, Xiao-Li Fan, Rong-Chang Zeng, Lan-Yue Cui, Shuo-Qi Li, Fen Zhang, and Qing-Kun He et al. 2019. "Corrosion Resistance of In-situ Growth of Nano-sized Mg(OH)$_2$ on Micro-arc Oxidized Magnesium Alloy AZ31: Influence of EDTA." *Journal of Materials Science & Technology* 35 (6): 1088–98. https://doi.org/10.1016/j.jmst.2019.01.006.

Li, Hua, Feng Peng, Donghui Wang, Yuqin Qiao, Demin Xu, and Xuanyong Liu. 2018. "Layered Double Hydroxide/Poly-dopamine Composite Coating with Surface Heparinization on Mg Alloys: Improved Anticorrosion, Endothelialization and Hemocompatibility." *Biomaterials Science* 6 (7): 1846–58. https://doi.org/10.1039/C8BM00298C

Li, Jianan, Peng Cao, Xiaonong Zhang, Shaoxiang Zhang, and Y. H. He. 2010. "In Vitro Degradation and Cell Attachment of a PLGA Coated Biodegradable Mg-6Zn Based Alloy." *Journal of Materials Science* 45 (22): 6038–45. https://doi.org/10.1007/s10853-010-4688-9

Li, Jianfang, Xiaojing He, Ruiqiang Hang, Xiaobo Huang, Xiangyu Zhang, and Bin Tang. 2017. "Fabrication and Corrosion Behavior of TiO$_2$ Nanotubes on AZ91D Magnesium Alloy." *Ceramics International* 43 (16): 13683–88. https://doi.org/10.1016/j.ceramint.2017.07.079

Li, Jing-an, Li Chen, Xue-qi Zhang, and Shao-kang Guan. 2020. "Enhancing Biocompatibility and Corrosion Resistance of Biodegradable Mg-Zn-Y-Nd Alloy by Preparing PDA/HA Coating for Potential Application of Cardiovascular Biomaterials." *Materials Science and Engineering C* 109: 110607. https://doi.org/10.1016/j.msec.2019.110607

Li, Xuan, Chenglin Chu, Lei Liu, Xiaokai Liu, Jing Bai, Chao Guo, Feng Xue, Pinghua Lin, and Paul K. Chu. 2015. "Biodegradable Poly-lactic Acid-based Composite Reinforced Unidirectionally with High-strength Magnesium Alloy Wires." *Biomaterials* 49: 135–44. https://doi.org/10.1016/j.biomaterials.2015.01.060

Li, Nola, Y. D. Li, Yanbo Wang, Ming Li, Yanling Cheng, Yuanhao Wu, and Yufeng Zheng. 2013. "Corrosion Resistance and Cytotoxicity of a MgF$_2$ Coating on Biomedical Mg-1Ca Alloy via Vacuum Evaporation Deposition Method." *Surface and Interface Analysis* 45 (8): 1217–22. https://doi.org/10.1002/sia.5257

Li, Yang, Xuqiang Liu, Lili Tan, Ling Ren, Peng Wan, Yongqiang Hao, Xinhua Qu, Ke Yang, and Kerong Dai. 2016. "Enoxacin-loaded Poly(lactic-co-glycolic acid) Coating on Porous Magnesium Scaffold as a Drug Delivery System: Antibacterial Properties and Inhibition of Osteoclastic Bone Resorption." *Journal of Materials Science & Technology* 32 (9): 865–73. https://doi.org/10.1016/j.jmst.2016.07.013.

Liang, J., P. Bala Srinivasan, C. Blawert, and W. Dietzel. 2009. "Comparison of Electrochemical Corrosion Behaviour of MgO and $ZrO_2$ Coatings on AM50 Magnesium Alloy Formed by Plasma Electrolytic Oxidation." *Corrosion Science* 51 (10): 2483–92. https://doi.org/10.1016/j.corsci.2009.06.034

Liangjian, Chen, Zhao Jun, Yu Kun, Chen Chang, Dai Yilong, Qiao Xueyan, and Yu Zhiming. 2015. "Improving of In Vitro Biodegradation Resistance in a Chitosan Coated Magnesium Bio-composite." *Rare Metal Materials and Engineering* 44 (8): 1862–65. https://doi.org/10.1016/S1875-5372(15)30114-4

Lin, Li-Han, Hung-Pang Lee, and Ming-Long Yeh. 2020. "Characterization of a Sandwich PLGA–Gallic Acid–PLGA Coating on Mg Alloy ZK60 for Bioresorbable Coronary Artery Stents." *Materials.* https://doi.org/10.3390/ma13235538

Lin, Xiao, Lili Tan, Peng Wan, Xiaoming Yu, Ke Yang, Zhuangqi Hu, Yangde Li, and Weirong Li. 2013. "Characterization of Micro-Arc Oxidation Coating Post-treated by Hydrofluoric Acid on Biodegradable ZK60 Magnesium Alloy." *Surface and Coatings Technology* 232: 899–905. https://doi.org/10.1016/j.surfcoat.2013.06.121

Lin, Kaili, Chengtie Wu, and Jiang Chang. 2014. "Advances in Synthesis of Calcium Phosphate Crystals with Controlled Size and Shape." *Acta Biomaterialia* 10 (10): 4071–4102. https://doi.org/10.1016/j.actbio.2014.06.017

Lin, Bingpeng, Mei Zhong, Chengdong Zheng, Lin Cao, Dengli Wang, Lina Wang, Jun Liang, and Baocheng Cao. 2015. "Preparation and Characterization of Dopamine-induced Biomimetic Hydroxyapatite Coatings on the AZ31 Magnesium Alloy." *Surface and Coatings Technology* 281: 82–88. https://doi.org/10.1016/j.surfcoat.2015.09.033

Liu, Chen, Zheng Ren, Yongdong Xu, Song Pang, Xinbing Zhao, and Ying Zhao. 2018. "Biodegradable Magnesium Alloys Developed as Bone Repair Materials: A Review." *Scanning* 2018 (March): 9216314. https://doi.org/10.1155/2018/9216314

Liu, Xiangmei, Qiuyue Yang, Zhaoyang Li, Wei Yuan, Yufeng Zheng, Zhenduo Cui, Xianjin Yang, Kelvin W. K. Yeung, and Shuilin Wu. 2018. "A Combined Coating Strategy Based on Atomic Layer Deposition for Enhancement of Corrosion Resistance of AZ31 Magnesium Alloy." *Applied Surface Science* 434: 1101–11. https://doi.org/10.1016/j.apsusc.2017.11.032

Liu, Xien, Wen Liu, Minseong Ko, Minjoon Park, Min Gyu Kim, Pilgun Oh, and Sujong Chae et al. 2015. "Metal (Ni, Co)–Metal Oxides/Graphene Nanocomposites as Multifunctional Electrocatalysts." *Advanced Functional Materials* 25 (36): 5799–5808. https://doi.org/10.1002/adfm.201502217

Liu, Yun, Yuan Zhang, Yan-Li Wang, Ya-Qiang Tian, and Lian-Sheng Chen. 2021. "Research Progress on Surface Protective Coatings of Biomedical Degradable Magnesium Alloys." *Journal of Alloys and Compounds* 885: 161001. https://doi.org/10.1016/j.jallcom.2021.161001

Mao, Lin, Guangyin Yuan, Jialin Niu, Yang Zong, and Wenjiang Ding. 2013. "In Vitro Degradation Behavior and Biocompatibility of Mg-Nd-Zn-Zr Alloy by Hydrofluoric Acid Treatment." *Materials Science and Engineering: C* 33 (1): 242–50. https://doi.org/10.1016/j.msec.2012.08.036

Maqsood, Muhammad Faheem, Mohsin Ali Raza, Faizan Ali Ghauri, Zaeem Ur Rehman, and Muhammad Tasadaq Ilyas. 2020. "Corrosion Study of Graphene Oxide Coatings on AZ31B Magnesium Alloy." *Journal of Coatings Technology and Research* 17 (5): 1321–29. https://doi.org/10.1007/s11998-020-00350-3

Nair, Lakshmi S., and Cato T. Laurencin. 2007. "Biodegradable Polymers as Biomaterials." *Progress in Polymer Science* 32 (8): 762–98. https://doi.org/10.1016/j.progpolymsci. 2007.05.017

Nudelman, Fabio, Koen Pieterse, Anne George, Paul H. H. Bomans, Heiner Friedrich, Laura J. Brylka, Peter A. J. Hilbers, Gijsbertus de With, and Nico A. J. M. Sommerdijk. 2010. "The Role of Collagen in Bone Apatite Formation in the Presence of Hydroxyapatite Nucleation Inhibitors." *Nature Materials* 9 (12): 1004–9. https://doi.org/10.1038/nmat2875

Ostrowski, Nicole J., Boeun Lee, Abhijit Roy, Madhumati Ramanathan, and Prashant N. Kumta. 2013. "Biodegradable Poly(lactide-*co*-glycolide) Coatings on Magnesium Alloys for Orthopedic Applications." *Journal of Materials Science: Materials in Medicine* 24 (1): 85–96. https://doi.org/10.1007/s10856-012-4773-5

Peng, Feng, Donghui Wang, Yaxin Tian, Huiliang Cao, Yuqin Qiao, and Xuanyong Liu. 2017. "Sealing the Pores of PEO Coating with Mg-Al Layered Double Hydroxide: Enhanced Corrosion Resistance, Cytocompatibility and Drug Delivery Ability." *Scientific Reports* 7 (1): 8167. https://doi.org/10.1038/s41598-017-08238-w

Peng, Feng, Donghui Wang, Dongdong Zhang, Bangcheng Yan, Huiliang Cao, Yuqin Qiao, and Xuanyong Liu. 2018. "PEO/Mg-Zn-Al LDH Composite Coating on Mg Alloy as a Zn/Mg Ion-release Platform with Multifunctions: Enhanced Corrosion Resistance, Osteogenic, and Antibacterial Activities." *ACS Biomaterials Science & Engineering* 4 (12): 4112–21. https://doi.org/10.1021/acsbiomaterials.8b01184

Peron, Mirco, Abdulla Bin Afif, Anup Dadlani, Filippo Berto, and Jan Torgersen. 2020. "Comparing Physiologically Relevant Corrosion Performances of Mg AZ31 Alloy Protected by ALD and Sputter Coated TiO$_2$." *Surface and Coatings Technology* 395: 125922. https://doi.org/10.1016/j.surfcoat.2020.125922

Plachá, Daniela, and Josef Jampilek. 2019. "Graphenic Materials for Biomedical Applications." *Nanomaterials* 9 (12): 1758. https://doi.org/10.3390/nano9121758

Ren, Yufu, Elham Babaie, and Sarit B Bhaduri. 2018. "Nanostructured Amorphous Magnesium Phosphate/Poly(lactic acid) Composite Coating for Enhanced Corrosion Resistance and Bioactivity of Biodegradable AZ31 Magnesium Alloy." *Progress in Organic Coatings* 118: 1–8. https://doi.org/10.1016/j.porgcoat.2018.01.014

Roman, Diana Larisa, Vasile Ostafe, and Adriana Isvoran. 2020. "Deeper Inside the Specificity of Lysozyme When Degrading Chitosan: A Structural Bioinformatics Study." *Journal of Molecular Graphics and Modelling* 100: 107676. https://doi.org/10.1016/j.jmgm.2020.107676

Sennerby, Lars, Amir Dasmah, Birgitta Larsson, and Mattias Iverhed. 2005. "Bone Tissue Responses to Surface-modified Zirconia Implants: A Histomorphometric and Removal Torque Study in the Rabbit." *Clinical Implant Dentistry and Related Research* 7 (s1): s13–20. https://doi.org/10.1111/j.1708-8208.2005.tb00070.x

Shi, Yong-Juan, Jia Pei, Jian Zhang, Jia-Lin Niu, Hua Zhang, Sheng-Rong Guo, Zhong-Hua Li, and Guang-Yin Yuan. 2017. "Enhanced Corrosion Resistance and Cytocompatibility of Biodegradable Mg Alloys by Introduction of Mg(OH)$_2$ Particles into Poly(L-lactic acid) Coating." *Scientific Reports* 7 (1): 41796. https://doi.org/10.1038/srep41796

Shuai, Cijun, Bing Wang, Shizhen Bin, Shuping Peng, and Chengde Gao. 2020. "TiO$_2$-induced In Situ Reaction in Graphene Oxide-reinforced AZ61 Biocomposites to Enhance the Interfacial Bonding." *ACS Applied Materials & Interfaces* 12 (20): 23464–73. https://doi.org/10.1021/acsami.0c04020

Singer, Ferdinand, Magdalena Schlesak, Caroline Mebert, Sarah Höhn, and Sannakaisa Virtanen. 2015. "Corrosion Properties of Polydopamine Coatings Formed in One-step Immersion Process on Magnesium." *ACS Applied Materials & Interfaces* 7 (48): 26758–66. https://doi.org/10.1021/acsami.5b08760

Singh, Navdeep, Uma Batra, Kamal Kumar, Neeraj Ahuja, and Anil Mahapatro. 2023. "Progress in Bioactive Surface Coatings on Biodegradable Mg Alloys: A Critical Review towards Clinical Translation." *Bioactive Materials* 19: 717–57. https://doi.org/10.1016/j.bioactmat.2022.05.009

Sun, Jin'e, Jingbo Wang, Hongfeng Jiang, Minfang Chen, Yanze Bi, and Debao Liu. 2013. "In Vivo Comparative Property Study of the Bioactivity of Coated Mg-3Zn-0.8Zr Alloy." *Materials Science and Engineering: C* 33 (6): 3263–72. https://doi.org/10.1016/j.msec.2013.04.006

Sun, Xiang, Qing-Song Yao, Yu-Chao Li, Fen Zhang, Rong-Chang Zeng, Yu-Hong Zou, and Shuo-Qi Li. 2020. "Biocorrosion Resistance and Biocompatibility of Mg-Al Layered Double Hydroxide/Poly(L-lactic acid) Hybrid Coating on Magnesium Alloy AZ31." *Frontiers of Materials Science* 14 (4): 426–41. https://doi.org/10.1007/s11706-020-0522-8

Sun, Wei, Guangdao Zhang, Lili Tan, Ke Yang, and Hongjun Ai. 2016. "The Fluoride Coated AZ31B Magnesium Alloy Improves Corrosion Resistance and Stimulates Bone Formation in Rabbit Model." *Materials Science and Engineering: C* 63: 506–11. https://doi.org/10.1016/j.msec.2016.03.016

Tan, Jesslyn K E, P Balan, and N Birbilis. 2021. "Advances in LDH Coatings on Mg Alloys for Biomedical Applications: A Corrosion Perspective." *Applied Clay Science* 202: 105948. https://doi.org/10.1016/j.clay.2020.105948

Tang, Yan, Fang Wu, Liang Fang, Ting Guan, Jia Hu, and ShuFang Zhang. 2019. "A Comparative Study and Optimization of Corrosion Resistance of ZnAl Layered Double Hydroxides Films Intercalated with Different Anions on AZ31 Mg Alloys." *Surface and Coatings Technology* 358: 594–603. https://doi.org/10.1016/j.surfcoat.2018.11.070

Tang, Xin, Xuan Zhang, Yingqi Chen, Wentai Zhang, Junyu Qian, Hanaa Soliman, and Ai Qu et al. 2020. "Ultraviolet Irradiation Assisted Liquid Phase Deposited Titanium Dioxide ($TiO_2$) Incorporated into Phytic Acid Coating on Magnesium for Slowing-down Biodegradation and Improving Osteo-compatibility." *Materials Science and Engineering: C* 108: 110487. https://doi.org/10.1016/j.msec.2019.110487

Tian, Peng, and Xuanyong Liu. 2015. "Surface Modification of Biodegradable Magnesium and Its Alloys for Biomedical Applications." *Regenerative Biomaterials* 2 (2): 135–51. https://doi.org/10.1093/rb/rbu013.

Tiwari, Himani, Neha Karki, Mintu Pal, Souvik Basak, Ravindra Kumar Verma, Rajaram Bal, Narain Datt Kandpal, Ganga Bisht, and Nanda Gopal Sahoo. 2019. "Functionalized Graphene Oxide as a Nanocarrier for Dual Drug Delivery Applications: The Synergistic Effect of Quercetin and Gefitinib against Ovarian Cancer Cells." *Colloids and Surfaces B: Biointerfaces* 178: 452–59. https://doi.org/10.1016/j.colsurfb.2019.03.037

Tong, Peiduo, Yulong Sheng, Ruiqing Hou, Mujahid Iqbal, Lan Chen, and Jingan Li. 2022. "Recent Progress on Coatings of Biomedical Magnesium Alloy." *Smart Materials in Medicine* 3: 104–16. https://doi.org/10.1016/j.smaim.2021.12.007

Wagman, Donald D., William H. Evans, Vivian B. Parker, Richard H. Schumm, Iva Halow, Sylvia M. Bailey, Kenneth L. Churney, and Ralph L. Nuttall. 1989. "The NBS Tables of Chemical Thermodynamic Properties: Selected Values for Inorganic and C1 and C2 Organic Substances in SI Units [J. Phys. Chem. Ref. Data 11, Suppl. 2 (1982)]." *Journal of Physical and Chemical Reference Data* 18 (4): 1807–12. https://doi.org/10.1063/1.555845

Wang, Shimeng, Lingxia Fu, Zhenggang Nai, Jun Liang, and Baocheng Cao. 2018. "Comparison of Corrosion Resistance and Cytocompatibility of MgO and $ZrO_2$ Coatings on AZ31 Magnesium Alloy Formed via Plasma Electrolytic Oxidation." *Coatings* 8 (12): 441. https://doi.org/10.3390/coatings8120441

Wang, Taolei, Chao Lin, Dan Batalu, Jingzhou Hu, and Wei Lu. 2021. "Tunable Microstructure and Morphology of the Self-assembly Hydroxyapatite Coatings on ZK60 Magnesium Alloy Substrates Using Hydrothermal Methods." *Coatings* 11 (1): 8. https://doi.org/10.3390/coatings11010008

Wang, Zhen-Lin, Yu-Hua Yan, Tao Wan, and Hui Yang. 2013. "Poly(L-lactic acid)/Hydroxyapatite/ Collagen Composite Coatings on AZ31 Magnesium Alloy for Biomedical Application." *Proceedings of the Institution of Mechanical Engineers, Part H: Journal of Engineering in Medicine* 227 (10): 1094–1103. https://doi.org/10.1177/0954411913493845

Wei, Zhongling, Peng Tian, Xuanyong Liu, and Bangxin Zhou. 2014. "Hemocompatibility and Selective Cell Fate of Polydopamine-assisted Heparinized PEO/PLLA Composite Coating on Biodegradable AZ31 Alloy." *Colloids and Surfaces B: Biointerfaces* 121: 451–60. https://doi.org/10.1016/j.colsurfb.2014.06.036

Wu, Guosong, Jamesh Mohammed Ibrahim, and Paul K. Chu. 2013. "Surface Design of Biodegradable Magnesium Alloys: A Review." *Surface and Coatings Technology* 233: 2–12. https://doi.org/10.1016/j.surfcoat.2012.10.009

Wu, Wei, Xiang Sun, Chun-Liu Zhu, Fen Zhang, Rong-Chang Zeng, Yu-Hong Zou, and Shuo-Qi Li. 2020. "Biocorrosion Resistance and Biocompatibility of Mg-Al Layered Double Hydroxide/poly-L-glutamic Acid Hybrid Coating on Magnesium Alloy AZ31." *Progress in Organic Coatings* 147: 105746. https://doi.org/10.1016/j.porgcoat.2020.105746

Xia, Meng-Ying, Yu Xie, Chen-Hao Yu, Ge-Yun Chen, Yuan-Hong Li, Ting Zhang, and Qiang Peng. 2019. "Graphene-based Nanomaterials: The Promising Active Agents for Antibiotics-independent Antibacterial Applications." *Journal of Controlled Release* 307: 16–31. https://doi.org/10.1016/j.jconrel.2019.06.011

Xiao, Xing, Haiying Yu, Qingsan Zhu, Guangyu Li, Yang Qu, and Rui Gu. 2013. "In Vivo Corrosion Resistance of Ca-P Coating on AZ60 Magnesium Alloy." *Journal of Bionic Engineering* 10 (2): 156–61. https://doi.org/10.1016/S1672-6529(13)60210-3

Xiong, Pan, Zhaojun Jia, Wenhao Zhou, Jianglong Yan, Pei Wang, Wei Yuan, Yangyang Li, Yan Cheng, Zhenpeng Guan, and Yufeng Zheng. 2019. "Osteogenic and PH Stimuli-responsive Self-healing Coating on Biomedical Mg-1Ca Alloy." *Acta Biomaterialia* 92: 336–50. https://doi.org/10.1016/j.actbio.2019.05.027

Xu, He, Yu-Wei Ge, Jia-Wei Lu, Qin-Fei Ke, Zhi-Qing Liu, Zhen-An Zhu, and Ya-Ping Guo. 2018. "Icariin Loaded-hollow Bioglass/Chitosan Therapeutic Scaffolds Promote Osteogenic Differentiation and Bone Regeneration." *Chemical Engineering Journal* 354: 285–94. https://doi.org/10.1016/j.cej.2018.08.022

Xu, Haitao, Tu Hu, Manle Wang, Yuxin Zheng, Hui Qin, Huiliang Cao, and Zhiquan An. 2020. "Degradability and Biocompatibility of Magnesium-MAO: The Consistency and Contradiction between In-Vitro and In-Vivo Outcomes." *Arabian Journal of Chemistry* 13 (1): 2795–2805. https://doi.org/10.1016/j.arabjc.2018.07.010

Xu, Liping, Feng Pan, Guoning Yu, Lei Yang, Erlin Zhang, and Ke Yang. 2009. "In Vitro and in Vivo Evaluation of the Surface Bioactivity of a Calcium Phosphate Coated Magnesium Alloy." *Biomaterials* 30 (8): 1512–23. https://doi.org/10.1016/j.biomaterials.2008.12.001

Xu, Ruizhen, Yi Shen, Jiangshan Zheng, Qiang Wen, Zhi Li, Xiongbo Yang, and Paul K Chu. 2017. "Effects of One-step Hydrothermal Treatment on the Surface Morphology and Corrosion Resistance of ZK60 Magnesium Alloy." *Surface and Coatings Technology* 309: 490–96. https://doi.org/10.1016/j.surfcoat.2016.11.111

Yang, Jingxin, Fuzhai Cui, and In Seop Lee. 2011. "Surface Modifications of Magnesium Alloys for Biomedical Applications." *Annals of Biomedical Engineering* 39 (7): 1857–71. https://doi.org/10.1007/s10439-011-0300-y

Yang, Zhilu, Qiufen Tu, Ying Zhu, Rifang Luo, Xin Li, Yichu Xie, Manfred F. Maitz, Jin Wang, and Nan Huang. 2012. "Mussel-inspired Coating of Polydopamine Directs Endothelial and Smooth Muscle Cell Fate for Re-endothelialization of Vascular Devices." *Advanced Healthcare Materials* 1 (5): 548–59. https://doi.org/10.1002/adhm.201200073

Yang, Qiuyue, Wei Yuan, Xiangmei Liu, Yufeng Zheng, Zhenduo Cui, Xianjin Yang, Haobo Pan, and Shuilin Wu. 2017. "Atomic Layer Deposited $ZrO_2$ Nanofilm on Mg-Sr Alloy for Enhanced Corrosion Resistance and Biocompatibility." *Acta Biomaterialia* 58: 515–26. https://doi.org/10.1016/j.actbio.2017.06.015

Yang, Yuyun, Kai Zheng, Ruifang Liang, Astrid Mainka, Nicola Taccardi, Judith A. Roether, Rainer Detsch, Wolfgang H. Goldmann, Sannakaisa Virtanen, and Aldo R. Boccaccini. 2018. "Cu-releasing Bioactive Glass/Polycaprolactone Coating on Mg with Antibacterial and Anticorrosive Properties for Bone Tissue Engineering." *Biomedical Materials* 13 (1): 15001. https://doi.org/10.1088/1748-605X/aa87f2

Yin, Z. Z., R. C. Zeng, L. Y. Cui, Y. H. Zou, S. Q. Li, and F. Zhang. 2017. "Progress on Phosphate Coatings on Biodegradable Magnesium Alloys." *Journal of Shandong University of Science and Technology(Natural Science)* 36 (2): 57–69. https://www.scopus.com/inward/record.uri?eid=2-s2.0-85051580629&partnerID=40&md5=b5082229bae852634922da78ccfa0036

Yu, Chi, Lan-Yue Cui, Yong-Feng Zhou, Zhuang-Zhuang Han, Xiao-Bo Chen, Rong-Chang Zeng, and Yu-Hong Zou et al. 2018. "Self-degradation of Micro-arc Oxidation/Chitosan Composite Coating on Mg-4Li-1Ca Alloy." *Surface and Coatings Technology* 344: 1–11. https://doi.org/10.1016/j.surfcoat.2018.03.007

Yu, Yang, Shi-Jie Zhu, Hao-Tian Dong, Xue-Qi Zhang, Jing-An Li, and Shao-Kang Guan. 2021. "A Novel MgF2/PDA/S-HA Coating on the Bio-degradable ZE21B Alloy for Better Multi-Functions on Cardiovascular Application." *Journal of Magnesium and Alloys* 11 (2): 1–11. https://doi.org/10.1016/j.jma.2021.06.015

Yuan, Bo, Hewei Chen, Rui Zhao, Xuangeng Deng, Guo Chen, Xiao Yang, and Zhanwen Xiao et al. 2022. "Construction of a Magnesium Hydroxide/Graphene Oxide/Hydroxyapatite Composite Coating on Mg-Ca-Zn-Ag Alloy to Inhibit Bacterial Infection and Promote Bone Regeneration." *Bioactive Materials* 18: 354–67. https://doi.org/10.1016/j.bioactmat.2022.02.030

Yuan, Tianwen, Jia Yu, Jun Cao, Fei Gao, Yueqi Zhu, Yingsheng Cheng, and Wenguo Cui. 2016. "Fabrication of a Delaying Biodegradable Magnesium Alloy-Based Esophageal Stent via Coating Elastic Polymer." *Materials* 9 (5): 384. https://doi.org/10.3390/ma9050384

Zeng, Rong-Chang, Li-Jun Liu, Kai-Jie Luo, Li Shen, Fen Zhang, and Yu-Hong Zou. 2015. "In Vitro Corrosion and Antibacterial Properties of Layer-by-layer Assembled GS/PSS Coating on AZ31 Magnesium Alloys." *Transactions of Nonferrous Metals Society of China* 25 (12): 4028–39. https://doi.org/10.1016/S1003-6326(15)64052-3

Zhang, Zhongyang, Lasse Hyldgaard Klausen, Menglin Chen, and Mingdong Dong. 2018. "Electroactive Scaffolds for Neurogenesis and Myogenesis: Graphene-based Nanomaterials." *Small* 14 (48): 1801983. https://doi.org/10.1002/smll.201801983

Zhang, Tingting, Zhongxian Liu, Yi An Zhu, Zhicheng Liu, Zhijun Sui, Kake Zhu, and Xinggui Zhou. 2020. "Dry Reforming of Methane on Ni-Fe-MgO Catalysts: Influence of Fe on Carbon-resistant Property and Kinetics." *Applied Catalysis B: Environmental* 264 (May): 118497. https://doi.org/10.1016/j.apcatb.2019.118497

Zhang, Lei, Jia Pei, Haodong Wang, Yongjuan Shi, Jialin Niu, Feng Yuan, Hua Huang, Hua Zhang, and Guangyin Yuan. 2017. "Facile Preparation of Poly(lactic acid)/Brushite Bilayer Coating on Biodegradable Magnesium Alloys with Multiple Functionalities for Orthopedic Application." *ACS Applied Materials & Interfaces* 9 (11): 9437–48. https://doi.org/10.1021/acsami.7b00209

Zhang, Dongdong, Feng Peng, Ji Tan, and Xuanyong Liu. 2019. "In-situ Growth of Layered Double Hydroxide Films on Biomedical Magnesium Alloy by Transforming Metal Oxyhydroxide." *Applied Surface Science* 496: 143690. https://doi.org/10.1016/j.apsusc.2019.143690

Zhang, Keru, Xing Tang, Juan Zhang, Wei Lu, Xia Lin, Yu Zhang, Bin Tian, Hua Yang, and Haibing He. 2014. "PEG–PLGA Copolymers: Their Structure and Structure-influenced Drug Delivery Applications." *Journal of Controlled Release* 183: 77–86. https://doi.org/10.1016/j.jconrel.2014.03.026

Zhang, Zhao-Qi, Yong-Xin Yang, Jing-An Li, Rong-Chang Zeng, and Shao-Kang Guan. 2021. "Advances in Coatings on Magnesium Alloys for Cardiovascular Stents: A Review." *Bioactive Materials* 6 (12): 4729–57. https://doi.org/10.1016/j.bioactmat.2021.04.044

Zhang, Xiaoyong, Jilei Yin, Cheng Peng, Weiqing Hu, Zhiyong Zhu, Wenxin Li, Chunhai Fan, and Qing Huang. 2011. "Distribution and Biocompatibility Studies of Graphene Oxide in Mice after Intravenous Administration." *Carbon* 49 (3): 986–95. https://doi.org/10.1016/j.carbon.2010.11.005

Zhao, Zhanyong, Peikang Bai, Wenbo Du, Bin Liu, Duo Pan, Rajib Das, Chuntai Liu, and Zhanhu Guo. 2020. "An Overview of Graphene and Its Derivatives Reinforced Metal Matrix Composites: Preparation, Properties and Applications." *Carbon* 170: 302–26. https://doi.org/10.1016/j.carbon.2020.08.040

Zhao, Yun, Yangping Chen, Wei Wang, Zhiyu Zhou, Shuxin Shi, Wei Li, Minfang Chen, and Ze Li. 2020. "One-Step In Situ Synthesis of Nano Silver–Hydrotalcite Coating for Enhanced Antibacterial and Degradation Property of Magnesium Alloys." *Materials Letters* 265: 127349. https://doi.org/10.1016/j.matlet.2020.127349

Zhao, Jun, Liang-jian Chen, Kun Yu, Chang Chen, Yi-long Dai, Xue-yan Qiao, Yang Yan, and Zhi-ming Yu. 2015. "Effects of Chitosan Coating on Biocompatibility of Mg–6%Zn–10%Ca$_3$(PO$_4$)$_2$ Implant." *Transactions of Nonferrous Metals Society of China* 25 (3): 824–31. https://doi.org/10.1016/S1003-6326(15)63669-X

Zhao, Yanbin, Zhao Zhang, Liqian Shi, Fen Zhang, Shuoqi Li, and Rongchang Zeng. 2019. "Corrosion Resistance of a Self-Healing Multilayer Film Based on SiO$_2$ and CeO$_2$ Nanoparticles Layer-by-layer Assembly on Mg Alloys." *Materials Letters* 237: 14–18. https://doi.org/10.1016/j.matlet.2018.11.069

Zhao, Nan, and Donghui Zhu. 2014. "Collagen Self-assembly on Orthopedic Magnesium Biomaterials Surface and Subsequent Bone Cell Attachment." *PLoS One* 9 (10): e110420. https://doi.org/10.1371/journal.pone.0110420

Zheng, Qiyao, Jun Li, Wei Yuan, Xiangmei Liu, Lei Tan, Yufeng Zheng, Kelvin Wai Kwok Yeung, and Shuilin Wu. 2019. "Metal–Organic Frameworks Incorporated Polycaprolactone Film for Enhanced Corrosion Resistance and Biocompatibility of Mg Alloy." *ACS Sustainable Chemistry & Engineering* 7 (21): 18114–24. https://doi.org/10.1021/acssuschemeng.9b05196

Zhou, Wuchao, Zhenrong Hu, Taolei Wang, Guangzheng Yang, Weihong Xi, Yanzi Gan, Wei Lu, and Jingzhou Hu. 2020. "Enhanced Corrosion Resistance and Bioactivity of Mg Alloy Modified by Zn-Doped Nanowhisker Hydroxyapatite Coatings." *Colloids and Surfaces B: Biointerfaces* 186: 110710. https://doi.org/10.1016/j.colsurfb.2019.110710

Zhu, Yuwei, Wei Liu, and To Ngai. 2022. "Polymer Coatings on Magnesium-based Implants for Orthopedic Applications." *Journal of Polymer Science* 60 (1): 32–51. https://doi.org/10.1002/pol.20210578

Zhu, Liwei, Cong Peng, Kensuke Kuroda, and Masazumi Okido. 2019. "Hydrophilic Thin Films Formation on AZ31 Alloys by Hydrothermal Treatment in Silicate Containing Solution and the Evaluation of Corrosion Protection in Phosphate Buffered Saline." *Materials Research Express* 6 (11): 116424. https://doi.org/10.1088/2053-1591/ab4705

Zhu, Yanying, Guangming Wu, Yun-Hong Zhang, and Qing Zhao. 2011. "Growth and Characterization of Mg(OH)$_2$ Film on Magnesium Alloy AZ31." *Applied Surface Science* 257 (14): 6129–37. https://doi.org/10.1016/j.apsusc.2011.02.017

Zomorodian, A., I. A. Ribeiro, J. C. S. Fernandes, A. C. Matos, C. Santos, A. F. Bettencourt, and M. F. Montemor. 2017. "Biopolymeric Coatings for Delivery of Antibiotic and Controlled Degradation of Bioresorbable Mg AZ31 Alloys." *International Journal of Polymeric Materials and Polymeric Biomaterials* 66 (11): 533–43. https://doi.org/10.1080/00914037.2016.1252347

# 8 Corrosion Behavior of Mg Alloys in Simulated Body Fluids

*Umer Masood Chaudry and Tea-Sung Jun*
Incheon National University
and
Research Institute for Engineering and Technology
Incheon, Republic of Korea

*Hafiz Muhammad Rehan Tariq*
Incheon National University, Incheon, Republic of Korea

*Badar Zaman Minhas and Muhammad Atiq Ur Rehman*
Institute of Space Technology, Islamabad, Pakistan

## 8.1 INTRODUCTION

Magnesium and its alloys are promising candidate as biomaterials owning to its excellent biocompatibility in the physiological environment and superior regeneration ability of bone. The remarkable specific strength makes it an ideal candidate for load-bearing applications, such as in bone implants (Chaudry, Hamad, and Jun 2022, Chaudry, Noh, Han, Jaafreh et al. 2022, Chaudry, Noh, Han, Hamad et al. 2022, Masood Chaudry, Hamad, and Kim 2020b). Moreover, Young's modulus of magnesium has been reported to be approximately 45 GPa, a value that closely matches the modulus of bone, which bone minimizes the likelihood of stress shielding (Kirkland 2012). In addition to its superior strength, magnesium also exhibits favorable biocompatibility. When used as a biomaterial, it does not provoke adverse reactions or toxicity in living tissue. This property is due to natural occurrence of magnesium in the human body (Figure 8.1). Daily intake of magnesium for every adult human is recommended about 420 mg which is much greater than other bio-implanting candidates like iron and zinc. Thus, its use as a biomaterial reduces the likelihood of harmful effects compared to other foreign materials (Masood Chaudry, Tekumalla et al. 2022). Another advantage of magnesium as a biomaterial is its ability to gradually degrade and get absorbed by the body over time. This property arises from its good solubility in human plasma-like media (Chen, Xu et al. 2014). As such, magnesium-based biomaterials can be tailored to degrade at controlled rates, providing time for the body to heal and regenerate the

DOI: 10.1201/9781003400462-8

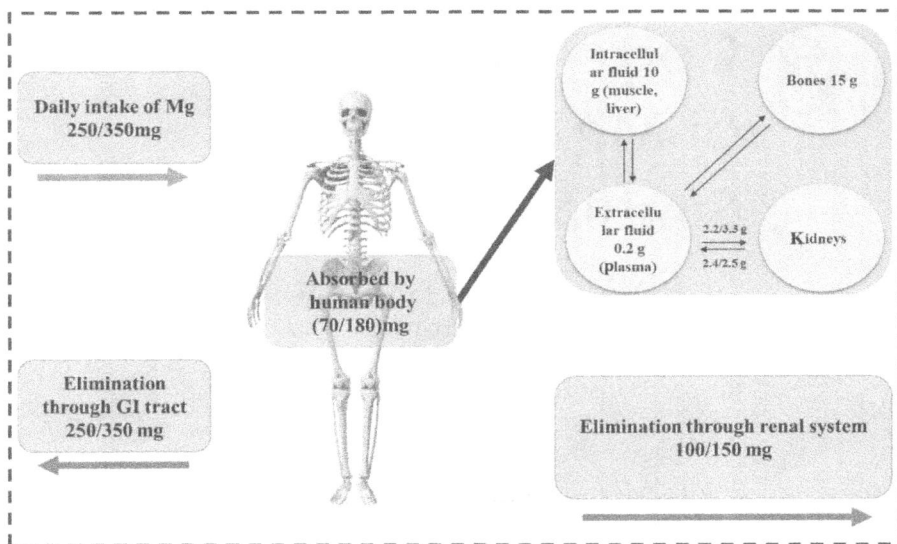

**FIGURE 8.1**   Mg absorption and elimination balance in human body (De Baaij, Hoenderop, and Bindels 2012).

affected tissue. In late 19th century, Edward C. Huse first introduced magnesium wires in medical field as a bandage to stop bleeding. Later on in early 20th century, Erwin Payr used fixator pins, nails, wires, and plates made of magnesium in the field of orthopedics. He also conducted notable research on the decomposition of magnesium and identified the factors that lead to its inherent corrosion (Riaz, Shabib, and Haider 2019). Despite investigations into the promising behavior of magnesium as an implant material beginning as early as 19th century, several fundamental challenges that prevent its global usage still persist. The main challenge that cause implant failure is the swift deterioration of magnesium in physiological environment that leads to a loss of mechanical potency.

## 8.2   ELECTROCHEMICAL CORROSION RESPONSE OF MAGNESIUM ALLOYS IN SIMULATED BODY FLUID

SBF is a solution that simulates the ionic composition of human blood plasma and is used to evaluate the corrosion behavior of metallic biomaterials. The SBF is composed of $NaCl$, $NaHCO_3$, $KCl$, $K_2HPO_4$, $MgCl_2$, $CaCl_2$, and $Na_2SO_4$. The pH of SBF is maintained at 7.4, which is the pH of human blood. The formation of a protective layer on the alloy surface is critical for their biocompatibility and biodegradability (Masood Chaudry et al. 2018; Witte 2010). The hydroxyapatite layer is formed by the reaction of Mg with SBF, which results in the precipitation of calcium phosphate on the alloy surface.

The corrosion rate (CR) of Mg alloys in SBF can be calculated using the following equation:

$$CR = \frac{\Delta W}{A \times t} \times 10^3$$

where $\Delta W$ is the weight loss of the Mg alloy, $A$ is the surface area of the Mg alloy, $t$ is the exposure time, and $10^3$ is the conversion factor from mg to g.

The corrosion behavior of Mg alloys in SBF can be evaluated using various electro-chemical techniques such as potentio-dynamic polarization, electrochemical impedance spectroscopy (EIS), and cyclic voltammetry (CV). Potentio-dynamic polarization is a technique that measures the current response of the Mg alloy to an applied potential. EIS measures the impedance of the Mg alloy at various frequencies, while CV measures the current response of the Mg alloy to a changing potential.

One important parameter to consider when evaluating the corrosion behavior of Mg alloys in SBF is the open-circuit potential (OCP). It predicts the affinity of the Mg alloy to corrode in SBF. A more negative OCP indicates a higher tendency for corrosion. The corrosion behavior of Mg alloys in SBF can be understood by the following equation:

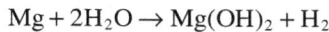

$$Mg + 2H_2O \rightarrow Mg(OH)_2 + H_2$$

The reaction shows the formation of magnesium hydroxide and hydrogen gas as a product of the reaction between Mg and water in SBF. The rate of this reaction determines the rate of corrosion of the Mg alloy in SBF. The presence of chloride ions in SBF can dissolve Mg and accelerate the corrosion process (Zengin et al. 2020). The following reaction occurs in the presence of chloride ions.

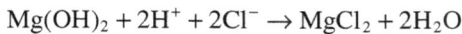

$$Mg(OH)_2 + 2H^+ + 2Cl^- \rightarrow MgCl_2 + 2H_2O$$

Besides other techniques, alloying magnesium with rare earth elements (RE) (like yttrium, gadolinium, lanthanum, etc.) and non-RE like elements (aluminum, zinc, calcium, etc.) is considered to be a most effective mechanism for improving its mechanical properties along with corrosion resistance (Chaudry, Noh, Hamad et al. 2022). Table 8.1 presents information on how the properties of Mg are impacted by varying alloying elements.

Most of the studies have shown that Mg alloys with higher amounts of Al and Zn exhibit better corrosion resistance in SBF due to the formation of a protective layer of Mg-Al and Mg-Zn compounds on their surface (Masood Chaudry, Farooq et al. 2022). More likely, the enhanced resistance to corrosion is attributed to the creation of a nonsoluble layer of $Al_2O_3$, rather than $Mg(OH)_2$, which can be dissolved in chloride solutions (Brar, Wong, and Manuel 2012). Zn addition in Mg-Al can also have the tendency to enhance the corrosion resistance. When the Mg-Al-Zn alloy is exposed to air or oxygen, it results in the formation of a thin layer of zinc oxide on the surface of the alloy. Zinc oxide is a stable and nonporous material that acts as a barrier to further corrosion, protecting the underlying alloy from corrosion

**TABLE 8.1**

**Effect of Alloying Elements on Magnesium Presented in Different Studies**

| Alloying Element | Improved Mechanical Properties | Improved Corrosion Resistance | References |
|---|---|---|---|
| Al | YS, UTS hardness, EL | $I_{corr}$, $E_{corr}$, mass loss | Pardo et al. 2008, Rahman, Pompa, and Haider 2015, Singh, Singh, and Das 2015, Wang, Shinohara, and Zhang 2010 |
| Zn | YS, UTS hardness, EL | $I_{corr}$, $E_{corr}$, mass loss | Cai et al. 2012, Gu et al. 2009, Zhang et al. 2011 |
| Ca | YS, UTS hardness, EL | $I_{corr}$, $E_{corr}$, mass loss | Bakhsheshi-Rad et al. 2014, Drynda et al. 2010 |
| RE | YS, UTS hardness, EL | $I_{corr}$, $E_{corr}$, mass loss | Cao et al. 2013, Ding et al. 2014, Zhao, Shi, and Xu 2013 |

damage. The addition of Zr to Mg-Zn alloys, resulting in ZK alloys, is a well-known technique for enhancing both mechanical properties and corrosion resistance (Li et al. 2022{Malik, 2022 #762)}(Chaudry and Hamad 2021). Moreover, the incorporation of RE into ZK alloys yields highly effective and significantly anticorrosive Mg alloys. It is worth mentioning that corrosion resistance of Mg is often improved by introducing Zn in amounts less than 5 wt% and Zr in levels less than 2 wt%. Savaedi et al. used EIS experiments in SBF solution to examine the biocorrosion resistance of hot-rolled pure Mg, ZK30, and ZEK300 alloys (Savaedi et al. 2022). The findings were evaluated using Nyquist plots (Figure 8.2(a)). The diameter of the semicircular arc in pure Mg was noticeably lower than in the other samples, which is an important finding. On the other hand, the semicircular arc width was significantly bigger in the ZK30 alloy, which also contains Zn and Zr in addition to Mg. By looking at the polarization curves shown in Figure 8.2(b), where the Tafel extrapolation method indicated corrosion current density ($i_{corr}$) values of 79 A/cm$^2$ for pure Mg and 32 A/cm$^2$ for ZK30, these findings were further supported.

Studying the Nyquist plot of the rolled ZEK300 alloy, it is possible to conclude that the addition of Ce to ZK30 favorably improved corrosion resistance, which is consistent with the results provided in Figure 8.2(b) ($i_{corr}$ = 30 A/cm$^2$). In fact, adding RE to magnesium alloys reduces galvanic corrosion and promotes the creation of a stable oxide coating at the corrosion interface. As a result, the ZEK300 alloy not only proved good thermal stability and strength at relatively high temperatures, but it also revealed remarkable biocorrosion resistance.

Apart from this, Ca also plays an important role and being a crucial mineral of bone, its alloying with Mg up to a certain content limit (0.6 wt%) can also result in better corrosion resistance as compared to pure magnesium. Above this limit there is a possibility of formation of $Mg_2Ca$ secondary phase which facilitates establishment of galvanic cell that lower the corrosion resistance (Chaudry et al. 2023, Datta et al. 2011, Han et al. 2022, Masood Chaudry, Hamad, and Kim 2020a).

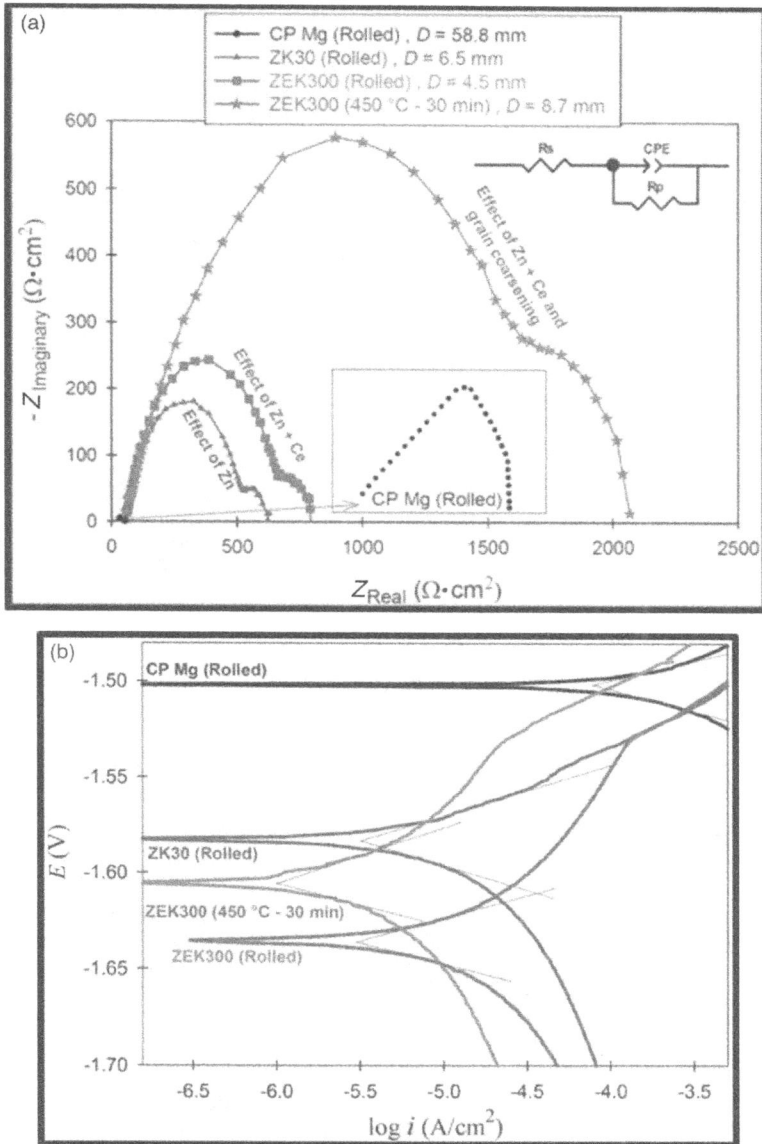

**FIGURE 8.2**   (a) Nyquist curves and (b) Tafel plots, respectively, for pure Mg, ZK30, ZEK300 Mg alloys (Savaedi et al. 2022).

The biological performance of magnesium-based alloy AZ91D in SBF at 37°C was studied by the analysis of electrochemical impedance spectroscopy (EIS) with immersion time. The main aim is to explore the possible ways to improve the corrosion resistance of the implants. The Bode plots for AZ91D alloy in SBF was conducted for 35 h, as shown in Figure 8.4 (a)–(c). The plots show capacitive region at intermediate

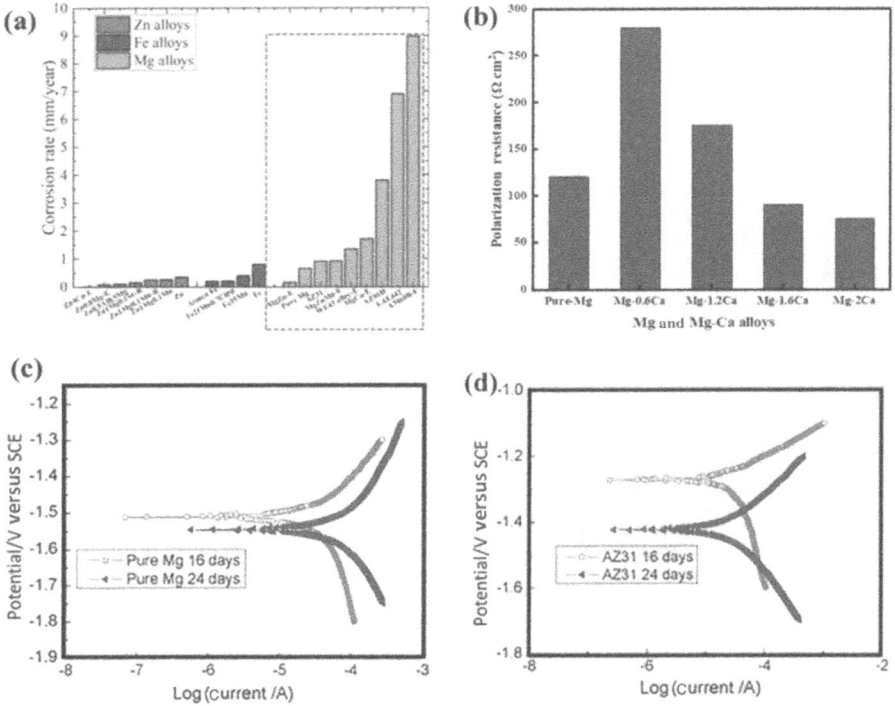

**FIGURE 8.3** (a) Comparison between corrosion rates of magnesium and other biomaterials. (b) Effect of Ca addition in Mg on polarization resistance. (c and d) Tafel curve of pure magnesium and AZ31 Mg alloy after immersing in SBF for 16 and 24 days, respectively (Chaudry, Hamad, and Kim 2019, Wan et al. 2008, Wen et al. 2009).

frequency, while at high and low frequencies it displayed resistive response. It can be observed that an increase in time of immersion, from 0 to 1.5 h (Figure 8.3 (a)), continuously increases the $|Z|$ value, while $\theta_{max}$ is nearly constant. However, at 2.0–10 h (Figure 8.3(b)), the impedance value increases but not sharply. At higher immersion time, 15–35 h (Figure 8.4(c)), an increase in the immersion time increases the $|Z|$ value, while $\theta_{max}$ gradually decreases with a concomitant shift to lower frequencies. This indicates that capacitance values of the surface are decreased. In Figure 8.4(d) the SEM image show smooth surface, while Figure 8.4(e) illustrates the microcrack formation which predicts the favorable region for the corrosive ion (El-Taib Heakal, Mohammed Fekry, and Ziad Fatayerji 2009, Heakal, Fekry, and Fatayerji 2009).

The EIS data is analyzed by the equivalent electric circuit (EECs). The Bode data were simulated by appropriate EECs as shown in Figure 8.4(f) and (g). Generally, the response of simple corroding metal in an aqueous solution is well recorded by the classic parallel resistor capacitor (R1C1) combination in series with the solution resistance ($R_s$) between the specimen and the RE. In this circuit, a charge transfer resistance (R1) is in parallel with the double-layer capacitance (C1), as shown in (Figure 8.4 (f)).

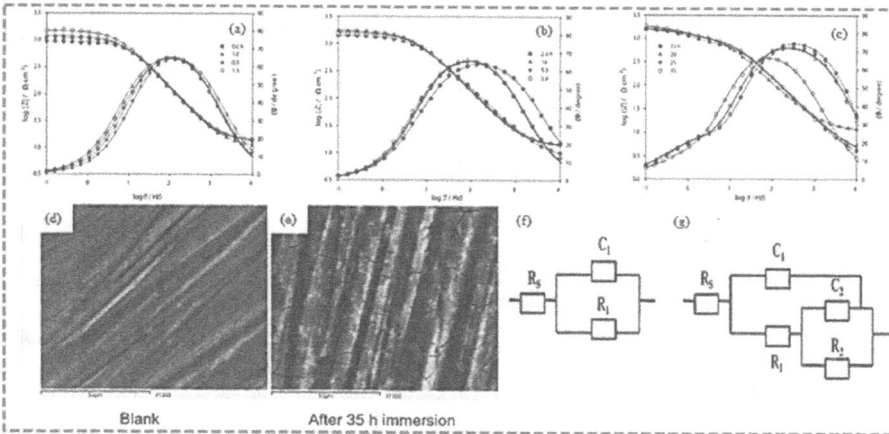

**FIGURE 8.4**  (a–c) Bode plots of AZ91D alloy over the immersion time in SBF at 37°C. (d and e) SEM image of AZ91D, bare and after 35 h in SBF. (f and g) Equivalent electric circuits used to fit EIS spectra, one-time constant and two-time constants for an electrode–electrolyte solution interface, respectively.

On the other hand, the Bode data with two-time constants in good agreement with the equivalent electric circuit consists of $R(C_1(R_1(C_2R_2)))$, as illustrated in Figure 8.4(g). The C1 is the capacitance of the outer layer and the faradaic reaction therein and C2 pertains to the inner layer, while R1 and R2 are the respective resistances of the outer and inner layers constituting the surface film, respectively (El-Taib Heakal, Mohammed Fekry, and Ziad Fatayerji 2009). The results show that EECs are in good agreement with the experimental data.

Alloying with RE elements can also increase the corrosion resistance of magnesium alloys like Mg-Al and Mg-Zn. High concentration of Ce in Mg-Al alloy generates $Al_{11}Ce_3$ phase which behaves like cathode of galvanic cell and helps to prevent the corrosion of magnesium. Moreover, alloying Mg with Gd (up to 10 wt%) can also improve the corrosion resistance by forming $Mg_5Gd$ phase (Zhang et al. 2016).

## 8.3  BIO-FRIENDLY COATINGS AND SURFACE MODIFICATION FOR Mg ALLOYS

Surface treatment has emerged as a cost-effective solution to control the degradation of Mg and its alloys. The goal of surface treatment is to improve their corrosion resistance by applying a biocompatible protective layer. Various coating techniques have been researched and employed to achieve the desired corrosion properties. There are many different bio-friendly coatings, through which Mg implants are protected in the human body fluid. Figure 8.3 shows the cathodic electrodeposition of hydroxy-apatite coating on AZ31 alloy (Ilican et al. 2008).

Mostly composite coatings (polymer and ceramic) are used on Mg implants. Table 8.2 provides a summary of the commonly used coatings for Mg and its alloys through different techniques.

**TABLE 8.2**

**Coatings for Mg and Its Alloys through Different Techniques**

| Coating Technique | Coatings | Substrates | Performance Indicator for CR | Bioactivity Indicator |
|---|---|---|---|---|
| Chemical conversion | $Ca_3(PO_4)_2$ | Pure Mg, AZ31, AZ61, Mg-Mn- Zn alloy, WE43 | $I_{corr}$ mass loss, Mg ion release, volume loss | Cell proliferation, in vivo mice, in vivo rabbits, Mg serum level |
| | $MgF_2$ | Pure Mg, ANd42, AZ31, LAE442, LANd442, LNd442, Mg/$Al_2O_3$ composite, Mg-Ca alloys, Nd2, ZK30, ZK60 | Charge transfer resistance, corrosion rate, $E_{corr}$, $H_2$ evolution, $I_{corr}$ mass loss, pH change, polarization resistance, volume loss | Cell proliferation, cell viability, hemocompatibility, in vivo rabbits |
| | $ZnCa_3(PO_4)_2$, $Sr_3(PO_4)_2$ | AZ31, pure Mg | $E_{corr}$, $H_2$ evolution, $I_{corr}$ | Cell proliferation, cell viability |
| MAO | $Ca_3(PO_4)_2$ | AZ31, AZ91, Mg-Zn-Ca alloy | $E_{corr}$, $H_2$ evolution, $I_{corr}$ polarization resistance | n/a |
| Anodization | Oxide layer | AM60, AZ31, AZ91, ZK60 | Charge transfer resistance, corrosion rate, $E_{corr}$, $I_{corr}$ Mg ion release, pH change | Cell proliferation, cell viability |
| | Fluoride layer | AZ31, WE43 | Corrosion rate, $E_{corr}$, $I_{corr}$ mass loss | n/a |
| Ion implantation | Zn, Ce, ZrN, Hf, Nd, Fe, Ca, Cr-O, Zr-O, N, Ta ion implantations | Pure Mg, AZ31, AZ91, Mg-Ca alloys, WE43, ZK60 | Charge transfer resistance, corrosion rate, $E_{corr}$, $I_{corr}$ Mg ion release, pH change, polarization resistance | Cell proliferation, cell viability |
| ECD | $Ca_3(PO_4)_2$ | AZ31, AZ91, Mg-Sr alloy, Mg-Zn-Ca alloy, Mg-2Zn, Mg-3Zn | Charge transfer resistance, corrosion rate, $E_{corr}$, $H_2$ evolution, $I_{corr}$ mass loss, pH change | Cell proliferation, cell viability |
| PVD | HA | AZ31, AZ91, Mg-1Ca | Charge transfer resistance, $E_{corr}$, $I_{corr}$ mass loss, polarization resistance | Cell proliferation, cell viability |

*Sources:* Carboneras, García-Alonso, and Escudero (2011), Chen, Nisbet et al. (2014), Chiu et al. (2007), Hiromoto and Yamamoto (2009), Li et al. (2017), Lin et al. (2017), Seitz et al. (2011), Xu et al. (2009), and Zeng et al. (2016).

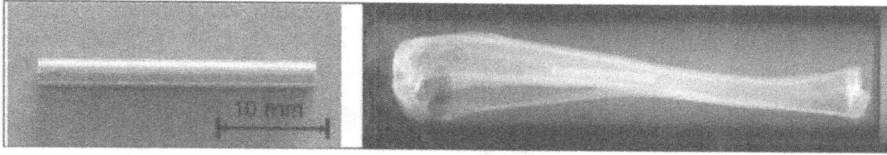

**FIGURE 8.5** Implant material and implant location. (a) Extruded magnesium pin. (b) Radiograph of implant location.

## 8.4  MAGNESIUM ALLOY AS A DEGRADABLE MATERIAL IN ORTHOPEDIC APPLICATIONS

In orthopedic research, magnesium implants are promising candidate. The main advantage of using magnesium as orthopedic implants is that it is nonallergic and a natural component of the body (Chaudry, Farooq et al. 2022). In order to examine, the chosen magnesium alloys appropriate for the use in orthopedic applications, in vivo studies in rabbit tibiae were done. All vivo tests were carried out under the ethic committee approval in accordance with German federal legislation. Five rabbits were used for each group. Extruded pins with 2.5 mm in diameter and 25 mm in length were implanted into both tibiae (Figure 8.5). Four tibiae remained without implant and served as control. The vivo alloy consisted of magnesium, the elements Li, Al and a rare earth composition metal (LAE442), yttrium and a rare earth composition metal (WE43), calcium (MgCa0.8), aluminum and calcium (AX30) or zinc, a rare earth composition metal, and zirconium (ZEK100). The detailed procedure is described elsewhere (Pearce et al. 2007). At the end of the observation period, the rabbits were euthanized, and the tibiae removed. The results indicated that the residual implants which contained calcium degraded faster than those containing rare earth alloys (Thomann et al. 2009).

## REFERENCES

Bakhsheshi-Rad, H. R., M. H. Idris, M. R. Abdul-Kadir, A. Ourdjini, M. Medraj, M. Daroonparvar, and E. Hamzah. 2014. "Mechanical and bio-corrosion properties of quaternary Mg-Ca-Mn-Zn alloys compared with binary Mg-Ca alloys." *Materials & Design* no. 53:283–92.

Brar, Harpreet S., Joey Wong, and Michele V. Manuel. 2012. "Investigation of the mechanical and degradation properties of Mg-Sr and Mg-Zn-Sr alloys for use as potential biodegradable implant materials." *Journal of the Mechanical Behavior of Biomedical Materials* no. 7:87–95.

Cai, Shuhua, Ting Lei, Nianfeng Li, and Fangfang Feng. 2012. "Effects of Zn on microstructure, mechanical properties and corrosion behavior of Mg-Zn alloys." *Materials Science and Engineering: C* no. 32 (8):2570–77.

Cao, Fuyong, Zhiming Shi, Guang-Ling Song, Ming Liu, and Andrej Atrens. 2013. "Corrosion behaviour in salt spray and in 3.5% NaCl solution saturated with Mg(OH)$_2$ of as-cast and solution heat-treated binary Mg-X alloys: X= Mn, Sn, Ca, Zn, Al, Zr, Si, Sr." *Corrosion Science* no. 76:60–97.

Carboneras, M., M. C. García-Alonso, and M. L. Escudero. 2011. "Biodegradation kinetics of modified magnesium-based materials in cell culture medium." *Corrosion Science* no. 53 (4):1433–39.

Chaudry, Umer Masood, Ameeq Farooq, Kaab bin Tayyab, Abdul Malik, Muhammad Kamran, Jung-Gu Kim, Chuan Li, Kotiba Hamad, and Tea-Sung Jun. 2022. "Corrosion behavior of AZ31 magnesium alloy with calcium addition." *Corrosion Science* no. 199:110205.

Chaudry, Umer Masood, and Kotiba Hamad. 2021. "Effect of calcium on the superplastic behavior of AZ31 magnesium alloy." *Materials Science and Engineering: A* no. 815:140874.

Chaudry, Umer Masood, Kotiba Hamad, and Tea-Sung Jun. 2022. "Investigating the microstructure, crystallographic texture and mechanical behavior of hot-rolled pure Mg and Mg-2Al-1Zn-1Ca alloy." *Crystals* no. 12 (10):1330.

Chaudry, Umer Masood, Kotiba Hamad, and Jung-Gu Kim. 2019. "On the ductility of magnesium based materials: A mini review." *Journal of Alloys and Compounds* no. 792:652–64.

Chaudry, Umer Masood, Gukin Han, Yeonju Noh, and Tea-Sung Jun. 2023. "Effect of Ca alloying and cryogenic temperature on the slip transmission across the grain boundary in pure Mg." *Journal of Alloys and Compounds* no. 950:169828.

Chaudry, Umer Masood, Yeonju Noh, Kotiba Hamad, and Tea-Sung Jun. 2022. "Effect of deformation temperature on the slip activity in pure Mg and AZX211." *Journal of Materials Research and Technology* no. 19:3406–20.

Chaudry, Umer Masood, Yeonju Noh, Gukin Han, Kotiba Hamad, and Tea-Sung Jun. 2022. "Effect of pre-twinning on microstructure and texture evolution in room and cryogenically deformed Mg-0.5 Ca alloy." *Journal of Physics: Conference Series* no. 2169:012009.

Chaudry, Umer Masood, Yeonju Noh, Gukin Han, Russlan Jaafreh, Tea-Sung Jun, and Kotiba Hamad. 2022. "Effect of CaO on structure and properties of AZ61 magnesium alloy." *Materials Science and Engineering: A* no. 844:143189.

Chen, Xiao Bo, David Russell Nisbet, Rachel W. Li, P. N. Smith, Trevor B. Abbott, Mark Alan Easton, D.-H. Zhang, and Nick Birbilis. 2014. "Controlling initial biodegradation of magnesium by a biocompatible strontium phosphate conversion coating." *Acta Biomaterialia* no. 10 (3):1463–74.

Chen, Yongjun, Zhigang Xu, Christopher Smith, and Jag Sankar. 2014. "Recent advances on the development of magnesium alloys for biodegradable implants." *Acta Biomaterialia* no. 10 (11):4561–73.

Chiu, K. Y., M. H. Wong, F. T. Cheng, and Hau Chung Man. 2007. "Characterization and corrosion studies of fluoride conversion coating on degradable Mg implants." *Surface and Coatings Technology* no. 202 (3):590–98.

Datta, Moni Kanchan, Da-Tren Chou, Daeho Hong, Partha Saha, Sung Jae Chung, Bouen Lee, Arif Sirinterlikci, Madhumati Ramanathan, Abhijit Roy, and Prashant N Kumta. 2011. "Structure and thermal stability of biodegradable Mg-Zn-Ca based amorphous alloys synthesized by mechanical alloying." *Materials Science and Engineering: B* no. 176 (20):1637–43.

De Baaij, Jeroen H. F., Joost G. J. Hoenderop, and René J. M. Bindels. 2012. "Regulation of magnesium balance: Lessons learned from human genetic disease." *Clinical Kidney Journal* no. 5 (Suppl 1):i15–24.

Ding, Yunfei, Cuie Wen, Peter Hodgson, and Yuncang Li. 2014. "Effects of alloying elements on the corrosion behavior and biocompatibility of biodegradable magnesium alloys: A review." *Journal of Materials Chemistry B* no. 2 (14):1912–33.

Drynda, Andreas, Thomas Hassel, René Hoehn, Angela Perz, Friedrich-Wilhelm Bach, and Matthias Peuster. 2010. "Development and biocompatibility of a novel corrodible fluoride-coated magnesium–calcium alloy with improved degradation kinetics and adequate mechanical properties for cardiovascular applications." *Journal of Biomedical Materials Research Part A* no. 93 (2):763–75.

El-Taib Heakal, Fakiha, Amany Mohammed Fekry, and Mohammed Ziad Fatayerji. 2009. "Electrochemical behavior of AZ91D magnesium alloy in phosphate medium: Part I: Effect of pH." *Journal of Applied Electrochemistry* no. 39:583–91.

Gu, Xuenan, Yufeng Zheng, Yan Cheng, Shengping Zhong, and Tingfei Xi. 2009. "In vitro corrosion and biocompatibility of binary magnesium alloys." *Biomaterials* no. 30 (4):484–98.

Han, Gukin, Yeonju Noh, Umer Masood Chaudry, Sung Hyuk Park, Kotiba Hamad, and Tea-Sung Jun. 2022. "{10–12} Extension twinning activity and compression behavior of pure Mg and Mg-0.5 Ca alloy at cryogenic temperature." *Materials Science and Engineering: A* no. 831:142189.

Heakal, F. El-Taib, A. M. Fekry, and M. Z. Fatayerji. 2009. "Influence of halides on the dissolution and passivation behavior of AZ91D magnesium alloy in aqueous solutions." *Electrochimica Acta* no. 54 (5):1545–57.

Hiromoto, Sachiko, and Akiko Yamamoto. 2009. "High corrosion resistance of magnesium coated with hydroxyapatite directly synthesized in an aqueous solution." *Electrochimica Acta* no. 54 (27):7085–93.

Ilican, Saliha, Yasemin Caglar, Mujdat Caglar, and Fahrettin Yakuphanoglu. 2008. "Structural, optical and electrical properties of F-doped ZnO nanorod semiconductor thin films deposited by sol–gel process." *Applied Surface Science* no. 255 (5):2353–59.

Kirkland, Nicholas Travis. 2012. "Magnesium biomaterials: Past, present and future." *Corrosion Engineering, Science and Technology* no. 47 (5):322–28.

Li, Chuan, Abdul Malik, Faisal Nazeer, Umer Masood Chaudry, Jianyu Long, and Yangwei Wang. 2022. "A strong, ductile and in-plane tensile isotropic Mg-0.5 Zn-0.5 Y-0.15 Si alloy." *Journal of Materials Research and Technology* no. 20:3344–54.

Li, Zhen, Sun Shizhao, Minfang Chen, Bradley Dean Fahlman, Debao Liu, and Hongwei Bi. 2017. "In vitro and in vivo corrosion, mechanical properties and biocompatibility evaluation of MgF2-coated Mg-Zn-Zr alloy as cancellous screws." *Materials Science and Engineering: C* no. 75:1268–80.

Lin, Da-Jun, Fei-Yi Hung, Ming-Long Yeh, Hung-Pang Lee, and Truan-Sheng Lui. 2017. "Development of a novel micro-textured surface using duplex surface modification for biomedical Mg alloy applications." *Materials Letters* no. 206:9–12.

Masood Chaudry, Umer, Ameeq Farooq, Abdul Malik, Muhammad Nabeel, Muhammad Sufyan, Asima Tayyeb, Sumbal Asif, Aqil Inam, Ahmed Elbalaawy, and Eslam Hafez. 2022. "Biodegradable properties of AZ31-0.5 Ca magnesium alloy." *Materials Technology* no. 37 (12):2230–41.

Masood Chaudry, Umer, Kotiba Hamad, and Jung-Gu Kim. 2020a. "A further improvement in the room-temperature formability of magnesium alloy sheets by pre-stretching." *Materials* no. 13 (11):2633.

Masood Chaudry, Umer, Kotiba Hamad, and Jung-Gu Kim. 2020b. "Optimisation of structure for enhancing the room-temperature stretch formability of magnesium alloy." *Philosophical Magazine Letters* no. 100 (10):461–67.

Masood Chaudry, Umer, Tae Hoo Kim, Sang Duck Park, Ye Sik Kim, Kotiba Hamad, and Jung-Gu Kim. 2018. "On the high formability of AZ31-0.5 Ca magnesium alloy." *Materials* no. 11 (11):2201.

Masood Chaudry, Umer, Sravya Tekumalla, Manoj Gupta, Tea-Sung Jun, and Kotiba Hamad. 2022. "Designing highly ductile magnesium alloys: Current status and future challenges." *Critical Reviews in Solid State and Materials Sciences* no. 47 (2):194–281.

Pardo, A., M. C. Merino, A. Ef Coy, R. Arrabal, F. Viejo, and E. Matykina. 2008. "Corrosion behaviour of magnesium/aluminium alloys in 3.5 wt.% NaCl." *Corrosion Science* no. 50 (3):823–34.

Pearce, A. I., R. G. Richards, S. Milz, E. Schneider, and S. G. Pearce. 2007. "Animal models for implant biomaterial research in bone: A review." *European Cells & Materials* no. 13 (1):1–10.

Rahman, Zia Ur, Luis Pompa, and Waseem Haider. 2015. "Electrochemical characterization and in-vitro bio-assessment of AZ31B and AZ91E alloys as biodegradable implant materials." *Journal of Materials Science: Materials in Medicine* no. 26:1–11.

Riaz, Usman, Ishraq Shabib, and Waseem Haider. 2019. "The current trends of Mg alloys in biomedical applications: A review." *Journal of Biomedical Materials Research Part B: Applied Biomaterials* no. 107 (6):1970–96.

Savaedi, Zeinab, Hamed Mirzadeh, Rouhollah Mehdinavaz Aghdam, and Reza Mahmudi. 2022. "Thermal stability, grain growth kinetics, mechanical properties, and biocorrosion resistance of pure Mg, ZK30, and ZEK300 alloys: A comparative study." *Materials Today Communications* no. 33:104825.

Seitz, Jan-Marten, Kelly Collier, Eric Wulf, Dirk Bormann, and Friedrich-Wilhelm Bach. 2011. "Comparison of the corrosion behavior of coated and uncoated magnesium alloys in an in vitro corrosion environment." *Advanced Engineering Materials* no. 13 (9):B313–23.

Singh, I. B., M. Singh, and S. Das. 2015. "A comparative corrosion behavior of Mg, AZ31 and AZ91 alloys in 3.5% NaCl solution." *Journal of Magnesium and Alloys* no. 3 (2):142–48.

Thomann, M., Ch Krause, D. Bormann, N. von der Höh, H. Windhagen, and A. Meyer-Lindenberg. 2009. "Comparison of the resorbable magnesium: Alloys LAE442 and MgCa0.8 concerning their mechanical properties, their progress of degradation and the bone-implant-contact after 12 months implantation duration in a rabbit model." *Materialwissenschaft Und Werkstofftechnik* no. 40 (1–2):82–87.

Wan, Yizao, Guangyao Xiong, Honglin Luo, Fang He, Yuan Huang, and Xiaoshong Zhou. 2008. "Preparation and characterization of a new biomedical magnesium–calcium alloy." *Materials & Design* no. 29 (10):2034–37.

Wang, Lei, Tadashi Shinohara, and Bo-Ping Zhang. 2010. "Corrosion behavior of Mg, AZ31, and AZ91 alloys in dilute NaCl solutions." *Journal of Solid State Electrochemistry* no. 14:1897–1907.

Wen, Zhaohui, Changjun Wu, Changsong Dai, and Feixia Yang. 2009. "Corrosion behaviors of Mg and its alloys with different Al contents in a modified simulated body fluid." *Journal of Alloys and Compounds* no. 488 (1):392–99.

Witte, Frank. 2010. "The history of biodegradable magnesium implants: A review." *Acta Biomaterialia* no. 6 (5):1680–92.

Xu, Liping, Feng Pan, Guoning Yu, Lei Yang, Erlin Zhang, and Ke Yang. 2009. "In vitro and in vivo evaluation of the surface bioactivity of a calcium phosphate coated magnesium alloy." *Biomaterials* no. 30 (8):1512–23.

Zhao, Xu, Ling-ling Shi, and Jian Xu. 2013. "A comparison of corrosion behavior in saline environment: Rare earth metals (Y, Nd, Gd, Dy) for alloying of biodegradable magnesium alloys." *Journal of Materials Science & Technology* no. 29 (9):781–87.

Zeng, Rong-Chang, Yan HU, Fen Zhang, Yuan-Ding Huang, Zhen-Lin Wang, Shuo-Qi Li, and En-Hou Han. 2016. "Corrosion resistance of cerium-doped zinc calcium phosphate chemical conversion coatings on AZ31 magnesium alloy." *Transactions of Nonferrous Metals Society of China* no. 26 (2):472–83.

Zengin, Huseyin, Yunus Turen, Hayrettin Ahlatci, and Yavuz Sun. 2020. "Microstructure, mechanical properties and corrosion resistance of as-cast and as-extruded Mg-4Zn-1La magnesium alloy." *Rare Metals* no. 39:909–17.

Zhang, Xiaobo, Zhixin Ba, Zhangzhong Wang, and Yajun Xue. 2016. "Microstructures and corrosion behavior of biodegradable Mg-6Gd-xZn-0.4 Zr alloys with and without long period stacking ordered structure." *Corrosion Science* no. 105:68–77.

Zhang, Baoping, Yunlong Hou, Xiaodan Wang, Yin Wang, and Lin Geng. 2011. "Mechanical properties, degradation performance and cytotoxicity of Mg-Zn-Ca biomedical alloys with different compositions." *Materials Science and Engineering: C* no. 31 (8):1667–73.

# 9 Reuse, Remanufacturing, and Recycling of Mg Alloys

*Sagar V. Wankhede and Akbar Ahmad*
Symbiosis Skills and Professional University Pune, India

*Pralhad Pesode*
Dr. Vishwanath Karad MIT World Peace University,
Pune, India

*Manoj Mugale*
Cleveland State University, Cleveland, USA

## 9.1 INTRODUCTION

Magnesium alloys are among the more lightweight metals used in everyday life. It has a lot of beneficial physical and mechanical properties as well, including high specific strength, enhanced conductivity and vibration resistance. They may also be easily recycled, chopped, and shaped, and they are also reasonably priced. Magnesium alloys have been praised as both environmentally classic building materials and benign technical materials for the twenty-first century because of their usefulness as building/biomedical applications materials [1–4]. Future usage of these materials will be difficult due to their strong electrochemical interactions, which render them corrosive in saltwater, moist environments, acids, and related organic/inorganic salts [5, 6]. At the moment, they are widely utilized in the following industries: portable computers, optical equipment, electronic communications, defense, automotive components, and aeroplanes [7, 8]. Defensive surface management is therefore required in their applications [9–11]. By covering metals with a protective layer, corrosion can be prevented. The protective coatings serve as a barrier between the applied metal and the corrosive environment. The coatings will occasionally act as sacrificial anodes. Some of the frequently employed coating application methods include metal cladding, PVD coatings, laser cladding, electroless plating, oxygen fuel with high-velocity spraying, plasma spraying, electroplating, anodizing, and friction stir processing (FSP) [12]. Advanced technologies were created between organic and conversion deposition, and both were used widely. The electroplating technique is the most cutting-edge technology for all materials due to its exceptional wear resistance, solderability, and corrosion resistance.

Magnesium alloy electroplating, on the other hand, is still in its infancy and has not made enough progress. There are two basic reasons why electroplating

DOI: 10.1201/9781003400462-9

magnesium alloys are challenging [13]. First, a powerful chemical reaction occurs and is followed by the rapid production of pores and an uneven oxide coating on their surface. The quality of the coatings generated without particular pre- and post-processing could deteriorate, and the microstructure of magnesium alloys would significantly affect electroplating [1]. Nonetheless, the low corrosion rate of Mg alloys remains a challenge, limiting their application in circumstances when high corrosion resistance is required.

The development of lightweight materials technology has been prompted by the growing demand for low-density structural materials like land/air travel. To comply with upcoming pollution requirements, the car sector is increasingly looking for stronger and lighter materials. A key strategy for decreasing emissions and saving energy and materials is to lighten the typical automobile. Many automotive parts are now made using magnesium instead of aluminium since it is 100% recyclable, 33% lighter, and has one of the highest strength-to-weight ratios of other regularly used metal [14]. For the past ten years, at a rate of 15% annually, the demand for these components has increased the output of magnesium die castings [15]. For automotive applications, over 70% of all magnesium die casting is done [16].

Since its invention in the nineteenth century, magnesium, the lightest construction metal, has seen a huge growth in use. In 1916, the first commercial magnesium production was noted in Germany [17]; nevertheless, due to a dearth of markets, the global magnesium production was just 300 tons [18]. The magnesium industry did not experience considerable growth until the Second World War. Magnesium production climbed to 237,000 tons globally by the end of 1943 [18]. Two years later, usage of magnesium had drastically decreased to 50,000 tons [18]. About 366,900 tons of magnesium were used up in the year 2000, and it took another 30 years for yearly production to return its 1945 level. The Yearbook-2004 of U.S. Geological Survey Minerals estimates that 584,000 metric tons of primary magnesium were produced globally in 2004 [19].

## 9.2   SOURCES OF MAGNESIUM SCRAP

### 9.2.1   DIE-CASTING SCRAP

In a normal die-casting operation, 41% of the magnesium lost is Class 1 garbage, 5% are dross/returns each and 36% are runners, gates, and trim scrap, according to the International Magnesium Association (IMA) [20]. Natural Resources Canada estimates that about 110,700 tons of magnesium were used in 2000 by the die-casting industry, or 30% of all primary magnesium produced globally [21].

According to the source in the previous sentence, the world produced 22,693 tons of Class 1 magnesium scrap, 2,768 tons of magnesium dross/returns each, and 19,926 tons of magnesium trim scrap, runners, and gates in 2000 (based on IMA numbers). The classification scheme for scrap magnesium is shown in Table 9.1 [22].

### 9.2.2   POST-CONSUMER SCRAP

It includes materials from telecommunications, electronics, automotive, computer industries, and audio. Due to the recent expansion of magnesium use in the massive

**TABLE 9.1**
**Categories of Magnesium Scrap**

| Mg Scrap Classes | Characterization |
| --- | --- |
| Class 1A | Clean, high-quality scrap without contaminants |
| Class 1B | Pristine scrap having a large surface area compared to weight |
| Class 2 | Clear-up scrap with steel or aluminium inserts. No brass or copper impurities |
| Class 3 | Turnings and swarfs that are clean, dry, and uncontaminated |
| Class 4 | Residues free of flux |
| Class 5 | Scrap painted or coated with or without aluminized or steel inlays. No brass or copper |
| Class 6 | Swarfs and turnings that are greasy or wet |
| Class 7 | Metal scrap that is unclean and contaminated (such as post-consumer scrap) could include Si (Al alloys, shot blasting), Cu-contaminated alloys, Ni coatings, magnesium-free sweepings |
| Class 8 | Flux-containing waste products from recycling magnesium |

*Source:* Reference [22].

automobile market, the amount of post-consumer magnesium scrap is constantly rising. Earlier, magnesium recycling from scrapped or "end-of-life" automobiles was not particularly progressed. Germany and Japan did not have any quantitative data on the recycling of magnesium from vehicle shredder scrap in 1992 [23]. Inefficiency and high prices are the two main reasons why magnesium recycling from shredder refuse is lacking. This is because metal recovery is constrained by the use of coatings composed of magnesium to avoid corrosion and the fact that the majority of recycling of magnesium has been done by handpicking.

### 9.2.2.1 Effect of Impurities in Magnesium

The creation of various magnesium alloys involves the use of eight primary alloying ingredients. Each element promotes distinct qualities in the magnesium at a particular concentration. Yet, the introduction of contaminants into the metal as a result of recycling can have a significant impact on the characteristics of magnesium. If these modifications are significant, the magnesium may no longer meet the standards for the intended purpose. Intermetallic and inclusions of magnesium oxide are the two impurities that are most frequently found in magnesium. Even in modest concentrations, intermetallics can significantly impair the corrosion resistance of magnesium and quickly reduce the parameters below what is needed. Intermetallics, which comprise iron, nickel, or cobalt, have the biggest effect on reducing magnesium's corrosion resistance.

Due to the substantial electrochemical potential difference between these elements and magnesium, small electrochemical cells form on the surface. Due to the extensive usage of iron-bearing machinery in the foundry, iron occurs in intermetallic inclusions most frequently among the three mentioned elements. However, some intermetallics can strengthen the magnesium by preventing or slowing the movement of dislocations as persistent stress is applied. Unfortunately, this causes the magnesium to harden substantially, leading to a large drop in ductility. Certain magnesium alloy systems have shown dwindlings in ductility of up to 50%. Magnesium oxide inclusions lessen the material's ductility and ultimate tensile strength (UTS), but they boost its yield strength (YS). Almost linear is the negative connection between the UTS and magnesium oxide content. The threshold concentration of oxide that must be present before the UTS falls below ASTM requirements has been determined to be 500 ppm. Magnesium's UTS and ductility both decline as particle size rises. Surprisingly, the YS of magnesium showed a slight increase with increasing oxide concentration due to the particles' ability to prevent dislocations. Magnesium oxide inclusions have a similar electrochemical potential as magnesium, hence they do not impact the magnesium's resistance to corrosion.

Magnesium oxide has also been proven to make magnesium less machinable and fluid by making it more viscous and increasing tool wear. Flux and magnesium silicate inclusions are two additional nonmetallic inclusions that may have an impact on the characteristics of magnesium. Because of the introduction of fluxless refining processes, flux inclusions are now uncommon. Yet, their presence on the magnesium surface may cause corrosion to dramatically rise. It has been discovered that magnesium silicate impurities can reduce the metal's ductility by up to 40% without affecting its strength.

## 9.3 REFINING TECHNOLOGIES FOR MAGNESIUM

Due to the increasing need for magnesium in the automotive die-casting industry, recycling of the metal has taken on greater significance. Currently, die-casting processes solely recycle high-grade magnesium scrap (Class 1) using flux or fluxless refining. This is because the variety of scrap generated during die casting cannot be sufficiently cleaned using current refining technology. Due to the excessive handling and soiled nature of the starting material, magnesium recycling of scrap classes 2–8 is not seen as an economical choice. To turn the magnesium back into a usable product from these classes, substantial preprocessing, chemical alterations, and refinement processes are needed. The methods are uneconomical because the procedures for processing these classes are complicated.

Thus, there is a growing need for more efficient magnesium refining systems for the recycling of all sorts of scrap as a result of the increased usage of magnesium and the accumulation of scrap. There are two types of refining technologies: flux-based and fluxless.

### 9.3.1 FLUX REFINING TECHNOLOGIES

The most popular and yet relatively old way of processing magnesium scrap is flux refining. It uses two separate fluxes to remove impurities from the underlying metal and stop surface oxidation. A cover flux is a flux that prevents the magnesium surface from oxidizing. Simple cover fluxes are made up of fluoroborate salts, boric acid, and sulfuric chemicals. It just takes a tiny amount of flux, typically 1 wt% of the total charge if the melt's cleanliness is high (Class 1), to ensure proper fluxing. A secondary flux is needed to refine the underlying metal because a cover flux will not clean the magnesium beneath it.

The primary function of the secondary flux in the refining process is to break up and agglomerate oxide particles, films, and skins that form during melting as well as to agglomerate nonmetallic impurities contained within the original metal. This flux may selectively wet tiny magnesium oxide skins to help remove them. It can also coat either solid or liquid surfaces. The flux should have a higher density because liquid magnesium has such a low specific gravity. Higher refining efficiency results from greater mixing capabilities with the liquid magnesium as a result. Also, to guarantee maximum contact between the flux and the magnesium metal, the flux is often applied to the melt surface while the magnesium is slowly churned with an impeller. The flux is allowed to settle and gather as a sludge at the bottom of the crucible once the correct inclusion composition has been achieved. The stirring is then halted. Flux removal from the crucible's bottom is known as sludging, and it is done on a regular basis (Figure 9.1).

A typical flux used in the refining of magnesium contains approximately 49 wt% anhydrous $MgCl_2$, 27 wt% KCl, 20 wt% $BaCl_2$, and 4 wt% $CaF_2$ [14]. Yet, the type of magnesium alloy being made has a significant impact on the flux's chemical makeup. An adequate amount of time must be allotted for settling in order to successfully eliminate the wetted inclusions. The process variables charge size, charge cleanliness, and flux addition all affect how long the charge actually settles. In the process of refining magnesium, the melt's temperature is also important. The best interaction between a liquid flux and molten metal has been discovered to occur at 705°C [24].

However, the critical temperature varies slightly depending on the type of alloy and the related flux. The purity of the feed material has a significant impact on the amount of flux needed for refining. The flux required for crude magnesium has been calculated to be 7–8% of the magnesium weight [25]. The quantity of flux needed rises as the magnesium's purity declines. This is especially true when melting magnesium scrap that includes casting sand, lubricants, and scrap with a high surface-to-volume ratio. In order to cover the surface of the scrap and better agglomerate the impurities, the flux will first be melted before the charge is added if the magnesium scrap is extremely unclean. In order to get rid of impurities like iron and silicon when the

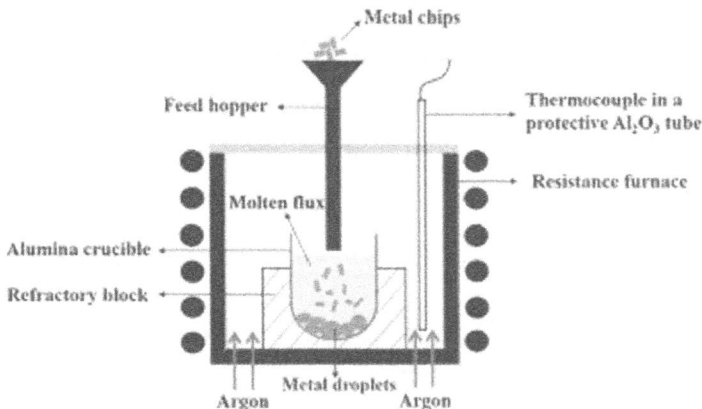

**FIGURE 9.1** Schematic of the experimental setup for the coalescence tests [90].

magnesium metal is polluted with them, additives are added to the flux. The additives must create intermetallic compounds with the metallic impurities in order to function as refiners. The possibility of intermetallic production is primarily influenced by three variables: electronegativity, ionization potential, and ionic radii. Boron and manganese chloride ($MnCl_2$) have been discovered to be efficient additions for the removal of iron from magnesium [26]. Magnesium also uses beryllium, in the form of a chloride, to purify iron. Because of its limited solubility in magnesium, beryllium is a very alluring refiner. Yet, due to its high toxicity, hardly many businesses use it. Following that, the intermetallics are precipitated from the magnesium and gathered in the sludge at the crucible's bottom. Although titanium chlorides and titanium remove both silicon and iron from the melt, zinc chloride or cobalt chloride is employed to remove silicon. The use of metallic additions, however, cannot remove all metallic species from the magnesium melt. This happens as a result of the strong interaction that certain species, like copper and nickel, have with magnesium.

Once the magnesium has been processed to the required standards, it is either pumped or tilt-poured into a holding/casting furnace. In this secondary furnace, molten magnesium is shielded from oxidation by a cover gas of variable composition. A gas combination containing sulfur hexafluoride is the most typical cover gas employed. After that, the magnesium solidifies into substantial ingots. Flux refining's key benefit is its capacity to clean up filthy magnesium scrap. The technique is a reasonably cost-effective method for refining magnesium because of the cheap initial capital cost of the equipment. Yet, the likelihood of including more contaminants increases when a flux is added to the magnesium melt.

Large flux inclusions can occasionally become trapped in the magnesium, degrading some of its physical characteristics. Due to this, the characteristics of magnesium degrade past the chemical and physical limits established for die-casting material. Moreover, the possibility of important alloying elements becoming trapped and leading to subpar alloying agent recoveries is increased by the addition of chlorides to the magnesium melt. Moreover, the majority of cover fluxes containing chlorides, particularly $MgCl_2$, are very hygroscopic. The likelihood of hydrogen absorption into the magnesium melt increases when water is trapped, and this is thought to be the main cause of the microporosity and microshrinkage seen in final castings [27]. In addition, the salt's chloride can combine with the dissolved hydrogen to form vapors of hydrochloric acid, which can quickly destroy steel furnace equipment. Inert gas sparging must be used to get rid of the hydrogen or other dissolved gases. Furthermore, magnesium is frequently trapped inside the globules that are created when oxides are wetted and absorbed. High melt losses arise from this, and extra procedures are needed to recover the magnesium from the flux. Also, it is unknown how used flux is disposed of or whether any of it may be recycled back into the process. It is obvious that flux-based refining methods are not the best option for refining magnesium.

### 9.3.2 FLUXLESS REFINING TECHNOLOGIES

Any other processes for refining magnesium that do not include the use of a salt flux are included in fluxless refining. In some fluxless processes, molten salt can still be used as a heating medium in the refining furnace. Salt however does little to clean out contaminants from the magnesium. Although there are several fluxless methods, using flux is still the most common technique in the industry for refining.

### 9.3.3  SALT FURNACE TECHNOLOGY

Particle adhesion and sedimentation brought on by convection in the salt bath are used in this Norsk Hydro method for melting and refining magnesium to purify the metal. The fundamental benefit of this method is that it can refine all scrap classes of magnesium with a relatively good recovery rate, excluding utilized fluxes and sludge [28]. High-purity magnesium alloys may be produced utilizing Class 1–2 scrap, thanks to increased process control. However, because of the intricacy of the furnace, the equipment's initial cost is more than that for flux refining. Moreover, a lot of waste materials (such as dross and spent salt) are created. A cover gas must be used because $MgCl_2$ is not used to protect the metal. This is an issue because the magnesium industry is currently progressively transitioning away from sulfur hexa-fluoride and toward alternative gases.

### 9.3.4  INERT GAS AND FILTER REFINING

This technology involves shredding, heating, and charging magnesium scrap into an enclosed crucible for melting. Argon sparging, settling, and filtering processes are used to purify the magnesium melt. As it is pumped from the crucible to the casting area, the magnesium is filtered. To prevent oxidation, an SF6 mixture is employed to shield the melt. The Dow Chemical Company employs procedures to refine the majority of its die-casting scrap (Class 1) in order to create very clean magnesium melt because argon gas sparging successfully removes the tiny inclusions and filter-ing effectively removes the larger ones. The resulting inclusion count was $65/cm^2$, and the use of argon sparging also decreased the amount of dissolved gases in the magnesium melt [27].

The important benefits of the process are that it requires only a mixer, filter, and sparger, resulting in a minimal initial investment cost. This enables recycling to be done inside. The equipment's survival can be increased through proper care and cleaning. The method can produce high-purity magnesium alloys at a reasonable recovery rate because it does not need salts. Moreover, the chemical makeup can be effectively adjusted. However, because big inclusions can rather quickly clog the filter, only Class 1 scrap can be purified using this method. Regular stoppages would result from this, and the filtration equipment's lifespan would be shortened, rais-ing processing expenses. Sulfur dioxide or gases containing hexafluoride must also be employed to shield the magnesium's surface. Another illustration of a fluxless method to produce pure magnesium from recovered die-casting debris is Rauch's recycling furnace [28]. A mixture of nitrogen gas and sulfur dioxide with a concen-tration of 0.2–0.5% is employed to protect the melt surface [28]. The actual furnace has three major chambers and burns gas. The first chamber is where the scrap mag-nesium is melted, while the second and third chambers are where the magnesium is refined. The three refinement processes used to remove impurities from the magne-sium include settling and filtering, as well as nitrogen or argon sparging.

### 9.3.5 Vacuum Distillation Refining

Vacuum distillation is a fascinating solution for recycling various kinds of scrap magnesium. By using this process, magnesium scrap will be converted into very-high-purity magnesium which will be used in the semiconductor sector [29]. According to some sources, vacuum distillation can increase the metal's purity by about 500 times with just one more step [29]. The output of conventional vacuum distillation technologies is modest, and they are intermittent. Moreover, the fine, compressed magnesium is very pyrophoric. Its usefulness for applications in the recycling industry is therefore quite low. Nevertheless, distillation carried out under standard pressure is less difficult, continuous, and extremely productive.

### 9.3.6 Hydrometallurgy

Hydrometallurgy is a technique of recycling old slags and drosses. The process includes producing chlorides of magnesium and other alloying elements by reacting aqueous hydrochloric acid with either dross or slag. By reintroducing magnesium chloride to the electrolytic cells, the magnesium may be recycled, and the priceless alloying elements can then be obtained and sold. The processing of dirty magnesium waste produced by the primary and secondary magnesium industries, as well as the ability to recover and market precious metals, are advantages of this processing. The main drawback is that the processing is uneconomical if the waste product contains too little precious metal due to the high processing costs. Also, because the Mg units must be returned to the electrolysis cell as $MgCl_2$, the majority of the magnesium value is lost.

## 9.4   COATING AND POSTPROCESSING TECHNIQUES FOR MAGNESIUM ALLOY

The literature study shows that there is not a single postprocessing strategy that can be applied to every coating techniques. The postprocessing procedure must be adjusted to the coating method's material, resource, and composition. This study will provide an inside look at various tactics for meeting the protective coatings. Another thing to remember is that coating techniques are significantly influenced by the microstructure of alloys. There were several methods for surface modification, including the friction stir process technique, laser cladding, and the sol–gel approach. The postprocessing methods using different coating technologies are described in the next section.

One of the most affordable and technically feasible methods for creating composite coatings is electrodeposition. The mechanical characteristics of coatings have been improved by using PC (pulse current) electrodeposition techniques [30]. The good composite coating can be employed in micro-drives that enhances mechanical properties [31]. The deposition properties, including hardness, porosity, and electric conductivity, are improved by pulse plating. Using pulse electrodeposition, a number of alloys, including nickel, copper, zinc, and nickel–iron, were created and their increased special features were disclosed.

Using pulse electrodeposition methods, the nanocomposite coating was studied [32]. The technology is commercially viable due to its low cost and greater control over the features and the structure of the coating. The corrosion resistance of PC coatings was found to be better than that of DC electrodeposited coatings which investigated the effects of microstructural, micro-hardness, and duty cycle characteristics on PC electrodeposition of steel basis materials [33]. The best corrosion resistance is found on the coated substrate with the lowest duty cycle. Al 7075 alloys' corrosion and wear characteristics were examined by using the PMC deposition technique [34]. The outcome demonstrates that the rate of corrosion of base materials with coatings is lower than that of the untreated Al 7075 alloy.

The impacts of SiC, $Si_3N_4$, and $Al_2O_3$ on the microstructural characteristics of electroplated nickel were studied [35] and it was concluded that micro-hardness has been increased by $Si_3N_4$ coatings. For Al alloy corrosion resistance, silica-based hybrid nanocomposite coatings were studied [36] and it was found that hybrid coatings advances methods of surface processing [37, 38]. To create a protective covering for magnesium alloys, the copper was coated using an electroplating procedure. Magnesium alloys could be coated with nanoparticles via an electrophoretic deposition process. Boron, silicon, phosphorous oxide, and aluminum nanoparticles were attempted as coating materials [39]. Utilizing the electrodeposition technique, an impact of the aluminum coating on AZ91D magnesium alloy was examined [40]. According to the study, magnesium alloy with an aluminum coating has strong adhesive strength and increases the substrate material's resistance to corrosion. Using a cold spraying approach, the impact of $Mg_{17}Al_{12}$ coating and Al on AZ91D magnesium alloy was investigated [41]. According to the study, the coating's hardness is greatly increased by intermetallics, and the Mg alloy's corrosion resistance is enhanced by pure aluminium. The corrosion performance of alloy AZ91 is enhanced by the various types of PVD deposition and plasma postprocessing. Utilizing the plasma CVD process using radio frequency, a diamond-like carbon film coating was produced to increase the corrosion and wear resistance of magnesium alloys. For the goal of protecting the surfaces of these alloys, pure zinc and $Zn_5Al$ coatings on AZ91 Mg alloys and AA7022 Al alloys were applied using the cold gas spray technique [42]. The dip deposition technique's sol–gel approach might be used to create CeO and $ZrO_2$ coatings on the magnesium alloys. The sol–gel technique using zirconium oxide with incorporated $CeO_2$ increases the corrosion resistance of magnesium alloys [40]. The laser surface melting increases the corrosion resistance of the Mg alloys like AZ61, AZ31, and WE [43, 44]. For the purpose of post-treating magnesium alloys, a number of surface modification techniques, including laser surface alloying, laser melting, laser cladding, and laser shock peening, were explored worldwide [45, 46]. The research demonstrates that several laser surface modification methods greatly enhance the surface characteristics of magnesium alloys [47, 48]. The corrosion resistance of AZ91D alloys is only slightly enhanced by the LSM approach [49]. The Zr-Al-Ni-Cu based coating applied to the pure Mg substrate using the laser cladding technology increased its resistance to corrosion and wear. Silver layer was applied to the Mg alloys using electroless deposition and organic coating techniques.

The PVD approach was successfully used to create a unique MGlue-TiMgN coating that protects the Mg alloys from corrosion and wear [46]. To increase corrosion resistance, copper sheets were electrolessly plated onto the surface of magnesium alloys. To improve the corrosion performance of pure magnesium metal, calcium phosphate was coated on the metal using the solution chemistry technique [1]. The microstructure of the magnesium alloy is altered by the nucleation of aluminium-rich particles caused by the aqueous copper deposition, according to research on the influence of magnesium alloy microstructure on the process of aqueous coating deposition [47].

Ni-Zr-Al was attempted to be coated onto AZ91 HP Mg alloy utilizing a laser cladding process. It was found that deposition improves wear/corrosion resistance and hardness. The protective anodic oxide layer on magnesium alloys was created using the micro-arc anodic oxidation (MAO) technique. By using the laser cladding process, it is possible to coat magnesium substrates with multiple layers of Ni, Cu, and Al. By using a laser cladding process, a multilayer coating of Ti-Ni-Al on AZ91HP Mg alloy can be produced. The wear/corrosion resistance and hardness of coatings are improved by the presence of $Ti_2Ni$ intermetallic [32].

The effects of heat processing on the corrosion resistance of AZ91D magnesium alloy for biodegradable implant applications were studied [48]. Investigations were done into how heat processing affected the corrosion properties of the magnesium alloy AZ31B H24 [49]. According to the study, the twinned microstructure had a higher rate of corrosion than the untwined one. Investigations into the AZ91D Mg alloys' susceptibility to stress corrosion cracking were conducted in physiological fluid simulations as well as in the air at various strain rates. Fractographic analyses reveal that the crack is primarily transgranular with a few tiny, isolated cracks. Arc ion cladding was used to cover AZ91 Mg alloys in a carbon layer that resembled a diamond.

When a composite coating made of styrene-acrylic emulsion and graphite was applied on the AZ91D alloy through anodic deposition [50], the corrosion resistance of the magnesium was found to have increased. Polymers have also been applied to magnesium metal coatings. Polymers were attempted to be used to magnesium alloys [51]. By using micro-arc oxidation, the impact of anodic coatings on magnesium alloys was studied [52]. In comparison to untreated specimens, anodic specimens treated with sodium borate solutions corrode less quickly. The technique using deionized water as a mineralizer was successful in synthesizing protective coatings on AZ31 Mg alloy [53]. Using electroless deposition directly onto acetic acid pickled AZ91D, the impact of Ni-B coating on AZ91D alloys was investigated [54]. According to the analysis, various coating reactions predominate at various stages of the plating process. By using a straightforward immersion approach, the vanadium coating on the ZE41 alloys was examined [55]. A vanadia coating improves the corrosion resistance of magnesium alloy, according to the study. Silane was attempted to be coated on magnesium alloys. The magnesium alloys received a silane coating using a dip coating technique. According to the study, silane coating increases the Mg alloy's ability to resist corrosion.

The dip coating process used sol–gel technique to deposit titanium oxide on AZ31 alloy [56]. A viable path has recently opened up for the development of an aluminum protective coating on magnesium alloys to improve their corrosion and wear qualities. Using fluidized bed CVD method, the coating of Al on Mg alloys was studied [57]. The impact of the aluminum coating on the corrosion and micro-hardness characteristics of AZ91D magnesium alloys was investigated [58]. For 1.5 hours, the aluminum coating on the AZ91D Mg alloy was created at 420°C. The microstructure investigation reveals that coated surfaces contain phases.

In comparison to uncoated AZ91D alloys, coated surfaces with rich b phases increased the surface hardness and corrosion resistance of AZ91D alloys. By using a laser cladding approach, the wear and corrosion performance of a magnesium alloy was improved [59]. The results show that the modified specimen's wear rate is much lower than that of the base materials. The application of aluminum powder coatings using the laser cladding method on ZE41 and WE43 Mg alloy was investigated [60]. The findings show that the presence of $Al_3Mg_2$ and $Al_{12}Mg_{17}$ intermetallic, generated as a result of laser cladding operation, increased the hardness.

Moreover, the magnesium alloys' corrosion resistance was improved by the aluminum powder coating. The research shows that the formation of tough secondary phase particles and a thick oxide layer by the Al-Cu alloy coating increased the wear and corrosion resistance. The effects of an $Al + Al_2O_3$ composite powder coating on the laser-clad AZ91D Mg alloy were investigated [61]. As a result of the homogeneous distribution of $Al_2O_3$ particles on the protected surface, the protective coating of $Al + Al_2O_3$ enhances wear resistance, according to the results. The laser cladding approach was also used by many researchers to layer aluminum on magnesium alloys. Researchers are drawn to the thermal spraying of aluminum coating on magnesium alloys, and numerous attempts have been made to use this technique [62].

Porosities in the protective coatings must be eliminated, which is a difficult task. The main disadvantage of thermal spray coating on magnesium alloy is porosity, which adversely affects the corrosion/wear performance and mechanical characteristics [9, 39, 42]. Thermal spraying approach was used to perform cold rolling on an aluminum-coated Mg-Li alloy [63]. The sealing of tiny channels between the surface and the substrate in the sprayed layer is what causes the impact of mild rolling. The magnesium-based surface nanocomposite was created by the FSP approach [13]. CNTs were successfully incorporated into an AZ31 Mg alloy by using the FSP approach.

An investigation of the impact of FSP on AZ31B magnesium alloy surface modification was carried out [64]. For the AZ61 alloy, the two-pass FSP combined with the quick heating sink results in a nanograined microstructure. Using FSP, the deterioration behavior of the AZ31B Mg alloy was examined [65]. The beneficial effect is anticipated to be more pronounced for magnesium alloys with high volumes of secondary phase particles that cause galvanic corrosion. Using FSP created ultrafine-grain-reinforced AZ91 Mg alloy composites with nanosized SiC and $Al_2O_3$ particles [66–68]. The outcome demonstrated that adding FSP passes improves fine grains, particle dispersion, and increases wear resistance, elongation, and hardness. Lastly, compared to coating quality, the laser cladding and thermal spraying processes have some drawbacks. They were unable to create coating surfaces without pores. To seal the porosities, further cold rolling is therefore required.

The FSP is recognized among the numerous surface modification techniques as a unique postprocessing procedure for alloys and metals. Aluminum alloys were the first materials utilized in the friction stir process. It has now been extended to ferrous alloys and nonferrous alloys such as magnesium alloys [69].

The materials for the friction stir tool would change based on the materials employed. The following are some important factors to consider while selecting tool materials (refer Table 9.2). The solid-state process, a unique technique for refining grains, is one of the advantages of FSP. Localized microstructure changes are possible and do not require additional heat input in place of frictional heat [69, 70].

**TABLE 9.2**
**Tool Materials for FSP**

| Materials Utilizing FSP | Tool Materials |
|---|---|
| Ni alloys | Cubic boron nitride that is polycrystalline |
| Low alloy steel | Polycrystalline cubic boron nitride with tungsten carbide |
| Stainless steel | Tungsten alloys, polycrystalline cubic boron nitride |
| Ti alloys | Ni alloys, tool steels, tungsten carbide tool steels, polycrystalline cubic boron nitride, tungsten alloys, and WC-Co |
| Cu alloys | Cubic boron nitride that is polycrystalline |
| Mg alloys | Polycrystalline cubic boron nitride with tungsten carbide |
| Al alloys | Polycrystalline cubic boron nitride, tungsten alloys |

*Source:* Reference [70].

FSP has some restrictions, including the requirement for stiff and durable fixtures, the formation of visible end holes, and the impossibility of filler welds. In comparison to existing post-spray processing, laser remelting was found to be a unique and effective postprocessing technique to enhance the performance of coated Mg alloy. The pharmaceutical industry has been more interested in using magnesium due to its remarkable properties as a biodegradable and biocompatible material, particularly when subjected to laser remelting [71–75]. The author's evidence suggests that optimization is required for the processing method's process parameters and postprocessing procedures [76–82].

Using the ultrasonic stir casting technique, it is possible to produce a uniform distribution of reinforcing powder particles during the process of manufacturing by adding cavitation to the liquid melting (Figure 9.2). Improved mechanical properties can be produced at a lower cost using environment-friendly approaches [83–88].

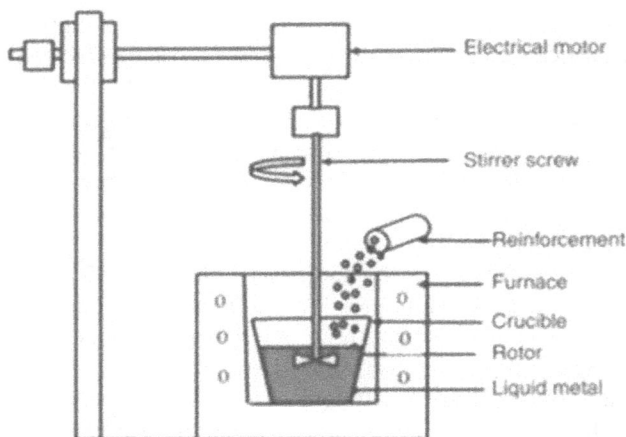

**FIGURE 9.2**   Block diagram of stir casting process [67].

## 9.5 CONCLUSION

The inability to efficiently separate, identify, and sort elements and components is what now prevents magnesium from being recycled to its full potential. Clean, properly sorted scrap is essential for recycling to be economical. In order for magnesium to continue to expand, all forms of magnesium scrap need to be recycled. More than half of the remaining low-grade magnesium scrap, such as turnings and thinner materials, cannot be treated economically, and only high-grade magnesium refuse, such as gates and failed castings, is currently recycled. This results from the variety of scrap produced not being sufficiently cleaned by present refining technology.

Through the use of effective refining methods, certain impurity elements associated with the recycling of magnesium scrap might cause embrittlement and poor corrosion resistance. The processing of low-grade magnesium scrap will be made easier with the development of enhanced sludging, evaporation, and filtering technologies, which can then be utilized to create magnesium alloys of the right caliber. As a result, there is an increasing demand for magnesium sorting and refining systems that are more efficient in order to recycle various forms of scrap.

Therefore, it can be concluded that the recycling market for magnesium, as it exists today, is fairly young. In particular, recycling low-grade scrap such turnings, dross, and end-of-life scrap is important. Impurities like nickel are typically removed by either producing a lower grade material that is appropriate only for steel desulfurization and aluminium alloying, or by diluting with pure magnesium, which inefficiently speeds up the process.

## REFERENCES

1. Gerashi, E., R. Alizadeh, and T. G. Langdon. 2022. "Effect of Crystallographic Texture and Twinning on the Corrosion Behavior of Mg Alloys: A Review." Journal of Magnesium & Alloys 10, no. 2: 313–25. https://doi.org/10.1016/j.jma.2021.09.009
2. Thakur, B., S. Barve, and P. Pesode. 2022. "Magnesium-based Nanocomposites for Biomedical Applications." In Advanced Materials for Biomechanical Applications, pp. 113–31. CRC Press.
3. _____. 2022. "Magnesium Alloy for Biomedical Applications." In Advanced Materials for Biomechanical Applications, pp. 133–58. CRC Press.
4. Pesode, P., S. Barve, S. V. Wankhede, and A. Chipade. 2023. "Metal Oxide Coating on Biodegradable Magnesium Alloys." 3c Empresa: Investigación y Pensamiento Crítico 12, no. 1: 392–421.
5. Maniam, K. K., and S. A. Paul. 2021. "A Review on the Electrodeposition of Aluminum and Aluminum Alloys in Ionic Liquids." Coatings 11, no. 1: 80. https://doi.org/10.3390/coatings11010080
6. Kumar, D., R. K. Phanden, and L. Thakur. 2021. "A Review on Environment Friendly and Lightweight Magnesium-based Metal Matrix Composites and Alloys." Materials Today: Proceedings 38: 359–64. https://doi.org/10.1016/j.matpr.2020.07.424
7. Wu, W., Z. Wang, S. Zang, X. Yu, H. Yang, and S. Chang. 2020. "Research Progress on Surface Treatments of Biodegradable Mg Alloys: A Review." ACS Omega 5, no. 2: 941–7. https://doi.org/10.1021/acsomega.9b03423
8. Rahman, M., Y. Li, and C. Wen. 2020. "HA Coating on Mg Alloys for Biomedical Applications: A Review." Journal of Magnesium & Alloys 8, no. 3: 929–43. https://doi.org/10.1016/j.jma.2020.05.003

9. Mohankumar, A., T. Duraisamy, D. Sampathkumar, S. Ranganathan, G. Balachandran, M. Kaliyamoorthy, M. Mariappan, and L. Mulugeta. 2022. "Optimization of Cold Spray Process Inputs to Minimize Porosity and Maximize Hardness of Metal Matrix Composite Coatings on AZ31B Magnesium Alloy." Journal of Nanomaterials 2022: 1–17. https://doi.org/10.1155/2022/7900150

10. Khodabakhshi, F., B. Marzbanrad, L. H. Shah, H. Jahed, and A. P. Gerlich. 2019. "Surface Modification of a Cold Gas Dynamic Spray-Deposited Titanium Coating on Aluminum Alloy by Using Friction-Stir Processing." Journal of Thermal Spray Technology 28, no. 6: 1185–98. https://doi.org/10.1007/s11666-019-00902-z

11. Zykova, A. P., S. Y. Tarasov, A. V. Chumaevskiy, and E. A. Kolubaev. 2020. "A Review of Friction Stir Processing of Structural Metallic Materials: Process, Properties, and Methods." Metals 10, no. 6: 772. https://doi.org/10.3390/met10060772

12. He, C., J. Wei, Y. Li, Z. Zhang, N. Tian, G. Qin, and L. Zuo. 2023. "Improvement of Microstructure and Fatigue Performance of Wire-Arc Additive Manufactured 4043 Aluminum Alloy Assisted by Interlayer Friction Stir Processing." Journal of Materials Science & Technology 133: 183–94. https://doi.org/10.1016/j.jmst.2022.07.001

13. Zhang, Z., A. Kitada, K. Fukami, and K. Murase. 2022. "Aluminum Electroplating on AZ31 Magnesium Alloy with Acetic Anhydride Pretreatment." Acta Metallurgica Sinica [English Letters] 35, no. 12: 1996–2006. https://doi.org/10.1007/s40195-022-01453-z

14. Scharf, C., and A. Ditze. 1998. Present State of Recycling of Magnesium and Its Alloys.

15. Luo, A. A. 2002. "Magnesium: Current and Potential Automotive Applications." JOM 54, no. 2: 42–8. https://doi.org/10.1007/BF02701073

16. Erickson, S. C. 1991. "Magnesium Gaining in Automotive Acceptance." Die Casting Engineer 35, no. 2: 18.

17. Wilson, C., K. Claus, M. Earlam, and J. Hillis. 1995. Magnesium and Magnesium Alloys: A Digest of Useful Technical Data. In Kirk-Othmer Encyclopedia of Chemical Technology, p. 1. McLean. PA: The International Magnesium Association.

18. Henstock, M. E. 1996. The Recycling of Nonferrous Metals. Ottawa, Ontario: International Council on Metals and the Environment.

19. US Geological Survey. 2004. "Magnesium – 2004." In U.S. Geological Survey Minerals Yearbook, pp. 46.1–6.

20. Brown, R. E. 2000. "Magnesium Recycling Yesterday, Today, Tomorrow." Recycling of Metals & Engineered Materials, 1: 1317–29.

21. Luo, A. A., N. R. Neelameggham, and R. S. Beals, eds. 2006. "Magnesium Technology." Proceedings of the Symposium Held during the TMS Annual Meeting in San Antonio, Texas, USA, March 12–16, 2006, vol. 2006. Minerals, Metals, & Materials Society.

22. Hanko, G., H. Antrekowitsch, and P. Ebner. 2002. "Recycling Automotive Magnesium Scrap." JOM 54, no. 2: 51–4. https://doi.org/10.1007/BF02701075

23. Sattler, H. P., and T. Yoshida. 1992. Recycling of Magnesium from Consumer Goods After Use.

24. Dalmijn, W. L., and J. A. Van Houwelingen. 1995. New Developments in the Processing of the Non-ferrous Metal Fraction of Car Scrap [No. CONF-951105]. Warrendale, PA: Minerals, Metals, & Materials Society.

25. Adamson, K. G., and D. S. Tawil. 1994. "Magnesium and Magnesium Alloys." In Corrosion, pp. 4–98. Butterworth-Heinemann.

26. Bowman, K. 1986. "Magnesium by the Magnetherm Process: Process Contamination and Fused Salt Refining." Light Metals 2: 1033–8.

27. _____. 2002. "Recycling Automotive Magnesium Scrap." JOM 54, no. 2: 51–4. https://doi.org/10.1007/BF02701075

28. Housh, S. E., and V. Petrovich. 1992. "Magnesium Refining: A Fluxless Alternative" [No. 920071]. SAE Technical Papers. https://doi.org/10.4271/920071

29. _____. 1998. Present State of Recycling of Magnesium and Its Alloys.

30. Odetola, P., P. Popoola, O. Popoola, and D. Delport. 2016. "Parametric Variables in Electrodeposition of Composite Coatings." Electrodeposition of Composite Materials. InTech. https://doi.org/10.5772/62010

31. Wu, Y., W. Qu, Z. Wang, and H. Zhuang. 2020. "Experimental Study on Brazing AZ31B Magnesium Alloy by Magnalium Alloys." Welding in the World 64, no. 1: 233–41. https://doi.org/10.1007/s40194-019-00809-x

32. Nguyen-Tri, P., T. A. Nguyen, P. Carriere, and C. Ngo Xuan. 2018. "Nanocomposite Coatings: Preparation, Characterization, Properties, and Applications." International Journal of Corrosion 2018: 1–19. https://doi.org/10.1155/2018/4749501

33. Kamnerdkhag, P., M. L. Free, A. A. Shah, and A. Rodchanarowan. 2017. "The Effects of Duty Cycles on Pulsed Current Electrodeposition of $ZnNiAl_2O_3$ Composite on Steel Substrate: Microstructures, Hardness and Corrosion Resistance." International Journal of Hydrogen Energy 42, no. 32: 20783–90. https://doi.org/10.1016/j.ijhydene.2017.06.049

34. Devaneyan, S. P., D. P. Pushpanathan, T. Senthilvelan, and R. Ganesh. 2018. "Enhanced Corrosion and Wear Behavior of Nano Titanium Carbide Reinforced Polyurethane PMC Coating on Aluminium 7075." Materials Today: Proceedings 5, no. 5: 11491–7. https://doi.org/10.1016/j.matpr.2018.02.116

35. Srivastava, M., V. K. William Grips, and K. S. Rajam. 2008. "Influence of SiC, $Si_3N_4$ and $Al_2O_3$ Particles on the Structure and Properties of Electrodeposited Ni." Materials Letters 62, no. 20: 3487–9. https://doi.org/10.1016/j.matlet.2008.03.008

36. Zandi-Zand, R., A. Ershad-Langroudi, and A. Rahimi. 2005. "Silica Based Organic–Inorganic Hybrid Nanocomposite Coatings for Corrosion Protection." Progress in Organic Coatings 53, no. 4: 286–91. https://doi.org/10.1016/j.porgcoat.2005.03.009

37. Veeramanikandan, K., S. Vignesh, B. P. Pitchia Krishnan, M. Mathanbabu, and M. Ashokkumar. 2021. "Investigation of $Al_2O_3$-Water Nano Fluid Flow through the Circular Tube." Materials Today: Proceedings 46: 8288–95. https://doi.org/10.1016/j.matpr.2021.03.253

38. Biswal, H. J., P. R. Vundavilli, and A. Gupta. 2022. "Fabrication and Characterization of Nickel Microtubes through Electroforming: Deposition Optimization Using Evolutionary Algorithms." Journal of Materials Engineering & Performance 31, no. 2: 1140–54.

39. Kannan, M., T. Duraisamy, T. Pattabi, and A. Mohankumar. 2022. "Investigate the Corrosion Properties of Stellite Coated on AZ91D Alloy by Plasma Spray Technique." Thermal Science 26, no. 2 Part A: 911–20. https://doi.org/10.2298/TSCI200722209K

40. Wang, J., J. Tang, and Y. He. 2010. "Top Coating of Low-Molecular Weight Polymer MALPB Used for Enhanced Protection on Anodized AZ31B Mg Alloys." Journal of Coatings Technology & Research 7, no. 6: 737–46. https://doi.org/10.1007/s11998-010-9258-1

41. Bu, H., M. Yandouzi, C. Lu, D. MacDonald, and B. Jodoin. 2012. "Cold Spray Blended Al+ $Mg_{17}Al_{12}$ Coating for Corrosion Protection of AZ91D Magnesium Alloy." Surface & Coatings Technology 207: 155–62. https://doi.org/10.1016/j.surfcoat.2012.06.050

42. Ashokkumar, M., D. Thirumalaikumarasamy, T. Sonar, S. Deepak, P. Vignesh, and M. Anbarasu. 2022. "An Overview of Cold Spray Coating in Additive Manufacturing, Component Repairing and Other Engineering Applications." Journal of the Mechanical Behavior of Materials 31, no. 1: 514–34. https://doi.org/10.1515/jmbm-2022-0056

43. Zandi Zand, R., V. Flexer, M. De Keersmaecker, K. Verbeken, and A. Adriaens. 2016. "Self-healing Silane Coatings of Cerium Salt Activated Nanoparticles." Materials & Corrosion 67, no. 7: 693–701. https://doi.org/10.1002/maco.201508670

44. McCarthy, C., and T. Vaughan. 2015. "Micromechanical Failure Analysis of Advanced Composite Materials." In Numerical Modelling of Failure in Advanced Composite Materials, pp. 379–409. Woodhead Publishing.

45. Wang, L., J. Zhou, J. Liang, and J. Chen. 2012. "Microstructure and Corrosion Behavior of Plasma Electrolytic Oxidation Coated Magnesium Alloy Pre-treated by Laser Surface Melting." Surface & Coatings Technology 206, no. 13: 3109–15. https://doi.org/10.1016/j.surfcoat.2011.12.040

46. Martin, I. T., B. Dressen, M. Boggs, Y. Liu, C. S. Henry, and E. R. Fisher. 2007. "Plasma Process. Polym 4/2007." Plasma Processes and Polymers 4, no. 4: 337.

47. Gray-Munro, J. E., and M. Strong. 2009. "The Mechanism of Deposition of Calcium Phosphate Coatings from Solution onto Magnesium Alloy AZ31. Journal of Biomedical Materials Research. Part A 90, no. 2: 339–50. https://doi.org/10.1002/jbm.a.32107

48. Guan, Y. C., W. Zhou, and H. Y. Zheng. 2009. "Effect of Laser Surface Melting on Corrosion Behaviour of AZ91D Mg Alloy in Simulated-modified Body Fluid." Journal of Applied Electrochemistry 39, no. 9: 1457–64. https://doi.org/10.1007/s10800-009-9825-2

49. Aung, N. N., and W. Zhou. 2010. "Effect of Grain Size and Twins on Corrosion Behaviour of AZ31B Magnesium Alloy." Corrosion Science 52, no. 2: 589–94. https://doi.org/10.1016/j.corsci.2009.10.018

50. Zhang, R., J. Liang, and Q. Wang. 2012. "Preparation and Characterization of Graphite-dispersed Styrene-acrylic Emulsion Composite Coating on Magnesium Alloy." Applied Surface Science 258, no. 10: 4360–4. https://doi.org/10.1016/j.apsusc.2011.12.113

51. Xu, L., and A. Yamamoto. 2012. "In Vitro Degradation of Biodegradable Polymer-coated Magnesium under Cell Culture Condition." Applied Surface Science 258, no. 17: 6353–8. https://doi.org/10.1016/j.apsusc.2012.03.036

52. Zhang, R. F., S. F. Zhang, Y. L. Shen, L. H. Zhang, T. Z. Liu, Y. Q. Zhang, and S. B. Guo. 2012. "Influence of Sodium Borate Concentration on Properties of Anodic Coatings Obtained by Micro Arc Oxidation on Magnesium Alloys." Applied Surface Science 258, no. 17: 6602–10. https://doi.org/10.1016/j.apsusc.2012.03.088

53. Zhu, Y., Q. Zhao, Y. H. Zhang, and G. Wu. 2012. "Hydrothermal Synthesis of Protective Coating on Magnesium Alloy Using De-ionized Water." Surface & Coatings Technology 206, no. 11–12: 2961–6. https://doi.org/10.1016/j.surfcoat.2011.12.029

54. Wang, Z. C., F. Jia, L. Yu, Z. B. Qi, Y. Tang, and G. L. Song. 2012. "Direct Electroless Nickel–Boron Plating on AZ91D Magnesium Alloy." Surface & Coatings Technology 206, no. 17: 3676–85. https://doi.org/10.1016/j.surfcoat.2012.03.020

55. Hamdy, A. S., and H. M. Hussien. 2013. "Deposition, Characterization and Electrochemical Properties of Permanganate-based Coating Treatments over ZE41 Mg-Zn-Rare Earth Alloy." International Journal of Electrochemical Science 8, no. 9: 11386–402. https://doi.org/10.1016/S1452-3981[23]13192-0

56. Amaravathy, P., S. Sowndarya, S. Sathyanarayanan, and N. Rajendran. 2014. "Novel Sol Gel Coating of $Nb_2O_5$ on Magnesium Alloy for Biomedical Applications." Surface & Coatings Technology 244: 131–41. https://doi.org/10.1016/j.surfcoat.2014.01.050

57. Christoglou, C., N. Voudouris, G. N. Angelopoulos, M. Pant, and W. Dahl. 2004. "Deposition of Aluminium on Magnesium by a CVD Process." Surface & Coatings Technology 184, no. 2–3: 149–55. https://doi.org/10.1016/j.surfcoat.2003.10.065

58. Zhu, L., and G. Song. 2006. "Improved Corrosion Resistance of AZ91D Magnesium Alloy by an Aluminium-alloyed Coating." Surface & Coatings Technology 200, no. 8: 2834–40. https://doi.org/10.1016/j.surfcoat.2004.11.042

59. Cui, Z., H. Yang, H. Wu, and B. Xu. 2012. "Laser Cladding Al-Si/$Al_2O_3$-$TiO_2$ Composite Coatings on AZ31B Magnesium Alloy." Journal of Wuhan University of Technology: Materials Science Edition 27, no. 6: 1042–7. https://doi.org/10.1007/s11595-012-0597-x

60. Ignat, S., P. Sallamand, D. Grevey, and M. Lambertin. 2004. "Magnesium Alloys Laser [Nd: YAG] Cladding and Alloying with Side Injection of Aluminium Powder." Applied Surface Science 225, no. 1–4: 124–34. https://doi.org/10.1016/j.apsusc.2003.09.043

61. Jun, Y., G. P. Sun, C. Liu, S. Q. Jia, S. J. Fang, and S. S. Jia. 2007. "Characterization and Wear Resistance of Laser Surface Cladding AZ91D Alloy with Al+ Al$_2$O$_3$." Journal of Materials Science 42, no. 10: 3607–12. https://doi.org/10.1007/s10853-006-0240-3

62. Mathanbabu, M., D. Thirumalaikumarasamy, P. Thirumal, and M. Ashokkumar. 2021. "Study on Thermal, Mechanical, Microstructural Properties and Failure Analyses of Lanthanum Zirconate Based Thermal Barrier Coatings: A Review." Materials Today: Proceedings 46: 7948–54. https://doi.org/10.1016/j.matpr.2021.02.672

63. _____. 2007. "Plasma Process. Polym 4/2007." Plasma Processes & Polymers 4, no. 4: 337–.

64. Joshi, S. S., S. M. Patil, S. Mazumder, S. Sharma, D. A. Riley, S. Dowden, R. Banerjee, and N. B. Dahotre. 2022. "Additive Friction Stir Deposition of AZ31B Magnesium Alloy." Journal of Magnesium & Alloys 10, no. 9: 2404–20. https://doi.org/10.1016/j.jma.2022.03.011

65. Bobby Kannan, M., W. Dietzel, and R. Zettler. 2011. "In Vitro Degradation Behaviour of a Friction Stir Processed Magnesium Alloy." Journal of Materials Science: Materials in Medicine 22, no. 11: 2397–401. https://doi.org/10.1007/s10856-011-4429-x

66. Arora, H. S., H. Singh, and B. K. Dhindaw. 2012. "Some Observations on Microstructural Changes in a Mg-based AE42 Alloy Subjected to Friction Stir Processing." Metallurgical & Materials Transactions B 43, no. 1: 92–108. https://doi.org/10.1007/s11663-011-9573-7

67. _____. 2023. "Investigation on Mechanical Properties of AZ31B Magnesium Alloy Manufactured by Stir Casting Process." Journal of the Mechanical Behavior of Biomedical Materials 138: 105641. https://doi.org/10.1016/j.jmbbm.2022.105641

68. _____. 2022. "Additive Manufacturing of Metallic Biomaterials and Its Biocompatibility." Materials Today: Proceedings. https://doi.org/10.1016/j.matpr.2022.11.248

69. Ashokkumar, M., D. Thirumalaikumarasamy, T. Sonar, M. Ivanov, S. Deepak, P. Rajangam, and R. Barathiraja. 2023. "Effect of Post-processing Treatments on Mechanical Performance of Cold Spray Coating: An Overview." Journal of the Mechanical Behavior of Materials 32, no. 1: 20220271. https://doi.org/10.1515/jmbm-2022-0271

70. Sharma, N., Z. A. Khan, and A. N. Siddiquee. 2017. "Friction Stir Welding of Aluminum to Copper: An Overview." Transactions of Nonferrous Metals Society of China 27, no. 10: 2113–36. https://doi.org/10.1016/S1003-6326[17]60238-3

71. Li, Y., Y. Guan, Z. Zhang, and S. Ynag. 2019. "Enhanced Bond Strength for Micro-arc Oxidation Coating on Magnesium Alloy via Laser Surface Microstructuring." Applied Surface Science 478: 866–71. https://doi.org/10.1016/j.apsusc.2019.02.041

72. _____. 2021. "Surface Modification of Titanium and Titanium Alloy by Plasma Electrolytic Oxidation Process for Biomedical Applications: A Review." Materials Today: Proceedings 46: 594–602. https://doi.org/10.1016/j.matpr.2020.11.294

73. Pesode, P. A., and S. B. Barve. 2021. "Recent Advances on the Antibacterial Coating on Titanium Implant by Micro-arc Oxidation Process." Materials Today: Proceedings 47: 5652–62. https://doi.org/10.1016/j.matpr.2021.03.702

74. Bär, F., L. Berger, L. Jauer, R. Kurtuldu, R. Schäublin, J. H. Schleifenbaum, and J. F. Löffler. 2019. "Laser Additive Manufacturing of Biodegradable Magnesium Alloy WE43: A Detailed Microstructure Analysis." Acta Biomaterialia 98: 36–49. https://doi.org/10.1016/j.actbio.2019.05.056

75. _____. 2020. "HA Coating on Mg Alloys for Biomedical Applications: A Review." Journal of Magnesium & Alloys 8, no. 3: 929–43. https://doi.org/10.1016/j.jma.2020.05.003

76. Kumar, L. G. S., D. Thirumalaikumarasamy, K. Karthikeyan, M. Mathanbabu, M. Ashokkumar, and C. S. Ramachandran. 2023. "An Overview of Recent Trends and Challenges of Post Treatments on Magnesium Alloys." Materials Today: Proceedings 78, no. 3: 700–07.

77. Eswaran, S. 2019. "Experimental Investigation of Solar Drier Integrated with HSU for Crops." Journal of Advanced Research in Dynamical & Control Systems 11, no. 12: 167–73.

78. Wankhede, S. V., and J. A. Hole. 2022. "MOORA and TOPSIS Based Selection of Input Parameter in Solar Powered Absorption Refrigeration System." International Journal of Ambient Energy 43, no. 1: 3396–401. https://doi.org/10.1080/01430750.2020. 1831600

79. Wankhede, S. V., J. A. Hole, and B. L. Patil. 2022. "Performance of Tetrafluoroethane [R134a]-Dimethyl Formamide [DMF] Diffusion Absorption Air Cooling System with Variable Power Input." International Journal of Ambient Energy 43, no. 1: 2019–25. https://doi.org/10.1080/01430750.2020.1722225

80. Patil, B., J. Hole, and S. Wankhede. 2017. "Parameters Affecting Productivity of Solar Still and Improvement Techniques: A Detailed Review." International Journal of Latest Technology in Engineering, Management & Applied Science 5, no. 2: 11–18.

81. Wankhede, S., P. Pesode, S. Pawar, and R. Lobo. 2023. "Comparison Study of GRA, COPRAS and MOORA for Ranking of Phase Change Material for Cooling System." Materials Today: Proceedings. https://doi.org/10.1016/j.matpr.2023.02.437

82. Pesode, P., S. Barve, S. V. Wankhede, D. R. Jadhav, and S. K. Pawar. 2023. "Titanium Alloy Selection for Biomedical Application Using Weighted Sum Model Methodology." Materials Today: Proceedings 72: 724–8. https://doi.org/10.1016/j.matpr.2022.08.494

83. Mathanbabu, M., D. Thirumalaikumarasamy, M. Tamilselvi, and S. Kumar. 2022. "Optimization of Plasma Spray Process Variables to Attain the Minimum Porosity and Maximum Hardness of the LZ/YSZ Thermal Barrier Coatings Utilizing the Response Surface Approach." Materials Research Express 9, no. 9: 096505. https://doi. org/10.1088/2053-1591/ac8857

84. Rajendran, P. R., T. Duraisamy, R. Chidambaram Seshadri, A. Mohankumar, S. Ranganathan, G. Balachandran, K. Murugan, and L. Renjith. 2022. "Optimisation of HVOF Spray Process Parameters to Achieve Minimum Porosity and Maximum Hardness in WC-10Ni-5Cr Coatings." Coatings 12, no. 3: 339. https://doi.org/10.3390/ coatings12030339

85. Mathanbabu, M., P. Mohanraj, N. Krishnan, K. T. Naveen, and S. Vijayb. 2019. "Design and Thermal Analysis of Ceramic Coated Diesel Engine Piston [$MgZrO_3$ and NiCrAl]." Ijariit Journal 4, no. 1: 148–156.

86. Sozhamannan, G. G., S. P. Balasivanandha, and V. S. K. Venkatagalapathy. 2012. "Effect of Processing Parameters on Metal Matrix Composites: Stir Casting Process." Journal of Surface Engineered Materials & Advanced Technology 2, no. 1: 16992.

87. Kumar, A., S. Kumar, and N. K. Mukhopadhyay. 2018. "Casting and Characterization of TiC Particulate Reinforced AZ91 Magnesium Alloy Metal Matrix Composite through Stir Casting Process." International Journal of Mechanical Engineering and Technology 9: 856–63.

88. Wankhede, S., P. Pesode, S. Gaikwad, S. Pawar, and A. Chipade. 2023. "Implementing Combinative Distance Base Assessment [Codas] for Selection of Natural Fibre for Long Lasting Composites." Materials Science Forum 1081: 41–8. https://doi.org/ 10.4028/p-4pd120

89. Wan, B., W. Li, F. Liu, T. Lu, S. Jin, K. Wang, A. Yi, J. Tian, and W. Chen. 2020. "Determination of Fluoride Component in the Multifunctional Refining Flux Used for Recycling Aluminum Scrap." Journal of Materials Research and Technology 9, no. 3: 3447–59.

# 10 Magnesium Alloys for Biomedical Applications
## *Future Scope and Challenges*

*Virendra Pratap Singh*
National Institute of Technology, Aizawl, India
and
IES College of Technology, Bhopal, India

*Vinyas Mahesh*
National Institute of Technology, Silchar, India

*Dineshkumar Harursampath*
Department of Aerospace Engineering, NMCAD Lab.,
Indian Institute of Science, Bengaluru, India

## 10.1 INTRODUCTION

At present, medical implants in health industries are in huge demand all over the globe. Approximately, 1.8–2.0 million artificial implant replacements have been successfully done worldwide. In case of atherosclerosis, more than 1 million stents (tube) have been effectively implanted in human arteries. From commercial point of view, the cardiovascular and endovascular stents were expected to exceed \$2,897.2 million in 2022 [1, 2]. The four basic types of biomaterials are polymers, metals, composites, and ceramics [3]. The metals show high fracture toughness and strength, which is suitable for high load-bearing capacity, compared to polymer and ceramics. Consequently, metallic implant materials like titanium alloys, stainless steels, and chromium–cobalt-based alloys found widespread use. Biomaterials must be biologically compatible. However, the by-product of corrosion of most traditional surgical alloys (i.e., Co-, Cr-, and Ni-based metals) leads to harmful effect to human body [4, 5], whereas Mg-based material's corrosion by-products leads to physiologically advantageous effect than detrimental. The majority of the magnesium in the adult human body is found in bone and muscle [6]. The U.S. FNB (Food and Nutrition Board) has recently reestablished the magnesium RDA for adults to 420 mg/day for males and 320 mg/day for females [7]. Any deficiency of Mg in dietary leads to osteoporosis risk [8]. Additionally, magnesium strongly make bond with phosphates. So, its existence affects the bone tissue mineralization by regulating the formation of hydroxyapatite (HA) (calcium phosphate) [9]. Any deficiency of magnesium leads to various major issues such as cardiac arrhythmias, constriction of the coronary

DOI: 10.1201/9781003400462-10

artery, atherosclerosis development, and high blood pressure [9]. Magnesium is therefore a popular ingredient in numerous medications and dietary supplements. Magnesium supplements have a broad therapeutic window and minimal adverse effects. Magnesium, along with potassium, calcium, and sodium, is effectively regulated by homeostatic mechanisms in the body, and there is no issue of toxicity [9]. In addition to its biocompatibility, magnesium is advantageous due to its mechanical properties. Compared to human calvarium bone density, i.e., 1.75 g/cm³, magnesium and its alloy have a density of 1.7 g/cm³. Pure magnesium has an elastic modulus of 45 GPa, whereas human bone fall into 40–57 GPa which is half of the $Ti_6Al_4V$ [10]. Thus, magnesium is appealing to orthopedic surgeons and researchers, despite the fact that some of the earliest orthopedic magnesium alloys failed and fell out of use. During early 20th century, magnesium alloys were first chosen as orthopedic biomaterials. Lambotte [11] reported the initial application of Mg in surgical procedures for traumatic injuries in 1907, when a pure magnesium plate fastened with gold-plated steel nails were used in a lower leg bone fracture. Lately, Witte et al. [12] performed cartilage restoration on subchondral bone replacement with AZ91 scaffolds. In vivo studies by Witte et al. [13], Zhang et al. [14], Duygulu et al. [15], and others indicated that the AZ31 alloy implant is advantageous to the formation of new biocompatible bone in animal studies. Wrought alloys probably are to be favored here over casting alloys as they generally contain lower alloying contents and feature higher strength and ductility. Table 10.1 lists some basic technological and biological aspects of selected alloying elements in magnesium. Figure 10.1 represents the position and stages of magnesium as a biomedical implant.

This chapter deals with various corrosion issues of Mg and its alloys, in order to comprehend the corrosion mechanism and protective capabilities of Mg alloys, significant advancements in the investigation of Mg alloys as materials used for implants, as well as the effect of various factors on the corrosion behavior of Mg alloys. Technical challenges based on previous existing research have also been discussed.

## 10.2   CORROSION IN BIOFLUIDS

Corrosion is a continuous phenomenon and is defined as the deterioration of the material surface due to its chemical, physical, and electrochemical interactions with its environment. Compared to natural environment, body fluids are more prompt to corrosion due to the fact that the corrosion rate depends on various factors such as pH value, protein and other body fluid, etc. [17].

### 10.2.1   CORROSION PHENOMENON IN Mg ALLOYS

The polarization curves for the two studied alloys in the three selected media are depicted in Figure 10.2. The purpose of polarization experiments is not to determine accurate corrosion rates. For this reason, hydrogen evolution and mass loss would help in estimation of corrosion rates [18, 19]. The purpose of this chapter is to compare, from a mechanistic standpoint, how corrosion varies (i) in different mediums and (ii) for different alloys [20].

**TABLE 10.1**

**Selection Criteria of Alloying Elements for Biomedical Magnesium Alloys**

| Element | Biological Aspects | Technological Aspects |
|---|---|---|
| Al | Risk factor in the development of Alzheimer's disease; can harm muscle fibers; reduces osteoclast activity | Strength and ductility (precipitation, solid-solution hardening, and grain refinement) as well as corrosion resistance and castability are enhanced |
| Ca | Calcium is the most common mineral in the human body and is closely controlled by homeostasis | Strength (precipitation, solid-solution hardening, grain refinement) and creep resistance are enhanced; castability is decreased |
| Li | Effects of possible teratogenic treatment | Reduces strength while enhancing formability/ductility (change to bcc lattice structure); decreases density and corrosion resistance |
| Mn | Trace element of vital importance to the metabolic cycle and immune system; neurotoxic in high concentrations | Improves ductility and strength (grain refinement); increases creep resistance; and, in combination with aluminum, increases corrosion resistance (precipitation that take iron) |
| Rare earth elements (Y) | Numerous rare earth elements demonstrate anticarcinogenic characteristics | Enhances high-temperature strength and creep resistance (precipitation, solid-solution hardening); enhances corrosion resistance (surface film); and decreases mechanical anisotropy (texture randomization) |
| Si | — | Lessens ductility, enhances creep resistance and high-temperature strength (precipitation), and decreases castability and corrosion resistance |
| Sr | — | Enhances ductility and tensile strength (grain refinement); enhances high-temperature strength and creep resistance |
| Zn | Essential chemical element (co-factor, immune system); neurotoxic at higher concentrations | Increases strength while decreasing ductility at high concentrations (precipitation, and solid-solution hardening); increases castability |
| Zr | — | In the absence of aluminum, increases strength, ductility, and high-temperature strength (solid grain refinement) |

*Source:* From Reference [16].

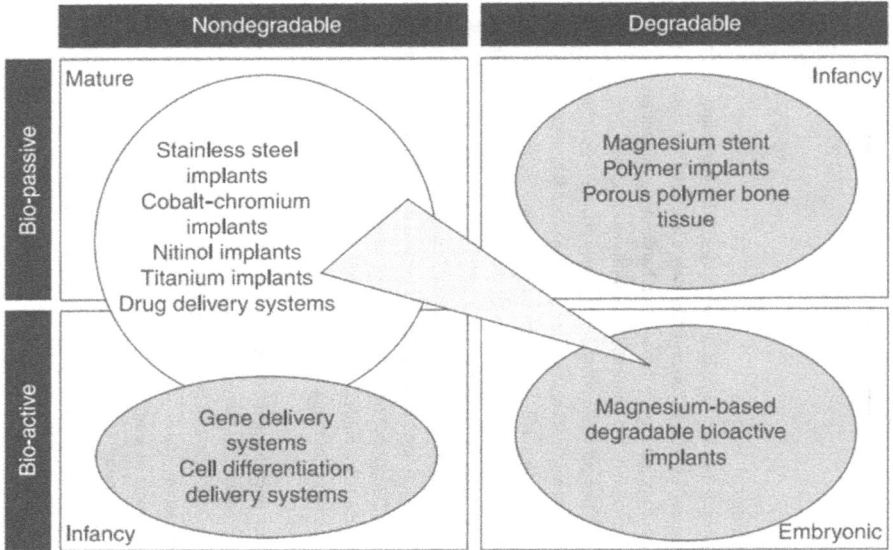

**FIGURE 10.1** The position of magnesium and stages of biomedical implants (indicated by an arrow) [16].

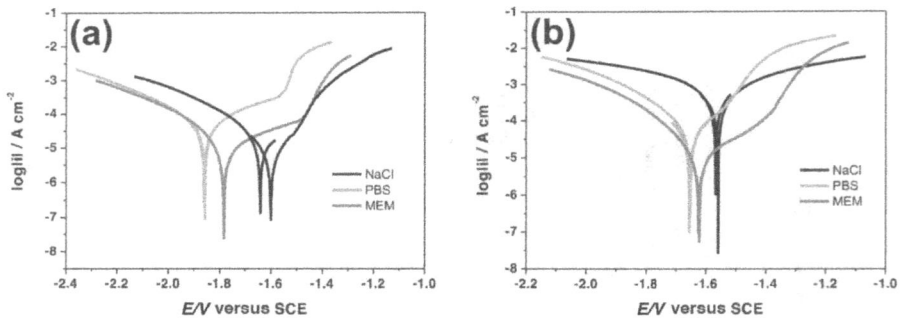

**FIGURE 10.2** Potentiodynamic polarization curves for various electrolytes (10 mM PBS, MEM, and 0.05 M NaCl) for (a) $Mg_1Ca$ and (b) $Mg_{10}Gd$ [21].

The corrosion mechanism in Mg alloys in an aqueous medium is characterized by the following partial reactions:

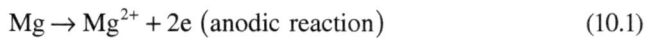

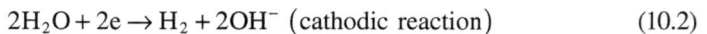

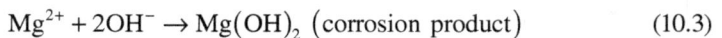

$$Mg \rightarrow Mg^{2+} + 2e \; (\text{anodic reaction}) \tag{10.1}$$

$$2H_2O + 2e \rightarrow H_2 + 2OH^- \; (\text{cathodic reaction}) \tag{10.2}$$

$$Mg^{2+} + 2OH^- \rightarrow Mg(OH)_2 \; (\text{corrosion product}) \tag{10.3}$$

## 10.3   TYPES OF CORROSION

In orthopedic biomaterial, various types of corrosion are observed such as fatigue, erosion, pitting, and galvanic corrosion. Fonta [22] identified various common types of corrosion: common corrosion, galvanic (bimetal) corrosion, pitting corrosion, crevice corrosion, intergranular corrosion, stress corrosion, and erosion corrosion. In addition, various other types of corrosion are also included like cavitation, fretting, fatigue corrosion, and hydrogen embrittlement [23]. The most prevalent types of corrosion that occur in Mg alloys in presence of SBFs are erosion corrosion, galvanic, pitting, and fatigue corrosion.

Three critical factors, including uneven microstructure, larger grain size, and secondary phase, leading to augmentation of corrosion in Mg implants and the percent involvement of each factor are specified for each manufacturing process, as shown in Figure 10.3(a).

### 10.3.1   CORROSION FATIGUE

Corrosion fatigue is a detrimental effect that occurs as an outcome of the contact between localized electrochemical reactions and irreversible cyclic permanent deformation compared to a passive or benign setting, in an aggressive environment. Corrosion fatigue is an important aspect in calculating the durability of implants subjected to variable (dynamic) load. For example, corrosion fatigue resistance must be considered when making material selection for bone implants and cardiac valves. Magnesium alloys have a significantly reduced fatigue life when exposed to aqueous solutions. Microstructure has a significant bearing on the fatigue life. Oxide and pores on the surface play a vital role in reduction of fatigue life. Porosity was found to decrease the fatigue life of Mg alloy due to its crack nucleation spots. The researchers suggest that this new material has the potential to be used in a variety of biomedical applications, including as an implant material for bone repair and regeneration. However, further studies are needed to fully evaluate its long-term biocompatibility and other properties before it can be used in clinical settings [25]. Gu et al. [26] studied the corrosion fatigue properties of WE43 and AZ91D in SBF. The die-cast AZ91D alloy's stress-life ($S-N$) behaviors under 37°C SBF and air testing are shown in Figure 10.3(b). As can be shown, the die-cast AZ91D alloy's fatigue limit is 50 MPa in air at $10^7$ cycles as opposed to 20 MPa at $10^6$ cycles performed in SBF conditions [26].

### 10.3.2   GALVANIC CORROSION

Galvanic or bimetallic corrosion occurs when two dissimilar metals, which have varying electrochemical potentials, are exposed to a conductive fluid environment, like interstitial fluid or serum. Galvanic corrosion is the main complication in using Mg alloys in aggressive environments, as Mg is the most reactive metal in the galvanic series [27]. Galvanic corrosion can happen between the intermetallic and matrix, even if they are the same type of metal. Figure 10.4 shows the galvanic corrosion representation in human body fluids (HBF). When a plate of Mg alloy

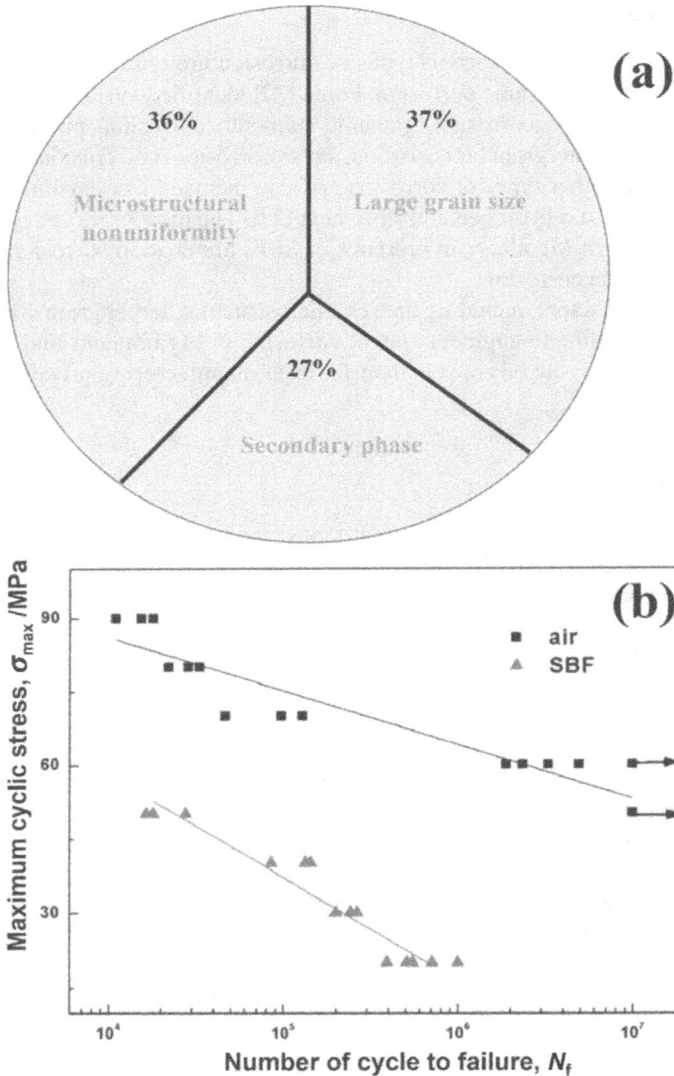

FIGURE 10.3    (a) Three critical factors, including uneven microstructure, larger grain size, and secondary phase, leading to augmentation of corrosion in Mg implants and the percent involvement of each factor is specified. (b) S–N curves for AZ91D at ambient temperature in SBF and air and at 37°C. The number of cycles was taken as $10^7$ cycles [24, 26].

screwed with stainless steel are implanted, the stainless steel screw behaves as a cathode because of its comparatively high potential, whereas the Mg alloy plate behaves as anode due to its lower potential. As stated previously, Lambotte [11] was the very first surgeon to implant Mg in orthopedic and other surgery. The application of pure Mg and gold-plated steel nails caused severe galvanic corrosion.

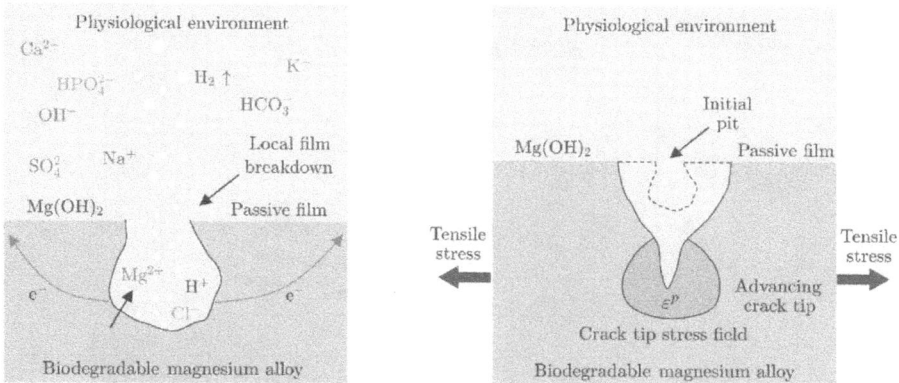

**FIGURE 10.4**   The schematic depicts pitting corrosion (*left*) and stress corrosion cracking (*right*) of magnesium alloys submerged in a physiological environment [24].

### 10.3.3   EROSION CORROSION

Dearnley [5] reported that after 17 years of implantation, a Cr-Co-Mo-based femoral head surface developed numerous scratches due to wear debris. Huang et al. [28] established that the amount of wear on AM60B and AZ91D improved as the vertical load increased, and it reduced as the frequency increased. The study investigated the effect of flow velocity on the corrosion behavior of AZ91D magnesium alloy in an elbow of a loop system. The researchers used electrochemical techniques to measure the corrosion rate and polarization curves of the alloy at various flow velocities. The results showed that the corrosion rate increased with increasing flow velocity, and the polarization curves indicated a more active corrosion behavior at higher velocities. The authors suggest that the increased turbulence and shear stress in the flow at higher velocities contribute to the increased corrosion rate. These findings have implications for the design and operation of loop systems that include AZ91D magnesium alloy components [29]. Over time, there was an increase in the speed at which mass was being lost. The contact between a matrix corrosion and wear led to severe pitting corrosion. The impact velocity affects the depth of pits.

### 10.3.4   PITTING CORROSION

Pitting corrosion occurs over the few surfaces of a material while the rest are unaffected. The microstructure of Al/Mg alloys is typically comprised of various intermetallic such as $\alpha$-matrix, $\beta(Mg_{17}Al_{12})$, and $Al_8Mn_5$, and they have potentials that are higher than the $\alpha$-matrix. Song [27] and Zeng et al. [30] provided the roles of intermetallic which play a significant function in the corrosion mechanism. The pitting corrosion is also the reason for fatigue and stress corrosion. Reifenrath et al. [31] determined in vitro that pitting corrosion were studied on AZ91, AZ91D and LAE442. It was seen that a uniform corrosion was found on LAE442 which exhibited scattered and severe pitting attack.

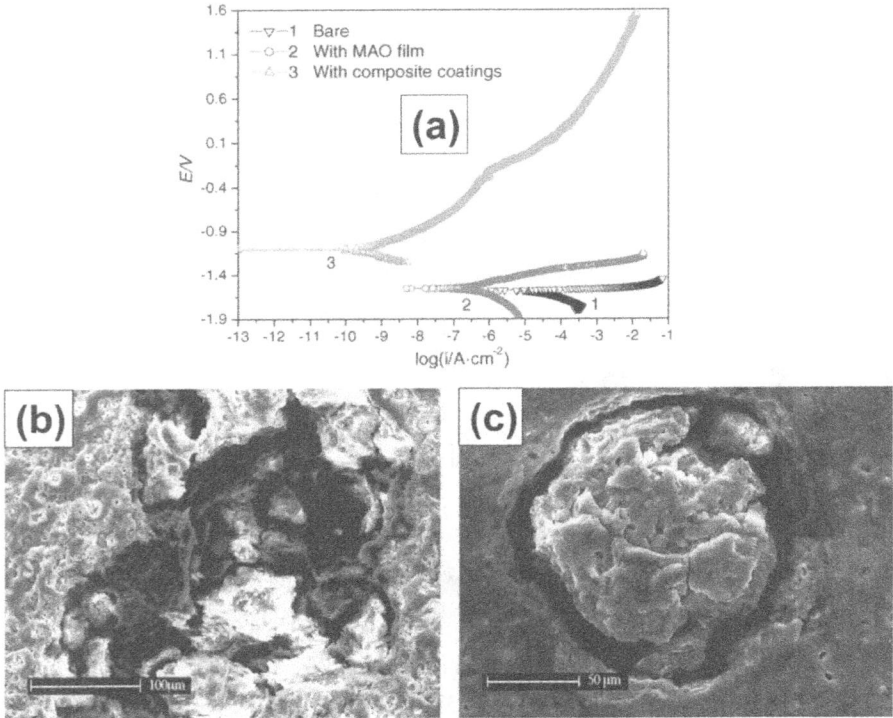

**FIGURE 10.5**  The behavior of (1) untreated AZ91D alloy, (2) AZ91D alloy with MAO film, and (3) AZ91D alloy with composite coatings were evaluated by plotting potentio-dynamic polarization curves in a 3.5% NaCl solution, (b) microstructure of MAO film, and (c) coating on AZ91D [32].

The formation of pitting corrosion of Mg alloy in $Cl^-$ comprising solution is crucial. The Tafel behavior in the anodic potentiodynamic polarization maps is shown in Figure 10.5(a). Diverse pitting corrosion behavior between the MAO film and composite coating is shown in Figure 10.5(b) and (c). When the polarization current gets to a definite value, the transitional corrosive would react with the MAO film, and several pits are established. The polarization current causes the corrosion products in pits to move out of the porous MAO film's structure and into solution. As a result, as seen in Figure 10.5(b), a sizable concave pit remains on the MAO surface. In addition, the sealing layer's blocking function prevented the corrosion products from dissolving, leaving the blocked pit structure as seen in Figure 10.5(c).

## 10.4  FACTOR AFFECTING CORROSION

The corrosion behavior of Mg alloys is mainly dependent on alloying element and its composition, heat treatment, corrosive media environment such as pH value variation, albumin, SBFs, etc. [30, 33]. Numerous internal and external factors affect the rate of corrosion directly or indirectly. Several of these factors are depicted in Figure 10.6.

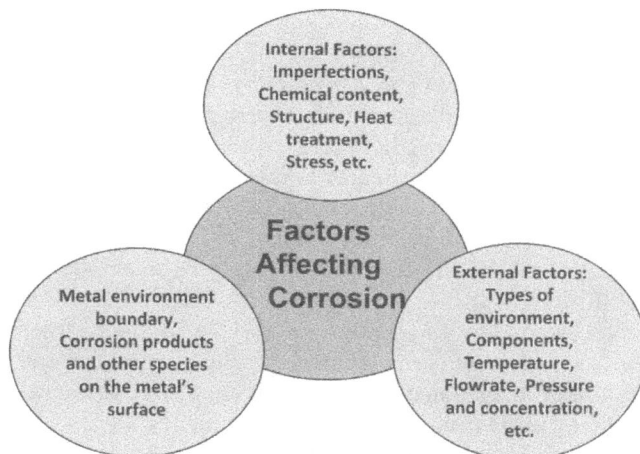

FIGURE 10.6 Various common factors affecting corrosion.

## 10.4.1 INFLUENCE OF MICROSTRUCTURE

The microstructure of magnesium alloys should be finer and more homogeneous. For instance, its microstructure is altered by rapid solidification rates. Hermann et al. [34] noted the reduction of $Mg_{17}Al_{12}$ and the creation of a prolonged solid solution containing Al of 9.6–23.4%. The repassivation behavior of Mg-Al alloys is improved by rapid solidification; this repassivation is greater for alloys having more Al content [35]. The literatures [30, 33] contain extensive debate, with an emphasis on the function of β-phases in Mg corrosion. To create a new magnesium alloy with enhanced properties for clinical applications, Mg was alloyed with Al, Cu, Bi, Fe, Cd, RE, Th, Li, Zr, Pb, Mn, Ni, Ag, Y, Cr, Si, Zn, and Sb, among others. These elements were incorporated into a different type of Mg-based alloys in order to suppress the Mg corrosion rate. Magnesium alloys with RE and Al elements, for instance, enhanced strength and corrosion resistance. However, aluminum has demonstrated toxicity, and RE elements are extremely costly. At times, Mg-Ca alloy was developed with the help of low-cost Ca with enhanced corrosion properties. Additionally, mechanical behavior was improved by adding Zn to Mg-Ca alloys. In developed alloys, the rate of corrosion was decreased by a factor of ~4 as the size of grain decreases [36, 37].

## 10.4.2 INFLUENCE OF HEAT TREATMENT

Microstructure and corrosion behavior of Mg alloys can be improved with the help of heat treatment. Heat treatment appears to be the most effective method for modifying the microstructure and, consequently, the corrosion behavior and mechanical behavior of Mg alloys without affecting their composition or shape. By precisely adjusting the heat treatment settings, a combination of corrosion resistance and mechanical performance can be obtained. The effects of heat treatments were used to improve the corrosion behavior, microstructure, and mechanical behavior of the most crucial biodegradable Mg alloys that can be treated with heat (Mg-Y, Mg-Gd, Mg-Zn, Mg-Al, Mg-Ag, and Mg-Nd) [38].

Aging causes aluminum atoms in Al/Mg alloys moving in the direction of the interfaces between grains and produce β-phase precipitation, thereby decreasing the concentration of Al within the α-Mg structure [30]. Typically, the corrosion rate of Al/Mg alloys in NaCl solutions decreases as they age. Liu et al. [39] examined the heat treatment effect (heating at a temperature of 413°C for a duration of 24 h as a means of treating the solution, henceforth aging at 216°C for 1, 5.5, and 12 h) on the corrosion behavior of AZ63 alloy. A two-week experiment in Tyrode's solution immersion of SBF revealed that the treated alloys have a corrosion rate roughly half of the unprocessed alloy. In addition, the variance in microstructure results in a change in microstructure of corrosion surface: pitting corrosion and narrow filamentous are exhibited in aged materials, whereas deep and homogeneous corrosion is observed in unprocessed materials.

After solution heat treatment, the alloy's uniform composition resulted in the development of a homogeneous protecting film. Considering this study, despite the presence of numerous intermetallic in the unprocessed alloy, shown in Figure 10.7(a), the volume fraction of intermetallic reduced significantly after solution treatment, shown in Figure 10.7(b). Immersion in Hank's solution caused the alloy to corrode uniformly, as shown in Figure 10.7(c), and a homogeneous protective corrosion coat developed on the surface of alloy, which could restrict the corrosion's expansion [38, 40].

### 10.4.3 EFFECT OF MANUFACTURING PROCESS

The corrosion behavior of Mg alloys is ascribed to the microstructure produced by numerous techniques. Hot extrusion and hot rolling can minimize the rate of

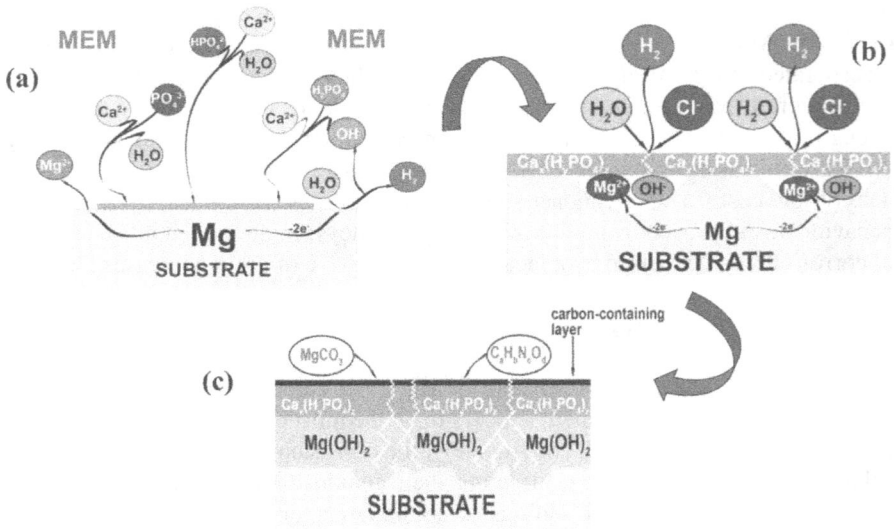

**FIGURE 10.7** The schematic illustrations of corrosion mechanism for Mg alloy (MA8) in the MEM. Three stages (a, b, and c) of the corrosion film evolution were exposed [38].

corrosion in magnesium–calcium alloys [41, 42]. As an illustration, the corrosion current densities of as-rolled, as-cast, and as-extruded Mg-1Ca alloys are 1.63, 12.56, and 1.74 mm/a, respectively, due to the creation of a finer microstructure during extrusion and rolling. Due to other factors like the lesser Cl⁻ ions concentration existing in bone, proteins, blood plasma, etc., the breakdown of Mg-1Ca alloy in vivo is significantly lower than the in vitro electrochemical testing.

### 10.4.4 INFLUENCE OF ALLOYING ELEMENTS

Due to a major corrosion problem, the lifetime is typically insufficient for a likely use of Mg alloys as biocompatible materials. Magnesium may be purified, alloyed, and produced using the right methods to increase its corrosion qualities. For instance, by lowering the concentrations of harmful elements like Cu, Fe, Co, and Ni, by obtaining a fine microstructure by adding other alloying elements like rare earths, Ca, Zr, and Sr among other things, corrosion resistance can be enhanced [42]. It is noteworthy [43] that Li can increase a MgLiAlRe alloy's resistance to corrosion by increasing the pH level to > 11.5. Witte et al. [13] in in vivo corrosion measurements showed that due to the degradation of the alloying elements in the Mg alloy, such as AZ91, AZ31, LAE442, and WE43, implants vary. In comparison to AZ31, AZ91, and WE43, LAE442 has a lower rate of corrosion.

The human body can tolerate various alloying elements such as Mn, Zn, and Ca, and may be a rare earth substance with extremely low levels of toxicity in small quantities, which might also delay biodegradation [43]. Potential biodegradable alloys include Mn/Zn containing Mg alloys, such as $Mg_2Zn_{0.2}Mn$, that have good mechanical performance [43]. The general corrosion behavior of Mg alloys in chloride-containing solutions is improved by the addition of calcium element [44]. Kannan et al. [45] considered in vitro deprivation of AZ91Ca (37 wt% Al, 50 wt% Mg, 0.5 wt% Zn, and 13 wt% Ca) and AZ61Ca (34 wt% Al, 55 wt% Mg, 1.0 wt% Zn, and 7 wt% Ca) in SBFs, and recommended that adding of Ca knowingly results in a higher corrosion rate of AZ91DCa alloy as compared to AZ91D alloy. However, it should be distinguished that the degree of calcium addition has a significant impact on the corrosion behavior of Mg alloys. There are some contradictory reports in this regard, as-cast $Mg_2Ca$, Mg-1Ca, and Mg-3Ca alloys have in vitro corrosion rates of 12.98 mm/a, 12.56 mm/a, and 25.00 mm/a, respectively, according to Li et al. [41]. In other words, a higher Ca concentration causes the creation of the intermetallic complex $Mg_2Ca$ to grow, which reduces the corrosion resistance of Mg-Ca alloys. The findings show that compared to other Mg-Ca alloys, Mg-1Ca alloy has greater corrosion resistance as a viable biocompatible material.

### 10.4.5 EFFECT OF ALBUMIN

Metallic corrosion is basically affected by human body proteins by altering cathodic and anodic processes, or both [41]. Liu et al. [46] suggested that the characteristics of corrosion process were changed as it comes in contact with implant's surfaces and proteins. The involvement of BSA (bovine serum albumin) dramatically alters the OC potential to a higher positive value in SBF and lean toward lower corrosion. Notably, the potentials are enhanced to greater values due to proteins below the oxygen line and above the hydrogen line, the purported stable area for hydrogen ions. Therefore, the $H_2$ generation and the corrosive mechanism are inhibited. In addition, Liu et al. [46] analyzed that the SBFs and SBFs containing 1 g/L BSA roughly doubled the corrosion resistance. An advanced BSA content reduces corrosion exposure, most likely as a result of the adsorbed BSA providing a more effective barrier between the electrolyte and the surface oxide film which significantly grow in potential. That makes sense since after being exposed to the SBF containing BSA in open circuit, samples have a surface coating made mostly of $Mg(OH)_2$, and albumin adsorbs completely, which multiplies quickly in a solution with $SO_4^{2-}$ or $Cl^-$, and the divalent $Mg^{2+}$ simply interrelating with BSA [46]. Furthermore, the newly created albumin film shows a corrosion-resistant film. Müller et al. [47] further projected that the possible passivation zone range for LAE442 and AZ31 was expanded in the presence of albumin.

### 10.4.6 EFFECT OF pH VALUE

The pH value of the solution has a significant effect on microstructure and corrosion behavior. Typically, Mg alloys undergo pitting corrosion in alkaline or neutral or salt solutions. When the pH level is greater than 11.5, corrosion occurs very infrequently. The rate of corrosion of β-phase is very small at pH values between 4 and 14 [48]. In acidic sodium chloride solutions, the rate of corrosion of die-cast and ingot AZ91 and extruded AM60 are greater than in neutral and highly alkaline solutions [49]. The typical biological pH in human blood, interstitial, and intracellular fluid is between 7.15 and 7.35, 7.0, and 6.8 [50]; therefore, enhanced surface corrosion of the Mg-implant can be anticipated in vivo. The data is derived from Xu et al. [51], Liu et al. [46], and Chen et al. [52]. The lower ellipse directs that materials were drenched in Hank's solutions or solutions containing 0.9% NaCl. Whereas the upper ellipse shows the capabilities of AZ91 absorbed in adapted SBFs. It has been demonstrated that the corrosion process of Mg alloys in Hank's solution or NaCl is alkalinization, and that the pH value rises to roughly 10.5 and goes with time, irrespective of the original pH in treatment solutions. There is no discernible difference in the increase in pH rate with mass fraction of $Cl^-$, nevertheless it appears to delay in Hank's solution and distilled water. But the transplanted tissue's pH level has been noted to be low, nearly 5.2 after implantation and then improves after 10–15 days [46]. This indicates that Mg implants will be subjected to an augmented occurrence during the commencing phase. On the short term, the acidic nature of SBF can root the development of a steady corrosion by-product film, but on the long term, it permits a more severe corrosion attack [46].

Ng et al. [53] studied the impact of pH value on corrosion of Mg degradable implant material. Figure 10.8(a) depicts the potentio-dynamic polarization curves for Mg in Hank's solution at various pH values. As the pH increases, the polarization curves demonstrate that the corrosion potential ($E_{corr}$) moves in the direction of current densities and nobler values where overpotentials decline. Figure 10.8(b) depicts the impedance data Nyquist maps of Mg in Hank's solution at various pH values. All Nyquist maps include two capacitive rings, i.e., at higher and lower frequencies, in addition to inductive characteristics at even lesser frequencies. At higher pH levels,

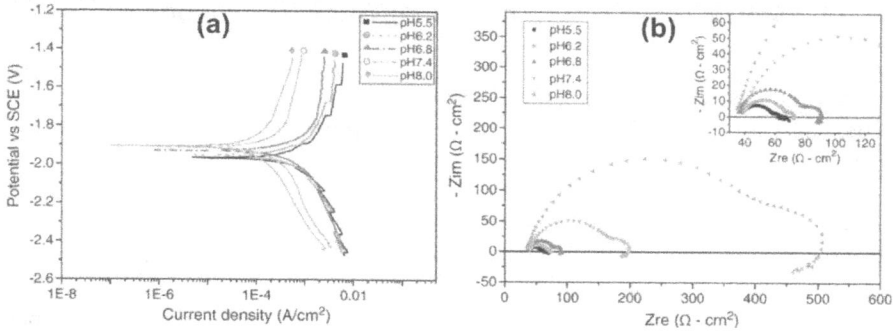

**FIGURE 10.8** Mg samples tested under different pH values in Hank's solution at 37°C: (a) Potentiodynamic polarization maps and (b) Nyquist maps of EIS data [53].

the capacitive loops and inductive characteristics can be observed more clearly than at lower pH levels [53, 54].

## 10.5 PROGRESS ON RESEARCH OF Mg ALLOYS AS BIOMATERIALS

In bioabsorbable stents, Mg alloys as biomaterials have made the most progress to date. The first Mg implant is a Mg coronary stent. The decomposable Mg stents, which are laser-sculpted from WE43 Mg alloy, have been produced and tested in trial run [55]. Animal experiments have been done followed by prior clinical uses. These Mg stents have the potential to overwhelm the restrictions of eternal metallic stents, including late stent thrombosis, chronic inflammation, artifacts, and extended antiplatelet therapy, when captured by multiclade computed tomography [56]. Kumar et al. [57] rooted 20 located Mg alloy tube stents with 10 mm length and an irregular strut width of 150–200 µm in 11 coronary arteries of 2.5–3.5 mm reference diameter in pigs. After 35 days, the mean neointimal area was 1.41 mm², and next 56 days, it was 2.71 mm². Biocorrosion of the strut began after 35 days, and extrapolation predicted that it would be ample in 98 days. Waksman et al. [56] implanted stents made of Mg or stainless steel in the coronary arteries of minipigs and domestic pigs. The outcomes demonstrated that Mg alloy stents remained unbroken after 3 days, but began to degrade after 28 days. There were no indications of stent particle thrombosis, embolization, fibrin deposition, or excessive inflammation. After 118 days, magnesium alloy stent segments had significantly less neointimal area than segments of stainless steel stent. In animal tests, these pure Mg stents degrade after one to three months without causing harm. Early clinical studies demonstrated the safety of Mg stents.

The aforementioned in vivo tests proved that Mg alloy implants appear to be a better option for stents; however, additional investigation is essential prior to replacing the existing pure metal standard. The difficulty lies in creating a stent with similar mechanical behaviors, a lesser corrosion rate, and antiproliferative or anti-inflammatory drugs.

### 10.5.1   STRATEGIES AND CHALLENGES FOR Mg ALLOYS AS ORTHOPEDIC MATERIAL IMPLANTS

For Mg implants to be used as a material for bone replacement, their corrosion properties must be improved. Normal methods of improvement include enhancing the material's behavior and searching for suitable plating.

#### 10.5.1.1   Enhancement of Intrinsic Materials Behavior

Various researchers have tried to develop magnesium-based porous metallic foam, which fulfills the properties of a bone and could be used as a favorable supported material. Surfaces with pores have been incorporated into subcutaneous, percutaneous, dental, and orthopedic implants to encourage tissue fusion [3]. Wen et al. [58] conducted compressive tests to investigate the mechanical characteristics of porous Mg with pore sizes ranging from 70 μm to 400 μm and a porosity of 35–55%. The outcomes revealed that maximum stress and Young's modulus increase as pore size and porosity decrease. The mechanical behavior of porous magnesium alloys was comparable to those of cancellate bone [58]. Yuan et al. [59] manufactured the Mg-based lotus-type porous material through metal/gas eutectic monodirectional cooling. This material has a consistent, porous structure that resembles lotus-type roots. It has been discovered that the mechanical properties of porous materials that are superior to those of traditional porous material developed by foaming or sintering [59]. Suitable selection of size of the pores can be suggestively enhanced by the connection between implant and native tissue [60]. Witte et al. [12] examined a cartilage restoration on AZ91 open-porous (75% porosity) scaffold utilized as bone replacement. The research revealed that over the first 12 weeks, this alloy disintegrated too fast in vivo to permit for effective cartilage healing upstairs the scaffold. Typically, the rate of corrosion increases as arc of pore increases. Increased contact surfaces with the corrosive fluid are the only approach to speed up the corrosion. Hence, slowing down corrosion through the pores is the first obstacle for porous magnesium. The second issue is the reduced fatigue life of materials with pores. Using additional biocompatible Mg alloys is one method for enhancing the efficiency of Mg scaffolds or the application of suitable coatings. Table 10.1 presents the most commonly used alloying elements as a biodegradable Mg alloys and its influence on the alloy's behavior. Figure 10.9 depicts the evolution of biocompatible Mg alloys based on strengthening capacity, toxicity, and deprivation rate [16, 61].

Hydroxyapatite (HA) is unsolvable in alkaline solution, soluble in acidic solutions, and to some extent soluble in purified water. Crystalline HA is the thermodynamically maximum sustainable form of calcium phosphate in bodily fluid. It energetically reacts with lipids, proteins, and other organic and inorganic substances [3]. HA's density influences its mechanical properties. The strength of a material increases as its density increases. On the basis of this knowledge, numerous HA-reinforced recyclable polymer composites, for instance, HA/polylactide and HA/polyhydroxybutyrate [3], have been developed. Tests in vitro demonstrated that the addition of nanoapatite to polyactive TM significantly rises the composites' capability to induce $Ca_3(PO_4)_2$ precipitation [3].

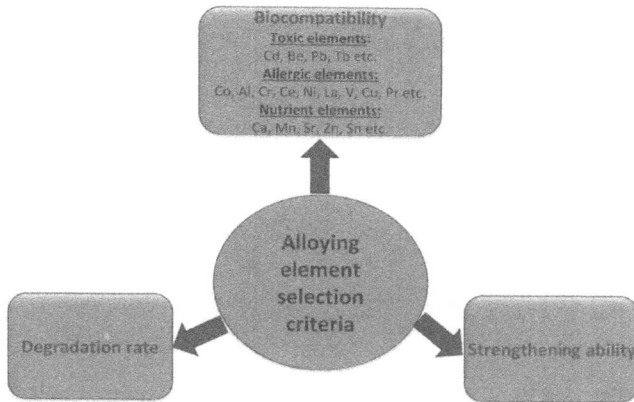

FIGURE 10.9  Alloy design of magnesium.

Witte et al. [62] examined in vitro the corrosion and mechanical behavior of MMC consisting HA particles as reinforcements and AZ91D as the matrix. In artificial seawater and cell solutions, HA particles stabilized the corrosion rate and showed an even corrosion attack, according to corrosion tests. The calcium phosphate ceramics' stable phases are extremely temperature and moisture dependent [3]. $CaCO_3$ was discovered on the surfaces of MMC-HA following a dip in artificial saltwater, whereas no $CaCO_3$ development was observed after submersion in cell solutions containing or lacking proteins. This analysis showed that the biomaterial MMC-HA is degradable with cytocompatibility and adaptable corrosion and mechanical behavior. One advantage of Mg/HA composites is the ability to regulate the rate of degradation.

### 10.5.1.2  Suitable Coating

Coating of Mg alloys is among the most important methods to advance the corrosion resistance. Additionally, surface treatments affect the mechanical behavior of implant material. Changes in the implant surface's structure and morphology can affect the integration behavior. It is difficult for researchers to develop a coating for Mg alloys for human body compatibility. The coating must adhere to Mg with sufficient force, possess high mechanical strength and hardness, be exceptionally strong, be environment-friendly, and be resistant to corrosion, fatigue, and wear. However, there are no such available coatings which fulfills the criteria of implant materials. The hardness and mechanical properties of metallic coatings, with chromate conversion coating, nickel electroless plating, and aluminium coating, are greater. However, it has harmful effect on human body. The nonmetallic coatings taken into consideration comprise conductive films, polymers, thermal spray coating, anodizing. etc. Guo et al. [63] used the zinc oxide/polypyrrole as a coating material on Mg alloys in orthopedic implant materials. The immersion and electrochemical tests discovered that the coating was significantly to decrease the rate of corrosion of the magnesium alloy. Various electrochemical corrosion results were shown in Figure 10.10(a)–(f).

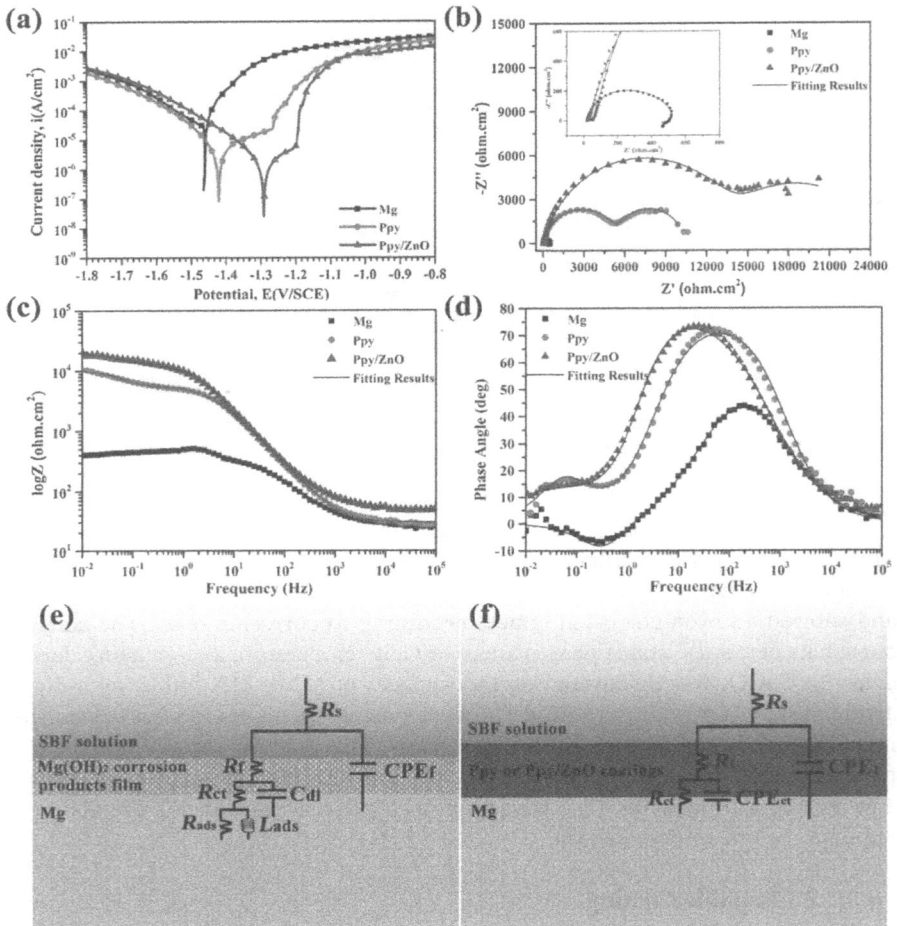

**FIGURE 10.10** Electrochemical corrosion behavior of various samples. (a) Polarization maps. (b) Nyquist maps. (c) Bode plots of log |Z|. (d) Bode plot of phase angle. (e) Equivalent circuits of uncoated magnesium alloy. (f) Equivalent circuits of coated magnesium alloys [63].

Zhang et al. [64] deposited an aluminum film on AZ91 using thermal spray. In order to ensure sufficient adhesion, a heat treatment at 450°C was performed. Owing to the atoms of Mg and Al diffusing, β-phase developed at the interface between matrix and coating. Thus, this layer possessed exceptional anticorrosion and anti-wear properties. Chiu et al. [65] examined the corrosion behavior of arc-sprayed aluminum coating. Due to the coating's high porosity, it was discovered that it lacked the ability to protect against corrosion. Corrosion resistance was enhanced through appropriate hot-pressing processes. Unfortunately, the release of aluminum ions from the Al coating during the corrosion process has negative effects on the human body. Ceramics-based biomaterials such as $TiO_2$, $Al_2O_3$, and ZrO show excellent structural and chemical stability, toughness, and mechanical strength. Zhang et al.

[66] coated AM60 magnesium alloy with $TiO_2$ using plasma spray technique. Due to the fact that there was galvanic corrosion between the coating and substrates, in Hank's solution, the corrosion resistance of AM60 with $TiO_2$ coating was not better than the alloy without the coating. After sealing the identical coating as $Na_2SiO_3$, the corrosion rate was remarkably decreased. The benefit of the thermal spray method is that Mg alloy coatings have poor surfaces and adherence and high porosity to the substrate. The porous coating's drawback is that it might encourage the development of soft tissue and could be loaded with substances that elute medications and coatings. Xin et al. [67, 68] successfully developed two coated layers of 1.5 μm thick $ZrO_2/Zr$ and 1 μm thick $Al_2O_3/Al$ on AZ91 using the plasma-based cathodic arc process. Al or Zr was used as an intermediate layer to prohibit O and Mg from coming into direct touch, thereby enhancing the adhesion of coatings to base metals. The outcomes demonstrate that such coatings have superior adhesion to the substrate material and enhance corrosion behavior. Nevertheless, electrolyte infiltration significantly degraded the coatings' shield after prolonged exposure to SBF due to the coatings' porous nature. Compared to plasma spray coatings, cathodic arc coatings are deeper, have flatter surfaces, and have superior adhesion strength to the base material. When soaked in SBF for an extended period of time, it is a common flaw for ceramic-coated films made using plasma techniques to lose their corrosion resistance if additional sealing is not employed. Furthermore, plasma technique poses health and safety concerns due to the dust, noise, fumes, and light radiation produced during treatment.

Microarc oxidation (MAO), or anodizing, is an electrolytic method that coats metals and their alloys in a protective oxide layer. The oxide film in this coating is porous, so it requires closure by an organic or other coating. As it is anodized, the coating can withstand wear and corrosion. Due to the fact that anodized Mg alloys are typically intended to be shielded by other protecting film, testing was typically not conducted on the anodized surfaces themselves, but rather on the coatings, film that accumulates on anodized surfaces. Therefore, evaluating a direct result of the anodizing coating's anticorrosion characteristics is extremely difficult. In Hank's solution, Kumar et al. [69] investigated the wear and corrosion resistance of AZ91D with and without MAO coating. This alloy is primarily made of $\beta$-$MgSiO_4$, $\delta$-$MgAl_{28}O_{40}$, $Mg_3Al_2Si_3O_{12}$, $(Mg_4Al_4)$ $(Al_4Si_2)O_{20}$, and spinel. In comparison to untreated AZ91D alloy, the wear and corrosion resistance of AZ91D in Hank's solution is significantly enhanced after MAO treatment. The results of the immersion test indicate that untreated AZ91D alloy mass loss is 15 times that of MAO alloys. The electrochemical corrosion test demonstrates that MAO surface treatment improves the corrosion potential of magnesium alloy from $-1.5786$ to $-0.43019$ V, reducing the corrosion current from $0.028703 \times 10^{-7}$ $A/cm^2$ to $2.0456 \times 10^{-7}$ $A/cm^2$. According to the results of lubricant sliding wear tests, the loss of mass for as-received AZ91D is 1.5 times that of MAO.

The aforementioned outcomes indicate that Mg alloys containing MAO have either excellent wear resistance or corrosion resistance. If a test is conducted in an interaction and combination of wear and corrosion environments, this may not be the case. A recent study conducted by Chen et al. [52] on AZ91 with MAO coating in 0.9% NaCl, 0.9% NaCl + 0.7 g/L $NaHCO_3$, and 0.9% NaCl + 0.35 g/L $NaHCO_3$

solutions demonstrates that micro-abrasive wear tests yield different results for wear resistance. Although MAO layer increased the corrosion resistance of AZ91, it also caused wear debris to accumulate, which reduced the AZ91 wear resistance with MAO layer in comparison to the substrate alloy. Consequently, it is essential to conduct additional evaluations of the anti-wear behavior of MAO coatings on magnesium alloys via numerous wear experiments. In a separate analysis, Kumar et al. [43] found that anodized commercially pure Mg in Hank's solution had not given off any hydrogen after a month. This indicates that the coating of MAO was successful in delaying magnesium biodegradation on the substrate. The electrochemical inhomogeneity caused by phase dissociation in the magnesium alloy is one of the greatest obstacles in making defender, corrosion-resistant anodic coatings on Mg. Under certain conditions, this crevice corrosion between the changed surface and the base underneath can cause a lot of damage, resulting in blister formation. Another problem is that anodic coatings can affected the wear resistance of Mg-2%Al-1%Zn [70], Mg alloys [71], and WE43-T6 [72]. The fatigue life of anodized metallic element goes down is typically caused by surface tensile tension brought on by oxidation, structural flaws in the oxide coating, and age-related base metal softening brought on by the heat generated during oxide film deposition [71]. Nevertheless, few researchers [73] assert that anodized and nonanodized coatings are identical and cannot be distinguished, excluding for a slight difference in the scattering range of data. Consequently, the existing fatigue statistics of anodized coatings are inconsistent. Many factors, including flaws in the raw material itself, stress between the substrate and coating, coating quality, etc., affect fatigue qualities in addition to load parameters like frequencies, load ratios, and machine kinds. The microstructural pores have a higher impact on fatigue characteristics, especially for cast Mg alloys. The distribution and size of pores produce scattering data. In this situation, evaluating the coating effect alone on fatigue life is extremely difficult.

### 10.5.2 Modification of Surfaces

#### 10.5.2.1 Ion Plating

Ion plating uses atomic-sized ionized particles called ions to form layer on the base metal while simultaneously bombarding it or bombarding it on a regular basis. Duygulu et al. [74] used ion plating to pure magnesium to achieve a well-adhered and thick Ti coating. The magnesium with the titanium coating's free corrosion potential ($E_{corr}$) in 0.9 wt% NaCl solution enlarged by 0.331 V is related to the uncoated magnesium (−1.638 V). The density of corrosion current of the magnesium with a Ti coating is $2.05 \times 10^{-5}$ A/cm$^2$, which is roughly a factor of ten or less than that of magnesium without a coating ($1.45 \times 10^{-4}$ A/cm$^2$). This indicates that Ti-coating can enhance the corrosion properties of Mg in SBFs. In addition, Kumar et al. [75] discovered that the creation of an interdiffusion film at the contact between the Ti layer and Mg alloy is shown by the steady rise in Ti content from the Mg substrate side via the interface to the Ti coating side. Notably, this result contradicts the findings of Duygulu et al. [74] regarding the Mg and Ti alloys bonding through diffusion. Figure 10.11(a) depicts the Ti-coated Mg microstructure in cross section. A uniform 10-μm thick Ti layer was observed. In addition, there are no pores throughout the entire

Ti-coating section, and there is no gap between the Ti-coating and Mg substrate, indicating a compact coating and strong edge bonding. Figure 10.11(b) depicts a Ti-coating fracture surface. A cleavage fracture is evidently present. On the fracture surface, there are also particles and pits, representing that intergranular decohesion has taken place. Nevertheless, there is no visible interface crack [75].

Figure 10.11(c) depicts the interface microstructure between the Mg substrate and Ti-coating under high magnification. Considering Figure 10.11(d), a line element scan was performed to unveil the Ti element dispersal across the edge. The line in Figure 10.11(c) indicates the line scanning location. It is evident from the Ti-element scanning profile that the content Ti increases steadily from Ti-coating side to the Mg-substrate side, indicating the formation of interface mutual diffusion between the Mg substrate and Ti-coating [75].

### 10.5.2.2  Mechanical Treatments

Mg alloy surfaces can be transformed mechanically using processes like shot peening, deep rolling, and roller burnishing [76]. The investigational results showed that residual compressive stresses caused by the procedure can counteract the negative effects of surface roughness, as evidenced by the fact that shot peened samples'

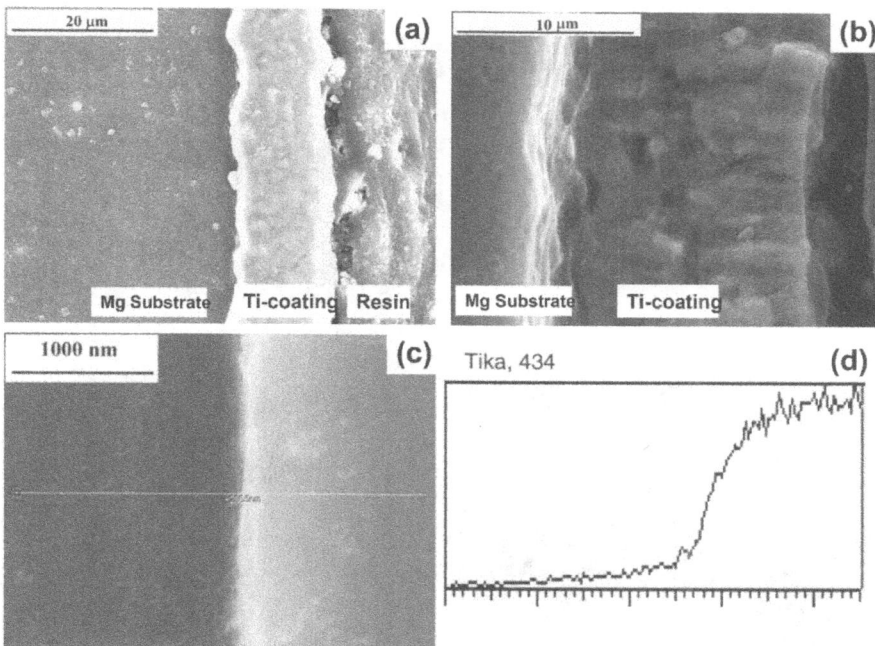

**FIGURE 10.11**    (a) No pore or crack was discovered in the microstructure of a Ti-coated pure Mg sample, confirming a dense Ti-coating. (b) Ti-coating fracture surface displaying a cleavage fracture. (c) High-definition microstructure Mg substrate and Ti-coating. (d) Ti-element line scan at the Ti-coating/Mg substrate contact as showed by yellow line in part (c) [75].

fatigue life is longer than that of the electropolished reference materials. Specifically, the fatigue life cycle extension brought about by the fatigue life is exceeded by the residual compressive stress field's ability to slow down the propagation of microcracks which was brought about by the earlier crack nucleation. He et al. [77] considered the outcome of 0.6 wt% Nd/Sc on the mechanical behavior of as-cast Mg-2Zn-0.2Zr alloy. The author found that the addition of 0.6% Sc in ZK20 improved UTS, i.e., 213 ± 1 MPa, and YS, i.e., 100 ± 4 MPa, is attained because of the precipitation strengthening of $\beta$-$(MgZn_2)$ precipitates [77]. Figure 10.12(a)–(d) demonstrated the tensile and conforming fracture behavior of composites.

The tissue development is promoted through rough surfaces. The question remains, nonetheless, as to whether these alloys' corrosion and corrosion fatigue life improved or degraded after undergoing mechanical treatments. It should be observed that at this moment, this surface treatment is not meant to be used with implanted materials. Consequently, it is crucial to look into the prospective uses in the bodily environment in more detail.

### 10.5.2.3 Laser- or Electron Beam–based Melting and Surface Cladding

Making use of high-intensity energy sources like electron and laser beams, it is possible to modify the surfaces of magnesium alloys. On the surface, a finer microstructure

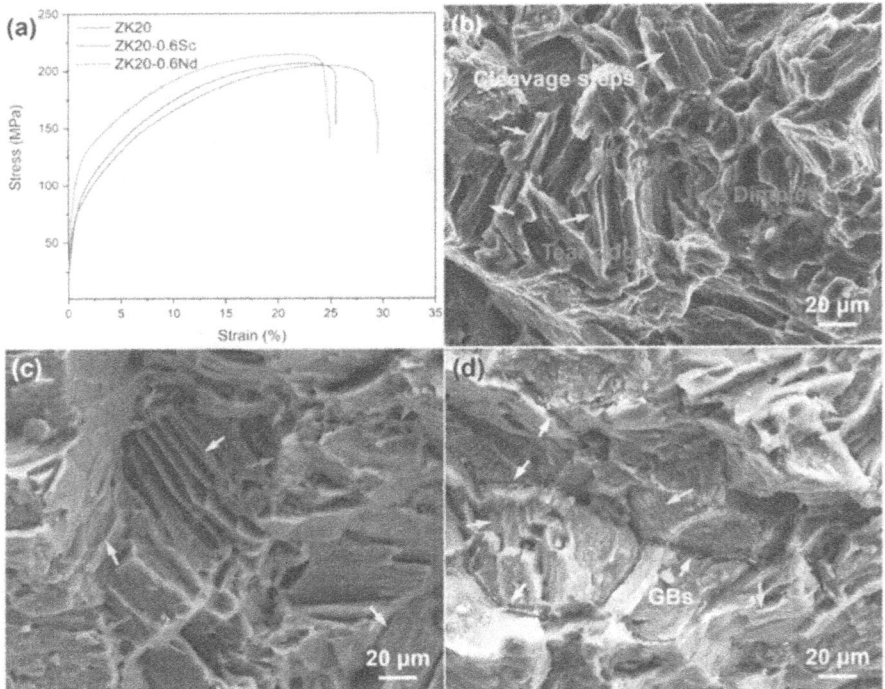

**FIGURE 10.12** (a) Stress–strain analysis of as-cast ZK20(–0.6Sc/Nd) alloys at room temperature; the fracture analysis of (b) ZK20, (c) ZK20-0.6Sc, and (d) ZK20-0.6Nd [77].

can be attained. Laser surface melting and cladding are useful methods for selectively enhancing magnesium alloys' corrosion resistance. Magnesium's resistance to corrosion in NaCl solutions is increased by laser-cladding aluminium layers [78]. Neubert et al. [79] described the laser cladding of Al- and Si-based eutectic alloy on Mg alloy (AS41) with C-short fibers composites. The clad coating's corrosion rate is approximately hundred times lesser than magnesium metals. Hao et al. [80] treated AZ91HP with a high current with pulsating electron beam, and the outcomes indicated a considerable potential for enhancing corrosion properties. Currently, almost nil research data is available for fatigue life with this technique. Pou-Álvarez et al. [81] considered the laser treatment of Mg alloy at various scale, i.e., nanosecond, picosecond, and femtosecond. They have done immersion test in NaCl solution and found various results. Figure 10.13 demonstrated the SEM microstructure after 26 h of immersion in NaCl solution.

Figure 10.13(a) demonstrates the corrosion by-products build-up on the base metal surface. Cross section in Figure 10.13(b) illustrates the metal's erosion during immersion. A closer inspection reveals the formation of a cracked and thus unshielded surface of corrosion by-products on the corroded material (Figure 10.13(c)).

Figures 10.13(e), (i), and (m) and Figure 10.13(f), (j), and (n) show that after 26 h of immersion, the laser-treated samples surface is hardly changed: top view and cross section, respectively. Cross section analyses at high resolution (Figure 10.13(g), (k), and (o)) expose the formation of a more compressed and complex corrosion by-products layer on the laser-treated metal. This behavior is explained by microstructural refining and homogeneity and oxidation of the external surface layers brought on by the laser treatment combined to create passivation in the material [82]. There are three

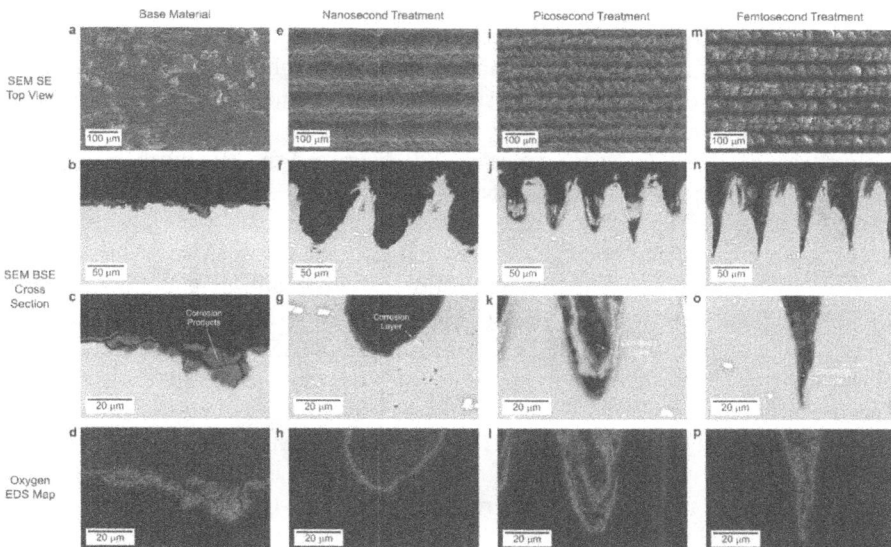

**FIGURE 10.13** Analysis of SEM microstructure of treated surfaces after immersion in NaCl solution for 26 h [81].

possible treatments: surface of nanosecond-treated demonstrates the most consistent surfacing by the corrosion by-products, which corresponds to the more reliable and consistent dispersal of the altered material coating, as deliberated previously. After immersion, the Mg and O ratio determined by top-view EDS examination enhanced to $2.35 \pm 0.02$, $1.80 \pm 0.06$, $1.71 \pm 0.04$, and $1.8 \pm 0.2$ for the parent material and femto-, pico-, and nanoseconds treatments, respectively. This demonstrates the deposition of $Mg(OH)_2$ constituting the corrosion by-products coatings shown in Figure 10.13 (c), (g), (k), (o), as established by the EDS analysis in Figure 10.13 (d), (h), (l), and (p).

### 10.5.2.4  Ion Implantation

In a study conducted by Liu et al. [83], the corrosion behavior of surgical AZ91 was investigated by implanting Ti ions. The study found that a blended together film was formed, and the surface-oxidized films primarily consisted of titanium oxide and a smaller amount of magnesium oxide. X-ray photoelectron spectroscopy (XPS) revealed that the oxide had three layers. The outer layer, which was 10 nm thick, was composed mainly of MgO and $TiO_2$ with a trace amount of $Mg(OH)_2$. The middle layers, which were 50 nm thick, primarily consisted of $TiO_2$ and MgO, with minor contributions from $MgAl_2O_4$ and TiO. The third layer was abundant in metallic Mg, Ti, Al, and Ti3Al. The study found that Ti ion implantation suggestively shifted the open-circuit potential (OCP) to a more positive potential and improved corrosion resistance at OCP in SBF at $37 \pm 1°C$, as determined by electrochemical experimentation. This improvement was due to a more compact surface oxide film, enhanced reoxidation on the implanted surface, and an increased $Mg_{17}Al_{12}$ phase. However, the authors did not provide information about the implanted coating microstructure and its adhesion to the substrate. It is important to note that ion-implanted coatings do not always enhance corrosion resistance. In a study conducted by Wan et al. [78], a zinc coating was prepared on Mg-Ca alloys by implanting $0.9 \times 10^{17}$ ions/cm$^2$ of zinc ions. Surprisingly, all Ti-implanted materials showed higher rate of corrosion than their unimplanted counterparts. This suggests that Zn is not a favorable element for the ion implantation of biomedical Mg-Ca alloys.

Furthermore, a study by Huang et al. [84] examined the effectiveness of nitrogen plasma immersion ion implantation on Ni-free ZrCuFeAl bulk metallic glass in terms of biocorrosion resistance. The researchers assessed the material's resistance to corrosion in simulated body fluid (SBF) and artificial saliva (AS).

The graph shown in Figure 10.14 illustrates the potentio-dynamic polarization curves of Ti and bulk metallic glass (BMG) samples, tested in two different solutions: simulated body fluid (SBF) and artificial saliva (AS), both with and without nitrogen plasma immersion ion implantation (N-PIII) treatment. The results indicate that the BMG samples had a higher corrosion potential ($E_{corr}$) and a lower corrosion current density ($I_{anod}$) compared to commercial biomedical Ti, irrespective of the test solution used. However, only the BMG samples exhibited evidence of pitting corrosion. Moreover, the N-PIII treatment significantly improved the corrosion resistance of BMG, as evidenced by the increased $E_{corr}$ and $E_{pit}$ (the pitting potential) and the decreased Ianod. In addition, the N-PIII treatment led to the formation of a protective nitride-containing oxide film ($ZrO_2/ZrN/Zr(N, O)$) with a thickness of approximately 15 nm on the Ni-free $Zr_{62.5}Cu_{22.5}Fe_5Al_{10}$ BMG samples. Therefore,

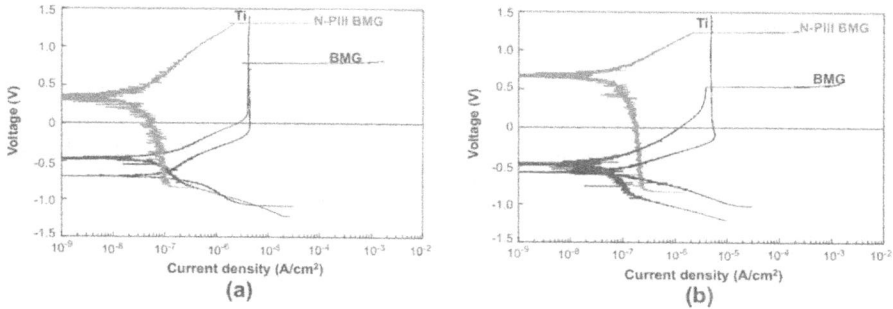

**FIGURE 10.14**   The electrochemical behavior of Ti and $Zr_{62.5}Cu_{22.5}Fe_5Al_{10}$ bulk metallic glasses (BMGs) were investigated using potentiodynamic polarization curves under different conditions. The experiments were conducted both with and without N-PIII treatment in two different environments, namely (a) AS and (b) SBF [84].

this Ni-free BMG alloy has a great potential for biomedical implants, and the proposed N-PIII treatment can further enhance its biocorrosion resistance, particularly against pitting corrosion [84].

## 10.6   CONCLUSION

The exploration of biodegradable materials made from magnesium is a new and important area of research for both academics and businesses. Despite its potential usefulness, there are three major scientific challenges that need to be addressed right away: strength and flexibility, controllable decomposition, and safety for use in living organisms. However, challenges present opportunities for growth. Magnesium alloys have already undergone clinical trials as biodegradable stents in orthopedic and trauma surgery, and they show promise as a replacement for current implant materials. Preliminary studies on MMC/HA suggest that it may be possible to create a biomaterial with adjustable mechanical and corrosive properties that is also compatible with living cells. A suitable bioactive coating should have properties such as resistance to corrosion, fatigue, and wear. Finally, these substitutes can be customized to meet the specific needs of individual patients.

## REFERENCES

1. Janssen, P., and T. Tailly. "New stent technologies." Urologic Clinics 49, no. 1 (2022): 185–196.
2. Im, S. H., D. H. Im, S. J. Park, Y. Jung, D.-H. Kim, and S. H. Kim. "Current status and future direction of metallic and polymeric materials for advanced vascular stents." Progress in Materials Science 126 (2022): 100922.
3. Shi, Donglu, ed. Biomaterials and tissue engineering. Springer Science+Business Media, 2004.
4. Upadhyay, D., M. A. Panchal, R. S. Dubey, and V. K. Srivastava. "Corrosion of alloys used in dentistry: A review." Materials Science and Engineering: A 432, no. 1–2 (2006): 1–11.

5. Dearnley, P. A. "A brief review of test methodologies for surface-engineered biomedical implant alloys." Surface and Coatings Technology 198, no. 1–3 (2005): 483–490.
6. Saris, N.-E. L., E. Mervaala, H. Karppanen, J. A. Khawaja, and A. Lewenstam. "Magnesium: an update on physiological, clinical and analytical aspects." Clinica Chimica Acta 294, no. 1–2 (2000): 1–26.
7. Institute of Medicine (US) Standing Committee on the Scientific Evaluation of Dietary Reference Intakes. Dietary reference intakes for calcium, phosphorus, magnesium, vitamin D, and fluoride. Washington, DC: National Academies Press, 1997.
8. Rude, R. K., H. E. Gruber, L. Y. Wei, A. Frausto, and B. G. Mills. "Magnesium deficiency: effect on bone and mineral metabolism in the mouse." Calcified Tissue International 72 (2003): 32–41.
9. Williams, D. "New interests in magnesium." Medical Device Technology 17, no. 3 (2006): 9–10.
10. Li, L., J. Gao, and Y. Wang. "Evaluation of cyto-toxicity and corrosion behavior of alkali-heat-treated magnesium in simulated body fluid." Surface and Coatings Technology 185, no. 1 (2004): 92–98.
11. Lambotte, A. "L'utilisation du magnesium comme materiel perdu dans l'osteosynthèse." Bull Mem Soc Nat Chir 28, no. 3 (1932): 1325–1334.
12. Witte, F., J. Fischer, J. Nellesen, H.-A. Crostack, V. Kaese, A. Pisch, F. Beckmann, and H. Windhagen. "In vitro and in vivo corrosion measurements of magnesium alloys." Biomaterials 27, no. 7 (2006): 1013–1018.
13. Witte, F., V. Kaese, H. Haferkamp, E. Switzer, A. Meyer-Lindenberg, C. J. Wirth, and H. Windhagen. "In vivo corrosion of four magnesium alloys and the associated bone response." Biomaterials 26, no. 17 (2005): 3557–3563.
14. Zhang, G. D., J. J. Huang, K. Yang, B. C. Zhang, and H. J. Ai, "Experimental study of in vivo implantation of a magnesium alloy at early stage." Acta Metallurgica Sinica 43, no. 11 (2007): 1186–1190.
15. Duygulu, O., R. A. Kaya, G. Oktay, and A. A. Kaya. "Investigation on the potential of magnesium alloy AZ31 as a bone implant." Materials Science Forum 546 (2007): 421–424.
16. Sillekens, W. H., and D. Bormann. "Biomedical applications of magnesium alloys." In Advances in wrought magnesium alloys, pp. 427–454. Woodhead Publishing, 2012.
17. Clark, G. C. F., and D. F. Williams. "The effects of proteins on metallic corrosion." Journal of Biomedical Materials Research 16, no. 2 (1982): 125–134.
18. Staiger, M. P., A. M. Pietak, J. Huadmai, and G. Dias. "Magnesium and its alloys as orthopedic biomaterials: a review." Biomaterials 27, no. 9 (2006): 1728–1734.
19. Yang, J., F. Cui, and I. S. Lee. "Surface modifications of magnesium alloys for biomedical applications." Annals of Biomedical Engineering 39 (2011): 1857–1871.
20. Singh, V. P., D. Kumar, R. P. Mahto, and B. Kuriachen. "Microstructural and mechanical behavior of friction-stir-welded AA6061-T6 and AZ31 alloys with improved electrochemical corrosion." Journal of Materials Engineering and Performance 32, no. 9 (2023): 4185–4204.
21. Neves, C. S., I. Sousa, M. A. Freitas, L. Moreira, C. Costa, J. P. Teixeira, and S. Fraga et al. "Insights into corrosion behaviour of uncoated Mg alloys for biomedical applications in different aqueous media." Journal of Materials Research and Technology 13 (2021): 1908–1922.
22. Fontana, M. G., and N. D. Greene. Corrosion engineering. McGraw-Hill, 2018.
23. Stephen D. Cramer and Bernard S. Covino, Jr. ASM handbook volume 13A: corrosion: fundamentals, testing and protection, p. 13. ASM International.
24. Kovacevic, S., W. Ali, E. Martínez-Pañeda, and J. L. Lorca. "Phase-field modeling of pitting and mechanically-assisted corrosion of Mg alloys for biomedical applications." Acta Biomaterialia 164 (2023): 641–658.

25. Razavi, M., M. H. Fathi, and M. Meratian. "Fabrication and characterization of magnesium–fluorapatite nanocomposite for biomedical applications." Materials Characterization 61, no. 12 (2010): 1363–1370.
26. Gu, X. N., W. R. Zhou, Y. F. Zheng, Y. Cheng, S. C. Wei, S. P. Zhong, T. F. Xi, and L. J. Chen. "Corrosion fatigue behaviors of two biomedical Mg alloys – AZ91D and WE43 – in simulated body fluid." Acta Biomaterialia 6, no. 12 (2010): 4605–4613.
27. Song, G. "Recent progress in corrosion and protection of magnesium alloys." Advanced Engineering Materials 7, no. 7 (2005): 563–586.
28. Huang, W., B. Hou, Y. Pang, and Z. Zhou. "Fretting wear behavior of AZ91D and AM60B magnesium alloys." Wear 260, no. 11–12 (2006): 1173–1178.
29. Jing, T. I. A. N., H.-L. Huang, Z.-Q. Pan, and Z. H. O. U. Hong. "Effect of flow velocity on corrosion behavior of AZ91D magnesium alloy at elbow of loop system." Transactions of Nonferrous Metals Society of China 26, no. 11 (2016): 2857–2867.
30. Zeng, R.-C., J. Zhang, W.-J. Huang, W. Dietzel, K. U. Kainer, C. Blawert, and K. E. Wei. "Review of studies on corrosion of magnesium alloys." Transactions of Nonferrous Metals Society of China 16 (2006): s763–s771.
31. Reifenrath, J., A. K. Marten, N. Angrisani, R. Eifler, and A. Weizbauer. "In vitro and in vivo corrosion of the novel magnesium alloy Mg-La-Nd-Zr: influence of the measurement technique and in vivo implant location." Biomedical Materials 10, no. 4 (2015): 045021.
32. Kumar, D., J. Jain, and N. N. Gosvami. "Anisotropy in nanoscale friction and wear of precipitate containing AZ91 magnesium alloy." Tribology Letters 67 (2019): 1–8.
33. Song, G. L., and A. Atrens. "Corrosion mechanisms of magnesium alloys." Advanced Engineering Materials 1, no. 1 (1999): 11–33.
34. Hermann, F., F. Sommer, H. Jones, and R. G. J. Edyvean. "Corrosion inhibition in magnesium–aluminium-based alloys induced by rapid solidification processing." Journal of Materials Science 24 (1989): 2369–2379.
35. Makar, G. L., J. Kruger, and K. Sieradzki. "Stress corrosion cracking of rapidly solidified magnesium–aluminum alloys." Corrosion Science 34, no. 8 (1993): 1311–1342.
36. Liao, J., M. Hotta, S.-I. Motoda, and T. Shinohara. "Atmospheric corrosion of two field-exposed AZ31B magnesium alloys with different grain size." Corrosion Science 71 (2013): 53–61.
37. Liao, J., M. Hotta, and N. Yamamoto. "Corrosion behavior of fine-grained AZ31B magnesium alloy." Corrosion Science 61 (2012): 208–214.
38. Gnedenkov, A. S., S. V. Lamaka, S. L. Sinebryukhov, D. V. Mashtalyar, V. S. Egorkin, I. M. Imshinetskiy, A. G. Zavidnaya, M. L. Zheludkevich, and S. V. Gnedenkov. "Electrochemical behaviour of the MA8 Mg alloy in minimum essential medium." Corrosion Science 168 (2020): 108552.
39. Liu, C., Y. Xin, G. Tang, and P. K. Chu. "Influence of heat treatment on degradation behavior of bio-degradable die-cast AZ63 magnesium alloy in simulated body fluid." Materials Science and Engineering: A 456, no. 1–2 (2007): 350–357.
40. Chen, J., S. Wei, L. Tan, and K. Yang. "Effects of solution treatment on mechanical properties and degradation of Mg-2Zn-0.5 Nd-0.5 Zr alloy." Materials Technology 34, no. 10 (2019): 592–601.
41. Kumar, D., J. Jain, and N. N. Gosvami. "Nanometer-thick base oil tribofilms with acrylamide additive as lubricants for AZ91 Mg alloy." ACS Applied Nano Materials 3, no. 10 (2020): 10551–10559.
42. Kim, J. J., and S. Han Do. "Recent development and applications of magnesium alloys in the Hyundai and Kia Motors Corporation." Materials Transactions 49, no. 5 (2008): 894–897.
43. Kumar, A., V. P. Singh, A. Nirala, R. C. Singh, R. Chaudhary, A.-H. I. Mourad, B. K. Sahoo, and D. Kumar. "Influence of tool rotational speed on mechanical and corrosion behaviour of friction stir processed AZ31/Al$_2$O$_3$ nanocomposite." Journal of Magnesium and Alloys 11, no. 7 (2023): 2585–2599.

44. Wu, G., Y. Fan, H. Gao, C. Zhai, and Y. P. Zhu. "The effect of Ca and rare earth elements on the microstructure, mechanical properties and corrosion behavior of AZ91D." Materials Science and Engineering: A 408, no. 1–2 (2005): 255–263.

45. Kannan, M. B., and R. K. S. Raman. "In vitro degradation and mechanical integrity of calcium-containing magnesium alloys in modified-simulated body fluid." Biomaterials 29, no. 15 (2008): 2306–2314.

46. Liu, C. L., Y. J. Wang, R. C. Zeng, X. M. Zhang, W. J. Huang, and P. K. Chu. "In vitro corrosion degradation behaviour of Mg-Ca alloy in the presence of albumin." Corrosion Science 52, no. 10 (2010): 3341–3347.

47. Müller, W. D., M. L. Nascimento, M. Zeddies, M. Córsico, L. M. Gassa, and M. A. F. L. de Mele. "Magnesium and its alloys as degradable biomaterials: corrosion studies using potentiodynamic and EIS electrochemical techniques." Materials Research 10 (2007): 5–10.

48. Froats, A., T. Kr Aune, D. Hawke, W. Unsworth, and J. Hillis. "Corrosion of magnesium and magnesium alloys." ASM Handbook 13 (1987): 740–754.

49. Kumar, D., J. Jain, and N. N. Gosvami. "In situ study of role of microstructure on anti-wear tribofilm formation on AZ91 magnesium alloy under zinc dialkyldithiophosphate containing lubricant." Advanced Engineering Materials 22, no. 8 (2020): 2000335.

50. Black, J. Biological performance of materials: fundamentals of biocompatibility. CRC Press, 2005.

51. Xu, L., E. Zhang, D. Yin, S. Zeng, and K. Yang. "In vitro corrosion behaviour of Mg alloys in a phosphate buffered solution for bone implant application." Journal of Materials Science: Materials in Medicine 19 (2008): 1017–1025.

52. Chen, J., and Z. Chen. "Extended Bayesian information criteria for model selection with large model spaces." Biometrika 95, no. 3 (2008): 759–771.

53. Ng, W. F., K. Y. Chiu, and F. T. Cheng. "Effect of pH on the in vitro corrosion rate of magnesium degradable implant material." Materials Science and Engineering: C 30, no. 6 (2010): 898–903.

54. Chaya, A., S. Yoshizawa, K. Verdelis, N. Myers, B. J. Costello, D.-T. Chou, S. Pal, S. Maiti, P. N. Kumta, and C. Sfeir. "In vivo study of magnesium plate and screw degradation and bone fracture healing." Acta Biomaterialia 18 (2015): 262–269.

55. Erne, P., M. Schier, and T. J. Resink. "The road to bioabsorbable stents: reaching clinical reality?" Cardiovascular and Interventional Radiology 29 (2006): 11–16.

56. Waksman, R. O. N., R. Pakala, R. Baffour, R. Seabron, D. Hellinga, and F. O. Tio. "Short-term effects of biocorrodible iron stents in porcine coronary arteries." Journal of Interventional Cardiology 21, no. 1 (2008): 15–20.

57. Kumar, D., S. Goel, N. N. Gosvami, and J. Jain. "Towards an improved understanding of plasticity, friction and wear mechanisms in precipitate containing AZ91 Mg alloy." Materialia 10 (2020): 100640.

58. Wen, C.'E., Y. Yamada, K. Shimojima, Y. Chino, H. Hosokawa, and M. Mabuchi. "Compressibility of porous magnesium foam: dependency on porosity and pore size." Materials Letters 58, no. 3–4 (2004): 357–360.

59. Yuan, L., L. Yanxiang, W. Jiang, and Z. Huawei. "Evaluation of porosity in lotus-type porous magnesium fabricated by metal/gas eutectic unidirectional solidification." Materials Science and Engineering: A 402, no. 1–2 (2005): 47–54.

60. Karageorgiou, V., and D. Kaplan. "Porosity of 3D biomaterial scaffolds and osteogenesis." Biomaterials 26, no. 27 (2005): 5474–5491.

61. Radha, R., and D. Sreekanth. "Insight of magnesium alloys and composites for orthopedic implant applications: a review." Journal of Magnesium and Alloys 5, no. 3 (2017): 286–312.

62. Witte, F., F. Feyerabend, P. Maier, J. Fischer, M. Störmer, C. Blawert, W. Dietzel, and N. Hort. "Biodegradable magnesium–hydroxyapatite metal matrix composites." Biomaterials 28, no. 13 (2007): 2163–2174.

63. Guo, Y., S. Jia, L. Qiao, Y. Su, R. Gu, G. Li, and J. Lian. "A multifunctional polypyrrole/zinc oxide composite coating on biodegradable magnesium alloys for orthopedic implants." Colloids and Surfaces B: Biointerfaces 194 (2020): 111186.
64. Zhang, J., Y. Wang, R. C. Zeng, and W. J. Huang. "Effects of post heat treatment on the interfacial characteristics of aluminum coated AZ91D magnesium alloy." Materials Science Forum 546 (2007): 529–532.
65. Chiu, L.-H., C.-C. Chen, and C.-F. Yang. "Improvement of corrosion properties in an aluminum-sprayed AZ31 magnesium alloy by a post-hot pressing and anodizing treatment." Surface and Coatings Technology 191, no. 2–3 (2005): 181–187.
66. Zhang, X. P., Z. P. Zhao, F. M. Wu, Y. L. Wang, and Jie Wu. "Corrosion and wear resistance of AZ91D magnesium alloy with and without microarc oxidation coating in Hank's solution." Journal of Materials Science 42 (2007): 8523–8528.
67. Xin, Y., C. Liu, W. Zhang, Jiang J., G. Tang, X. Tian, and P. K. Chu. "Electrochemical behavior Al$_2$O$_3$/Al coated surgical AZ91 magnesium alloy in simulated body fluids." Journal of the Electrochemical Society 155, no. 5 (2008): C178.
68. Xin, Y., C. Liu, X. Zhang, G. Tang, X. Tian, and P. K. Chu. "Corrosion behavior of biomedical AZ91 magnesium alloy in simulated body fluids." Journal of Materials Research 22, no. 7 (2007): 2004–2011.
69. Kumar, D., N. N. Gosvami, and J. Jain. "Influence of temperature on crystallographic orientation induced anisotropy of microscopic wear in an AZ91 Mg alloy." Tribology International 163 (2021): 107159.
70. Yerokhin, A. L., A. Shatrov, V. S. H. A. S. H. K. O. V. Samsonov, P. Shashkov, A. Leyland, and A. Matthews. "Fatigue properties of Keronite® coatings on a magnesium alloy." Surface and Coatings Technology 182, no. 1 (2004): 78–84.
71. Ogarevic, V. V., and R. I. Stephens. "Fatigue of magnesium alloys." Annual Review of Materials Science 20, no. 1 (1990): 141–177.
72. Eifert, A. J., J. P. Thomas, and R. G. Rateick, Jr. "Influence of anodization on the fatigue life of WE43A-T6 magnesium." Scripta Materialia 40, no. 8 (1999): 929–935.
73. Hsiao, H.-Y., and W.-T. Tsai. "Characterization of anodic films formed on AZ91D magnesium alloy." Surface and Coatings Technology 190, no. 2–3 (2005): 299–308.
74. Duygulu, O., A. A. Kaya, G. Oktay, and F. Ç. Şahin. "Diffusion bonding of magnesium, zirconium and titanium as implant material." Materials Science Forum 546 (2007): 417–420.
75. Kumar, D., J. Jain, and N. N. Gosvami. "Macroscale to nanoscale tribology of magnesium-based alloys: a review." Tribology Letters 70, no. 1 (2022): 27.
76. Sealy, M. P., Y. B. Guo, R. C. Caslaru, J. Sharkins, and D. Feldman. "Fatigue performance of biodegradable magnesium–calcium alloy processed by laser shock peening for orthopedic implants." International Journal of Fatigue 82 (2016): 428–436.
77. He, Y., R. Wang, C. Peng, Y. Feng, X. Wang, and Z. Cai. "Influence of 0.6 wt% Sc/Nd on the microstructure, mechanical property and in vitro biodegradation behavior of as-cast Mg-2Zn-0.2 Zr alloy." Journal of Alloys and Compounds 942 (2023): 168890.
78. Wan, Y. Z., G. Y. Xiong, H. L. Luo, F. He, Y. Huang, and Y. L. Wang. "Influence of zinc ion implantation on surface nanomechanical performance and corrosion resistance of biomedical magnesium–calcium alloys." Applied Surface Science 254, no. 17 (2008): 5514–5516.
79. Neubert, V., and A. Bakkar. "Effect of small Ca-additions on the corrosion resistance of AS41-Mg alloy." In Magnesium: Proceedings of the 6th International Conference Magnesium Alloys and Their Applications, pp. 638–645. Weinheim, FRG: Wiley-VCH Verlag GmbH & Co. KGaA, 2003.
80. Hao, S., B. Gao, A. Wu, J. Zou, Y. Qin, C. Dong, J. An, and Q. Guan. "Surface modification of steels and magnesium alloy by high current pulsed electron beam." Nuclear Instruments and Methods in Physics Research Section B: Beam Interactions with Materials and Atoms 240, no. 3 (2005): 646–652.

81. Pou-Álvarez, P., A. Riveiro, X. R. Nóvoa, M. Fernández-Arias, J. Del Val, R. Comesaña, M. Boutinguiza, F. Lusquiños, and J. Pou. "Nanosecond, picosecond and femtosecond laser surface treatment of magnesium alloy: role of pulse length." Surface and Coatings Technology 427 (2021): 127802.

82. Pou-Álvarez, P., A. Riveiro, X. R. Nóvoa, X. Jin, J. Del Val, R. Comesaña, and M. Boutinguiza et al. "Laser-guided corrosion control: a new approach to tailor the degradation of Mg-alloys." Small 17, no. 18 (2021): 2100924.

83. Liu, C., Y. Xin, X. Tian, J. Zhao, and P. K. Chu. "Corrosion resistance of titanium ion implanted AZ91 magnesium alloy." Journal of Vacuum Science & Technology A 25, no. 2 (2007): 334–339.

84. Huang, H.-H., H.-M. Huang, M.-C. Lin, W. Zhang, Y.-S. Sun, W. Kai, and P. K. Liaw. "Enhancing the bio-corrosion resistance of Ni-free ZrCuFeAl bulk metallic glass through nitrogen plasma immersion ion implantation." Journal of Alloys and Compounds 615 (2014): S660–S665.

# Index

Note: Locators in *italics* represent figures and **bold** indicate tables in the text.

For Product Safety Concerns and Information please contact our EU
representative GPSR@taylorandfrancis.com
Taylor & Francis Verlag GmbH, Kaufingerstraße 24, 80331 München, Germany

www.ingramcontent.com/pod-product-compliance
Lightning Source LLC
Chambersburg PA
CBHW060353220326
41598CB00023B/2907

* 9 7 8 1 0 3 2 5 0 9 5 8 7 *